Diagnostic and Therapeutic Advances in Alzheimer's Disease

Diagnostic and Therapeutic Advances in Alzheimer's Disease

Editor: Elena Poole

AMERICAN
MEDICAL PUBLISHERS
www.americanmedicalpublishers.com

AMERICAN
MEDICAL PUBLISHERS
www.americanmedicalpublishers.com

Cataloging-in-Publication Data

Diagnostic and therapeutic advances in Alzheimer's disease / edited by Elena Poole.
p. cm.
Includes bibliographical references and index.
ISBN 978-1-63927-658-5
1. Alzheimer's disease. 2. Alzheimer's disease--Diagnosis. 3. Alzheimer's disease--Treatment. I. Poole, Elena.
RC523 .D53 2023
616.831--dc23

American Medical Publishers,
41 Flatbush Avenue,
1st Floor, New York,
NY 11217, USA

ISBN 978-1-63927-658-5 (Hardback)

Contents

Preface

Alzheimer's disease (AD) refers to a type of neurologic condition, which causes the brain to shrink and brain cells to die over time. AD is the most frequent form of dementia in which a progressive loss in social, cognitive and behavioral abilities occurs that impairs a person's capacity to operate independently. The primary symptom of AD is forgetting recent events or discussions. A person with AD will have severe memory impairment, while losing the capacity to perform daily tasks, as the disease progress. Drug development for AD relies heavily on biomarkers and they can also be used to facilitate diagnosis, safety monitoring, demonstrating target engagement and supporting the modification of disease. AD is incurable due to its multifactorial and complex nature. Biomarkers aid in characterizing the baseline state, a therapy response or a disease process. This book is compiled in such a manner, that it will provide in-depth knowledge about the assessment and management of Alzheimer's disease. It presents researches and studies performed by experts across the globe.

Significant researches are present in this book. Intensive efforts have been employed by authors to make this book an outstanding discourse. This book contains the enlightening chapters which have been written on the basis of significant researches done by the experts.

Finally, I would also like to thank all the members involved in this book for being a team and meeting all the deadlines for the submission of their respective works. I would also like to thank my friends and family for being supportive in my efforts.

Editor

1

Epigenetic Factors in Late-Onset Alzheimer's Disease: *MTHFR* and *CTH* Gene Polymorphisms, Metabolic Transsulfuration and Methylation Pathways and B Vitamins

Gustavo C. Román [1,2,*,†], Oscar Mancera-Páez [3,4,†] and Camilo Bernal [3]

1 Department of Neurology, Methodist Neurological Institute, Institute for Academic Medicine Houston Methodist Research Institute, Houston Methodist Hospital, Houston, TX 77030, USA
2 Weill Cornell Medical College, Department of Neurology, Cornell University, New York, NY 10065, USA
3 Universidad Nacional de Colombia, Hospital Universitario Nacional, Faculty of Medicine, Department of Neurology, Bogotá ZC 57, Colombia; ogmancerap@unal.edu.co (O.M.-P.); camilobernalmd@hotmail.com (C.B.)
4 David Cabello International Alzheimer Disease Scholarship Fund, Houston Methodist Hospital, Houston, TX77030, USA
* Correspondence: GCRoman@HoustonMethodist.org
† These authors contributed equally to this work.

Abstract: DNA methylation and other epigenetic factors are important in the pathogenesis of late-onset Alzheimer's disease (LOAD). Methylenetetrahydrofolate reductase (*MTHFR*) gene mutations occur in most elderly patients with memory loss. MTHFR is critical for production of S-adenosyl-L-methionine (SAM), the principal methyl donor. A common mutation (1364T/T) of the cystathionine-γ-lyase (*CTH*) gene affects the enzyme that converts cystathionine to cysteine in the transsulfuration pathway causing plasma elevation of total homocysteine (tHcy) or hyperhomocysteinemia—a strong and independent risk factor for cognitive loss and AD. Other causes of hyperhomocysteinemia include aging, nutritional factors, and deficiencies of B vitamins. We emphasize the importance of supplementing vitamin B_{12} (methylcobalamin), vitamin B_9 (folic acid), vitamin B_6 (pyridoxine), and SAM to patients in early stages of LOAD.

Keywords: Alzheimer's disease; cystathionine-γ-lyase *CTH* gene; DNA methylation; epigenetics; epigenome-wide association study; methylome; methylenetetrahydrofolate reductase *MTHFR* gene; nutrition; S-adenosylmethionine; vitamin B complex

---

1. Introduction

Most genetic research on late-onset Alzheimer's disease (LOAD) has focused on genome-wide association studies (GWAS) that have provided low effect size results in general, with the exception of apolipoprotein E (ApoE) [1,2]. Studies of monozygotic twins with Alzheimer's disease (AD) showed discordance in onset and progression indicating a role for nongenetic factors in disease pathogenesis [3]. For these reasons, genetic research turned to epigenetic modifications using epigenome-wide association studies (EWAS) in the last few years [4,5]. Bonasio et al. [6] defined epigenetics as "the study of molecular signatures that provide a memory of previously experienced stimuli, without irreversible changes in the genetic information". Therefore, epigenetic refers to potentially heritable and nonheritable modifications in gene expression induced by environmental factors without changes in DNA base sequences [1]. These epigenetic processes include DNA methylation, histone modification and expression of long noncoding RNAs and noncoding microRNAs (miRNAs) that primarily repress target messenger RNAs (mRNAs) [7–10].

This review focuses on DNA methylation dynamics and other epigenetic changes, including the role of methylenetetrahydrofolate reductase (*MTHFR*) gene polymorphisms and its metabolic pathways particularly in aging and LOAD pathology [11]. We also review polymorphisms of the cystathionine-gamma(γ)-lyase (*CTH*) gene [12], the enzyme that converts cystathionine to cysteine in the transsulfuration pathway and is responsible for plasma elevation of total homocysteine (tHcy). The role of relevant nutritional factors including the B-vitamins folate, vitamin B_{12}, and vitamin B_6 status is summarized. Elevation of Hcy is important in oxidative stress contributing to the decrease of S-adenosyl-L-methionine (SAM) levels, which induce demethylation of DNA resulting in overexpression of genes involved in AD pathology such as presenilin (*PSEN1*) and beta-secretase (*BACE1*), the β-site amyloid precursor protein (APP)-cleaving enzyme that increases hypomethylation and $A\beta_{1\text{-}42}$ deposition [9]. Moreover, epigenetic markers have also been demonstrated to be critical regulatory factors of brain function [9], not only in AD but also in other neurodegenerative diseases [1,2] as well as in aging [9]. Experimental antiaging epigenetic interventions attempt to reverse age-related changes in DNA methylation [10].

2. DNA Methylation Studies

2.1. 5-Cytosine Methylation and DNA Methyltransferases

Methylation at the 5-position of the cytosine base (5mC) is considered a critical phase of epigenetic regulation in pathways related with neuronal development. Methylation and demethylation of cytosine-phosphate-guanine (CpG) islands is associated with alterations in local chromatin producing a long-term regulation of transcription tagging genome into active and inactive territories introducing a "masking" function [13]. Decreased levels of 5mC [1] and targeted mutations of DNA methyltransferases introduced into the germline produce severe developmental restriction [13] and finally a lethal phenotype in mice [14]. Cytosine base methylation occurs mainly at CpG dinucleotides [1]. Gene regulation is achieved by 5mC silencing gene expression via high-density CpG areas, known as CpG islands, which remain largely unmethylated [13]. In humans, genomic DNA methylation of cytosine results from the addition of a methyl group from SAM to the cytosine, catalyzed by DNA methyltransferases (DNMT1, DNMT3A, and DNMT3B) [9]. In addition to 5mC, hydroxymethylation at the 5-position of the cytosine base (5hmC) derived from the oxidation of methylated cytosines by ten-eleven translocation (TET) enzymes is another epigenetic regulatory mechanism, which is particularly abundant in the brain. The TET family of enzymes catalyzes Fe (II)- and alpha-ketoglutarate (α-KG)–dependent oxidation reactions, [9] and produces the initial step of oxidation of 5mC to 5hmC. TET enzymes also participate in the conversion of 5-formylcytosine (5fC) to 5-carboxylcytosine (5caC); this cycle ends when 5caC is excised by a thymine-DNA glycosylase (TDG) [9].

In humans, DNA methyltransferases are involved in tumor transformation and progression resulting in genome-wide hypomethylation of tumor cells and silencing of tumor-suppressor genes [15]; also, *DNMT3A* mutations have been associated with poor prognosis in acute myeloid leukemia [15]. *DNMT1* mutations occur in hereditary sensory and autonomic neuropathy type 1 (HSAN1) [15]. In mice, *DNMT1* mutations induce global hypomethylation along with cortical and hippocampal neuronal dysfunction causing neurodegeneration with severe deficits in learning, memory and behavior [16]. Hypomethylated excitatory neurons have postnatal maturation defects including abnormal dendritic arborization and impaired neuronal excitability [16]. Grossi et al. [17] used artificial neural network analysis to illustrate how low cobalamin; low folate and high Hcy are linked to AD. Low *PSEN1* methylation was linked to low folate levels and low promoter methylation of *BACE1* and *DNMT* genes. High levels of folate-vitamin B_{12} and low Hcy promoted methylation of genes required for DNA methylation reactions (*DNMT1*, *DNMT3A*, *DNMT3B*, and *MTHFR*) [18].

2.2. DNA Methylation in Alzheimer's Disease

Early studies of DNA methylation in LOAD from peripheral blood lymphocytes [19,20], brain biopsies and autopsy material [21–29] demonstrated variable results of cytosine methylation at CpG dinucleotides. Wang and coworkers [30] studied postmortem prefrontal cortex tissue and peripheral lymphocytes of AD patients and showed that specific loci in *MTHFR* gene promoter regions were hypermethylated compared to healthy controls. Ellison and collaborators [31] using gas chromatography/mass spectrometry found abnormal levels of 5mC and 5hmC in the superior and middle temporal gyri, hippocampus and parahippocampal gyrus in early stages of AD, as well as in frontotemporal lobe degeneration and Lewy body dementia; these global values returned to control levels as the disease progressed suggesting that methylation changes occur in early stages of neurodegenerative dementias. Chouliaras et al. [32] confirmed the presence of significant decreases in levels of 5mC and 5hmC in the hippocampus of AD patients compared with negative controls. Levels of 5mC were inversely proportional to the deposition of neurofibrillary tangles in the same hippocampal cells. Hernández et al. [33] studied DNA methylation patterns of cortical pyramidal layers in 32 brains of patients with LOAD demonstrating hypermethylation of synaptic genes and genes related to oxidative stress including *HOXA3, GSTP1, CXXC1-3* and *BIN1*.

One of the major problems of initial methylation studies was the small sample size. This was solved by De Jager and collaborators [4] utilizing one of the largest clinicopathological studies to date, the Religious Orders Study, with 708 brains to assess the methylation state of the brain's DNA correlated with AD pathology. Almost a half-million CpGs were interrogated including CpGs in the *ABCA7* and *BIN1* regions. The authors also identified genes whose RNA expression was altered in AD including *ANK1, CDH23, DIP2A, RHBDF2, RPL13, SERPINF1* and *SERPINF2*. *ANKYRIN* 1 (*ANK1*) and *RHOMBOID5* (*RHBDF2*) genes are involved in the protein tyrosine kinase 2-beta (*PTK2B*) gene network, a LOAD gene that is a key element of the calcium-induced signaling cascade involved in modulating the activation of microglia and macrophages, as well as in the transport of TNFα converting enzyme (ADAM17) from the cell surface.

Absence of *RHBDF2* in mice impacts the normal release of TNFα [4] activated astrocytes in the vicinity of neuritic plaques that overexpress *CADHERIN23* (*CDH23*) gene. DIP2A functions as a cell surface protein and connects directly to the known *SORTILIN RELATED RECEPTOR 1* (*SORL1*) susceptibility gene that is involved in the APP susceptibility network and amyloid processing [4]. Both *SERPIN PEPTIDASE INHIBITORS* (*SERPINF1* and *SERPINF2*) interact with elements of amyloid processing. *SERPINF1* mRNA expression is reduced in LOAD and when knocked-out in vitro leads to reduced neurite outgrowth [4].

A Religious Orders companion study by Lunnon and coworkers [5] found robust association between differences in methylation, mRNA levels, and Braak & Braak staging. The severity of Alzheimer's disease is defined in neuropathology by the presence of tau-based neurofibrillary tangles ranging from early stages (I and II) to extensive neocortical involvement in Braak & Braak stages V and VI in advanced disease. Dysregulation of DNA methylation occurred earlier in brain areas affected at onset by AD and appeared to have stronger effects (28.7%) than the combination of ApoE and other risk genes (13.9%) identified by GWAS [1,2], indicating the importance of epigenetic changes in AD. Additional studies by Yu et al. [34] confirmed the association of DNA methylation in *SORL1, ABCA7, HLA-DRB5, SLC24A4,* and *BIN1* genes with pathological diagnosis of AD including both Aβ load and tau tangle density. RNA expression of transcripts of *SORL1* and *ABCA7* was associated with tau tangle density, and the expression of *BIN1* was associated with Aβ load [34]. Moreover, Lunnon et al. [5] found hypermethylation of the *ANK1* gene in the entorhinal cortex, superior temporal gyrus and prefrontal cortex in LOAD. These findings confirm that AD involves significant disruption of DNA methylation. Epigenetic age-associated alterations of DNA methylation have also been reported in animal models of AD, in particular global DNA hypomethylation in the J20 model and DNA hypermethylation in the triple transgenic 3xTg-AD model [35].

3. miRNAs Epigenetic Effects

Long noncoding RNAs and noncoding microRNAs (miRNAs) that primarily repress target messenger RNAs (mRNAs) play a pivotal role in oncology, cardiovascular diseases and dementia [7,8]. In AD, the miRNA-125b is overexpressed enhancing neuronal apoptosis and tau phosphorylation by activation of cyclin-dependent kinase 5 (CDK5) and p35/25. *FORKHEAD BOX Q1 (FOXQ1)* is the direct target gene of miR-125b [7]. Patrick and coworkers [8] studied the role of miRNA-132, miRNA-129 and miRNA-99 in the dorsolateral prefrontal cortex of more than 500 brain samples demonstrating a small number of specific alterations on target genes such as *EP300* that encodes p300, a histone acetyltransferase that regulates transcription in the cortex of subjects with AD.

4. Transsulfuration Metabolic Pathways and Remethylation Defects

The metabolism of sulfur-containing amino acids in the transsulfuration pathway involves the transfer of the sulfur atom of methionine to serine to produce cysteine (Figure 1). Methionine first reacts with ATP to form S-adenosyl-L-methionine (SAM), then S-adenosyl-homocysteine (SAH) and finally, homocysteine. Plasma elevation of total homocysteine (tHcy) or hyperhomocysteinemia may result from congenital deficiency of cystathionine β-synthase (CBS) leading to homocystinuria, or more frequently from polymorphisms of the cystathionine γ lyase (*CTH*) gene (OMIM *607657; EC 4.4.1.1.) in chromosome 1 (1p31.1) [36]. CTH is the enzyme that converts cystathionine to cysteine, the last step in the transsulfuration pathway. Wang et al [12] demonstrated that a single nucleotide polymorphism (SNP), namely c.1364G > T in exon 12 of the *CTH* gene causes elevation of tHcy and cystathioninuria. Caucasian subjects homozygous for the *CTH* 1364T/T SNP showed elevation of tHcy that reached effects sizes similar to those caused by the 677C > T *MTHFR* gene polymorphism [12].

Closely related to the transsulfuration pathway are the remethylation defects resulting from the failure to convert homocysteine to the amino acid methionine (Figure 1). This pathway requires the integrity of the gene encoding methylenetetrahydrofolate reductase (*MTHFR*) required for the interaction of folate and cobalamin (vitamin B_{12}). Folate provides the methyl group required for the remethylation pathway (Figure 1) to finally produce SAM, the main methyl donor for epigenetic processes. The human *MTHFR* gene (OMIM *607093; EC 1.5.1.20) is localized in chromosome 1 (1p36.3) and it encodes for 5,10-methylenetetrahydrofolate reductase (MTHFR) [37]. This enzyme catalyzes the conversion of 5,10-methylenetetrahydrofolate to 5-methyltetrahydrofolate, a co-substrate with vitamin B_{12} for the remethylation of homocysteine to methionine [11]. Mutations of this gene occur in 10–15% of the population and the resulting MTHFR deficiency affects the production of methionine and SAM. Patients with AD have low levels of SAM in the CSF [38].

MTHFR gene polymorphisms cause enzyme thermolability and involve C-to-T substitution at nucleotide 667 and A-to-C at nucleotide 1298; these *MTHFR* mutations have been associated with homocystinuria, neural tube defects, preeclampsia, cleft lip and cleft palate, cerebrovascular disease, and psychiatric disorders including susceptibility to depression and schizophrenia [39,40]. Population-based international studies showed no increased risk of dementia in subjects with *MTHFR* polymorphisms [41,42]. In Japan, Nishiyama et al. [43] found a slight association of the *MTHFR*-C667T polymorphism with senile cognitive decline in men but not with AD. In Australia, a causal link between high tHcy and incident dementia was demonstrated [44] but the study lacked power to determine an effect of the *MTHFR*-C667T genotype. In contrast, de Lau and collaborators [45] in the normal elderly population of the Rotterdam Study observed that the *MTHFR*-C665T genotype was associated with elevated tHcy but not with cognitive loss or white matter lesions. In a small patient population in Tunisia [46], the *MTHFR*-A1298C mutation was associated with susceptibility to AD. As mentioned earlier, Román [11] found a very high frequency (above 90%) of *MTHFR* gene mutations in an elderly population attending a memory clinic in the USA, with diagnoses ranging from mild cognitive impairment (MCI) to LOAD; about 65% had single mutations; the *MTHFR*-C667T mutation was found in 58.5% of the patients and 41.5% had the *MTHFR*-A1298C mutation whereas 20% were compound heterozygous for both mutations [11].

MTHFR and Epigenetic Drift

In 2005, a multinational study of identical twins by Fraga and collaborators [47] first demonstrated that whereas DNA methylation and histone acetylation in young identical twins are indistinguishable, older identical twins showed substantial differences; epigenetic changes were up to four times greater than those of young twin pairs. The authors concluded that this "epigenetic drift" was associated with aging [47]. Epigenetic drift of identical twins with aging also occurs among a large number of animal species [48] following a non-Mendelian pattern. In identical twins with AD, the prognosis and onset of AD can differ by more than ten years [3,49,50]; young identical twin pairs are essentially indistinguishable in their epigenetic markings while older identical twin pairs show substantial variations. Breitner et al. [50] suggested that twins with a history of systemic infection developed AD at an earlier onset than their identical twin. Epigenetic drift can be caused by lifestyle, diet, infections, folate status, homocysteine status or toxic exposure [51]. Wang et al. [30] demonstrated that the *MTHFR* gene promoter in the brain displayed high interindividual variance in DNA methylation among twins. The methylation level of *MTHFR* and *APOE* in individuals 30 years of age apart decreased by 10.6%, whereas in patients with AD the methylation level increased by 6.8%. The epigenetic drift increases with age particularly in genes that play pivotal roles in removing β-amyloid such as *APOE* and among methylation genes such as *MTHFR* and *DNMT1* [9,52].

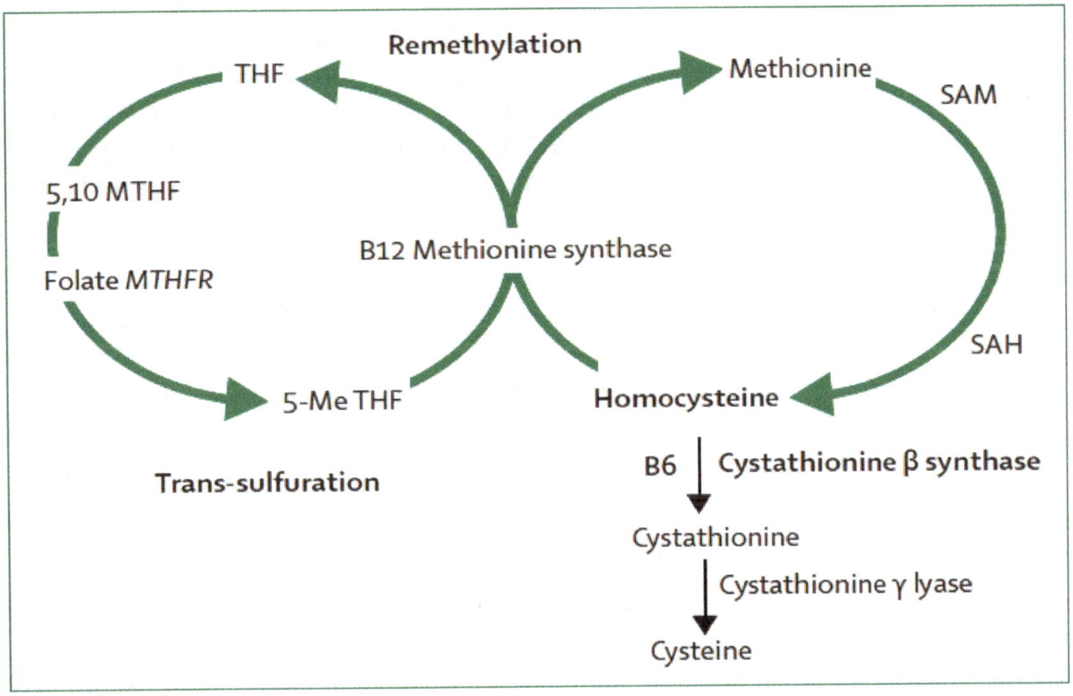

Figure 1. Homocysteine metabolism: B12 = cobalamin (vitamin B12). B6 = pyridoxine (vitamin B6). MTH = methylenetetrahydrofolate. MTHFR = methylenetetrahydrofolate reductase. SAM = S-adenosyl- methionine. SAH = S-adenosylhomocysteine. 5-Me THF = 5-methyl tetrahydrofolate. (From [53]).

5. Homocysteine (Hcy): A Risk Factor for Cognitive Loss and Dementia

Hcy is a sulfur-containing amino acid produced in the transsulfuration pathway (Figure 1) from the reaction of methionine with ATP to form SAM, then SAH and finally homocysteine. Homocystinuria due to congenital deficiency of the *CBS* gene causes hyperhomocysteinemia. Polymorphisms of the *CTH* and *MTHFR* genes are common genetic causes of hyperhomocysteinemia [38,39]. The remethylation pathway (Figure 1) involves reactions enzymatically mediated by MTHFR requiring as co-substrates the B-group vitamins folic acid (vitamin B_9) and cobalamin (vitamin B_{12}) for the remethylation of homocysteine to methionine. Pyridoxine (vitamin B_6) is required by CBS for the conversion of homocysteine to cysteine (Figure 1).

5.1. Hyperhomocysteinemia is an Independent Vascular Risk Factor

Elevation of plasma or serum tHcy (hyperhomocysteinemia) is an independent vascular risk factor linked to coronary disease, peripheral vascular disease, stroke and small-vessel cerebrovascular disease [53]. More importantly, elevated tHcy is considered a risk factor for dementia and cognitive decline in the elderly, particularly in association with low levels of folate and cobalamin [54,55]. A number of studies in cognitively normal elderly subjects, demonstrated that baseline tHcy is a strong and independent predictor of cognitive decline after observation periods ranging from 3 years (USA, $n = 321$ men [55] and Sydney, Australia, $n = 889$ [56]), 4 years (France, $n = 1241$) [57], 5 years (Wales, UK, $n = 32$) [58], 6 years (Norway, $n = 2189$) [59], 7 years (Finland $n = 274$) [60] and up to 10 years (UK, $n = 691$) [61]. In the Finland cohort [60], the magnetic resonance imaging (MRI) study demonstrated the association of higher baseline vitamin B_{12} and holotranscobalamin levels with a decreased rate of total brain volume loss during 8 years of the study period [62]. Increased tHcy levels were associated with faster rates of total brain volume loss and with progression of white matter hyperintensities among participants with hypertension (systolic blood pressure > 140 mm Hg) [62].

Regarding the risk of AD associated to elevated tHcy, in the Framingham Study, Seshadri and colleagues [63] demonstrated in elderly subjects (mean age, 76 years) that raised tHcy above 14 μmol/L nearly doubled the risk of LOAD over a period of 8 years. Similar findings were corroborated in two large Finnish [60,64] and Australian [65] cohorts. In 2008, Smith [66] performed a comprehensive review of cross-sectional and prospective studies involving >46,000 subjects and confirmed the association between elevated tHcy and cognitive deficit or dementia.

According to a recent international consensus statement [67], moderately raised homocysteine (>11 μmol/L) increases the relative risk of dementia in the elderly 1.15 to 2.5 fold, and the Population Attributable risk from 4.3 to 31% [67]. From the Public Health viewpoint, homocysteine-lowering treatment with B vitamins that markedly slows down the rate of brain atrophy and cognitive decline in the elderly offers the possibility that, in addition to folic acid fortification, mandatory methylcobalamin supplementation should also be considered for the prevention of LOAD [67].

5.2. Genetic and Nongenetic Causes of Hyperhomocysteinemia

Elevation of tHcy is caused by numerous factors including advancing age, diet, supplementation of B-vitamins, obstructive sleep apnea, smoking, *Helicobacter pylori* infection, and renal failure, among others [53,54]. As indicated earlier, both *CBS* gene polymorphisms and the C667T and the A1298C SNPs in the *MTHFR* gene decrease the activity of the MTHFR enzyme leading to hyperhomocysteinemia. Minagawa et al. [68] found that elevated Hcy inhibits the dimerization of ApoE3 and reduces ApoE3-mediated high-density lipoprotein (HDL) concentrations involved in degradation of soluble Aβ within microglia. ApoE4 was not affected; in patients with hyperhomocysteinemia the CSF levels of ApoE3 dimers were significantly lower than in controls. Minagawa and colleagues [68] suggested that the effects of elevated Hcy on ApoE3 contribute to the pathogenesis of AD. Smith and Refsum [54] reviewed the proposed mechanisms responsible for the harmful cognitive effects of hyperhomocysteinemia (Table 1). These include impaired endothelial function with reduced inducible nitric oxide synthase; augmented oxidative stress and decreased activity of key antioxidant enzymes; raised generation of the superoxide anion; alterations of lipid metabolism with increased cholesterol synthesis and reduced synthesis of apolipoprotein 1; and, carotid stenosis and induction of thrombosis [69,70].

Table 1. Harmful effects of homocysteine on vascular function and cognition (modified from Smith & Refsum [54]).

	Proposed Mechanisms
	Vascular Mechanisms
1	Impairs endothelial function reducing inducible NO synthase
2	NO-mediated endothelial dysfunction in brain vasculature
3	Causes a leaky blood-brain barrier
4	Induces thrombosis
5	Cerebrovascular ischemia leading to neuronal death and tau tangle deposition
6	Affects lipid metabolism increasing cholesterol synthesis
7	Reduces synthesis of apolipoprotein 1
8	Causes cerebral amyloid angiopathy
	Neuronal Mechanisms
1	Direct activation of NMDA receptor causes excitotoxic neuronal death
2	Homocysteic acid and cysteine sulfinic acid activate NMDA receptor causing neuronal death by excitotoxicity
3	Oxidative stress induced by generating superoxide and reactive oxygen species
4	Decreased activity of antioxidant enzymes
5	Formation and deposition of β-amyloid
6	Potentiates neurotoxic effects of β-amyloid by itself or via homocysteic acid
7	Activates tau kinases, such as Cdk5, causing tau tangle deposition
8	Triggers the cell cycle in neurons, leading to tangle formation and cell death
9	Causes DNA damage, limits DNA repair, leading to apoptosis
10	Increases SAH inhibiting methylation reactions, such as DNA cytosine methylation in promoters for amyloid genes, causing epigenetic effects
11	Inhibits PP2A activity leading to tau tangle deposition
12	Inhibits methylation of phosphatidyletanolamine
13	Stimulates endoplasmic reticulum stress response leading to amyloid formation
14	Activates the immune system
15	Decreases SAM-dependent synthesis of catecholamines and other neurotransmitters

Hyperhomocysteinemia induces a decrease in the SAM-dependent synthesis of catecholamines including dopamine, norepinephrine, and epinephrine, as well as non-catecholamine neurotransmitters such as melatonin and serotonin (5-HT) that contribute to development of depression [69]. Moreover, elevated tHcy produces two neurotoxic products, homocysteic acid (HCA) and cysteine sulfinic acid (CSA), which are agonists of the N-methyl-D-aspartate (NMDA) glutamate receptor, with neurotoxic effects on dopaminergic neurons derived from excessive Ca^{++} influx and reactive oxygen generation [70]. The beneficial effects of B-group vitamins on elevated tHcy will be reviewed next.

6. Folate Metabolism

Vitamin B_9 or folic acid (from the Latin *folium*, leaf) is abundantly found in green leafy vegetables. Folate is vital for cell development and growth given its role in numerous biochemical one-carbon (methyl-group, $-CH_3$) reactions, many of them critical for cognition. The Nun Study [71] first provided epidemiological and neuropathological data demonstrating that limited lifetime consumption of salads with low blood folate levels increased the risk of cognitive decline and dementia. Also, the severity of the atrophy in the neocortex and of the Alzheimer disease lesions were strongly correlated with low serum folate levels; none of 18 other nutrients, lipoproteins, or nutritional markers measured in the study correlated with the atrophy [71]. Further studies confirmed that normal cognitive scores were highly associated with elevated blood folate despite the neuropathological evidence of LOAD brain lesions [72].

The primary methyl-group donor for DNA methylation reactions is 5-methyl-tetrahydrofolate (CH_3-THF) required for the transformation of homocysteine into methionine mediated by methionine synthase with cobalamin (vitamin B_{12}) as a cosubstrate (Figure 1), leading to the synthesis of SAM.

Also, CH_3-THF is critical in the de novo purine synthesis to convert dUMP (deoxyuridylate) into dTMP (thymidylate) for DNA and RNA synthesis, DNA repair or replication. Several forms of cancer are associated with epigenetic differential methylation causing disturbances in nucleotide synthesis; for instance, hypermethylation may inhibit tumor suppressors. Folate, therefore, is a B-vitamin that plays an important role as a precursor in the epigenetic regulation of gene expression, DNA stability, DNA integrity and mutagenesis. Abnormal folate status has been associated with neural tube defects, cardiovascular and cerebrovascular diseases, cleft lip and palate, neurodegenerative diseases, schizophrenia and depression [40,73,74].

Telomeres and Folate Levels

Telomeres protect chromosomes from abnormal combination and degradation. The shortening of telomeres' cap serve as a signature of cell division history, acting as biomarker of aging. In peripheral leukocytes, short telomere length is associated with increased risk of cognitive decline and LOAD [75,76]. Low folate levels are associated with short telomeres due to DNA damage in the telomeric region. Telomere length is epigenetically regulated by DNA methylation and directly influenced by folate status, a process independent of DNA damage due to uracil incorporation. Shorter telomeres occur with age, infection, stress, and chronic diseases including LOAD [75].

Paul and collaborators [76] observed that decreased plasma folate concentration to <11.6 μmol/L was correlated with a decrease in mean telomere length. In this population, homozygous carriers of the *MTHFR*-C677T gene mutation showed decreased levels of plasma folate [77]. Decreased serum folate induces anomalous integration of uracil in place of thymidine in DNA [78], a mechanism corrected by folic acid supplementation. Troesch, Weber and Mohajeri [79] summarized the importance for the development of LOAD of reduced SAM-dependent methylation reactions due to genetic factors along with reduction of folate, vitamin B_6 and vitamin B_{12} levels. The resulting elevation of Hcy levels and the reduced capacity to synthetize, methylate and repair DNA, along with the impaired modulation of neurotransmission, appears to favor the development of AD particularly when combined with increased oxidative stress, particularly in ApoE ε4 carriers [80].

7. Vitamin B_{12} Deficiency and β-amyloid Deposition

Smith, Warren and Refsum [81] have recently provided a comprehensive review of vitamin B_{12}. Only bacteria can biosynthesize vitamin B_{12}; in humans B_{12} from the diet is a cofactor for the enzymes methionine synthase and L-methyl-malonyl-CoA mutase. B_{12} deficiency results in build-up of homocysteine and lack of interaction with folate that is trapped as CH_3-THF leading to depletion of tetrahydrofolates used in thymidylate and purine synthesis blocking DNA for the production of red cells in the bone marrow. B_{12} deficiency impedes cellular proliferation and protein synthesis and thereby causes development of megaloblastic anemia [81].

7.1. Clinical Manifestations of Vitamin B_{12} Deficiency

In 1920, pernicious anemia—a fatal form of a megaloblastic anemia—was successfully treated by adding liver to the diet. In 1955, Dorothy Hodgkin used crystallography to first identify the molecular structure of cyanocobalamin or vitamin B_{12} from the deep-red cyanide-containing pigment isolated from liver tissue. Pernicious anemia was the first disease to be identified as caused by vitamin B_{12} deficiency [81].

Stabler [82] reviewed the clinical manifestations of vitamin B_{12} deficiency. In addition to megaloblastic anemia, acidemia from elevation of serum methylmalonic acid (MMA), and methylmalonic aciduria, the neurological manifestations of pernicious anemia include memory loss and cognitive decline, visual disturbances from optic nerve neuropathy, burning and painful sensations in hands and feet from peripheral neuropathy, and spinal cord involvement with subacute combined degeneration resulting in loss of proprioception from dorsal column involvement and pyramidal tract symptoms such as paralysis and incontinence.

7.2. *Measuring Total Serum B_{12} Levels*

Dietary sources of B_{12} include liver, meat, fish, shellfish and dairy products; vegans are prone to B_{12} deficiency [81,82]. Vitamin B_{12} deficiency occurs from inborn metabolic errors, alterations of B_{12}-binding proteins including *haptocorrin* (HC) found in saliva, *intrinsic factor* (IF) produced by parietal cells in the stomach (pernicious anemia is associated with anti-parietal-cell and anti-IF auto-antibodies), and *transcobalamin* (TC), which binds B_{12} to facilitate uptake by the cells [81]. According to Stabler [82], measurement of total serum B_{12} levels is unsatisfactory because it reflects B_{12} that is bound to either HC or TC, and up to 60% of bound materials are cobalamin analogues (corrinoids). Therefore, "normal" total serum B_{12} levels can mask deficiency if serum contains relatively large amounts of cobalamin analogues [83]. Levels below 200 pg/mL usually indicate biochemical B_{12} insufficiency. Serum B_{12} < 350 pg/mL along with tHcy > 14 μmol/L indicate metabolic B_{12} deficiency [81,82]. For this reason, holotranscobalamin, MMA and tHcy levels should be included in the evaluation of a patient suspected of having B_{12} deficiency [83].

7.3. *Causes of Vitamin B_{12} Deficiency*

Other than pernicious anemia resulting from presence of anti-parietal-cell and anti-IF autoantibodies, other causes of B_{12} deficiency include atrophic body gastritis, *Helicobacter pylori* infection, malabsorption of vitamin B_{12}, gastrectomy, gastric bypass or other bariatric surgery, inflammatory bowel disease, tropical sprue, use of metformin, anticonvulsants, proton-pump inhibitors and other drugs to block stomach acid, and vegetarian diets low in meat and dairy products. Hemodialysis patients, nitrous oxide inhalation, and cholinesterase inhibitors in LOAD patients [84] also increase the risk of vitamin B_{12} deficiency.

Epidemiological studies have shown that prevalence of vitamin B_{12} deficiency increases with age [85,86], due to decreased saliva (e.g., dry eyes-dry mouth of Sjögren syndrome) [87] and gastric atrophy with deficits respectively of haptocorrin and intrinsic factor. Andrès and colleagues [88] have emphasized that as many as 20% of elderly people may have unrecognized B_{12} deficiency due to food-cobalamin malabsorption plus insufficient dietary intake. According to Spence [89], metabolic B_{12} deficiency occurs in 30% of vascular patients older than 71 years, increasing to as many as 40% in patients above age 80 years; these patients usually have plasma levels of tHcy >14 μmol/L resulting from B_{12} deficiency. Inadequate supply of B_{12} and folic acid is not only a strong and independent vascular risk factor particularly for subcortical ischemic small-vessel disease [90], a common and important contributor to cognitive impairment and memory complaints in the elderly, but also enhancing the development of LOAD [91]. Animal experimental data confirms the importance of B-vitamin deprivation in the expression of AD [92].

7.4. *Effects of B-Group Vitamins on Cognition: Negative Clinical Trials*

An international consensus [67] provided a comprehensive explanation of the negative results of meta-analyses [93] based on reviews of the results from a number of inadequately controlled clinical trials; most participants in those trials were enrolled in post-hoc studies which were not designed primarily to assess cognition. Usually, these were short-duration trials without baseline cognitive assessment and results were based on post-hoc brief cognitive assessments; only a few of these studies assessed the incidence of dementia or mild cognitive impairment.

In contrast, solid positive results were obtained in the Oxford Project to Investigate Memory and Ageing (OPTIMA) trial [94–96] that used comprehensive neuropsychological evaluations plus brain imaging end-points. The results of this trial indicate that supplementation of B_{12}, pyridoxine, and folic acid in subjects with MCI and hyperhomocysteinemia decreases tHcy resulting in improved episodic memory and global cognition [95], and most importantly, brain imaging demonstration of slowing of the progression of the brain atrophy in areas affected by AD [96]. Current recommendation is to provide oral supplementation of methylcobalamin 1000 μg/d, folic acid 800 μg/d and pyridoxine 100 mg/d.

8. SAM in Depression and Cognitive Loss

As described above (Figure 1) SAM is the main methyl-group donor for the methylation reactions reviewed here; as well as for synthesis of neurotransmitters, proteins, nucleic acids, phospholipids, and myelin. SAM has been used as an adjuvant for the treatment of depression [97]. Linnebank et al. [38] demonstrated a decrease of SAM in the cerebrospinal fluid (CSF) of patients with LOAD, affecting mainly ApoE ε4 carriers. According to Dayon et al. [98], plasma levels of one-carbon metabolites predicted cognitive decline. Despite the enhancing effects of SAM on antidepressants, no conclusive clinical trials of SAM have been reported [99].

9. Conclusions

It is established that the damaging effects of deficiencies of folate and cobalamin and the resulting elevation of tHcy contribute to the development of LOAD [67]. The numerous detrimental effects of elevated tHcy include, among others, endothelial and cerebrovascular damage of large-vessels as well as small-vessel disease [90]; activation of tau kinases; inhibition of methylation reactions; epigenetic effects on the β-amyloid pathway; reduced protein phosphatase-2A; and, impaired formation of phosphatidylcholine. Adequate supply of B-vitamins in the elderly, particularly in subjects with *MTHFR* and *CTH* gene mutations, appears to be critical to prevent the development of cognitive decline and to halt the progression of LOAD.

Author Contributions: Conceptualization, G.C.R. and O.M.-P.; methodology, G.C.R.; bibliographic investigation, G.C.R., O.M.-P. and C.B.; writing—original draft preparation, G.C.R., O.M.-P. and C.B.; writing—review and editing, G.C.R. and O.M.-P.; funding acquisition, G.C.R.

Acknowledgments: The authors would like to thank Houston Methodist Hospital for constant support to clinical research. Mancera-Páez was supported by the David Cabello International Alzheimer Disease Scholarship Fund. J David Spence, London, ON Canada provided valuable comments and bibliography.

References

1. Roubroeks, J.A.Y.; Smith, R.G.; van den Hove, D.L.A.; Lunnon, K. Epigenetics and DNA methylomic profiling in Alzheimer's disease and other neurodegenerative diseases. *J. Neurochem.* **2017**, *143*, 158–170. [CrossRef]
2. Millan, M.J. An epigenetic framework for neurodevelopmental disorders: From pathogenesis to potential therapy. *Neuropharmacology* **2013**, *68*, 2–82. [CrossRef] [PubMed]
3. Gatz, M.; Pedersen, N.L.; Berg, S.; Johansson, B.; Johansson, K.; Mortimer, J.A.; Posner, S.F.; Viitanen, M.; Winblad, B.; Ahlbom, A. Heritability for Alzheimer's disease: The study of dementia in Swedish twins. *J. Gerontol. A Biol. Sci. Med. Sci.* **1997**, *52*, M117–M125. [CrossRef] [PubMed]
4. De Jager, P.L.; Srivastava, G.; Lunnon, K.; Burgess, J.; Schalkwyk, L.C.; Yu, L.; Eaton, M.L.; Keenan, B.T.; Ernst, J.; McCabe, C.; et al. Alzheimer's disease: Early alterations in brain DNA methylation at *ANK1*, *BIN1*, *RHBDF2* and other loci. *Nat. Neurosci.* **2014**, *17*, 1156–1163. [CrossRef] [PubMed]
5. Lunnon, K.; Smith, R.; Hannon, E.; De Jager, P.L.; Srivastava, G.; Volta, M.; Troakes, C.; Al-Sarraj, S.; Burrage, J.; Macdonald, R.; et al. Methylomic profiling implicates cortical deregulation of *ANK1* in Alzheimer's disease. *Nat. Neurosci.* **2014**, *17*, 1164–1170. [CrossRef]
6. Bonasio, R.; Tu, S.; Reinberg, D. Molecular signals of epigenetic states. *Science* **2010**, *330*, 612–616. [CrossRef]
7. Ma, X.; Liu, L.; Meng, J. MicroRNA-125b promotes neurons cell apoptosis and tau phosphorylation in Alzheimer's disease. *Neurosci. Lett.* **2017**. [CrossRef] [PubMed]
8. Patrick, E.; Rajagopal, S.; Wong, H.A.; McCabe, C.; Xu, J.; Tang, A.; Imboywa, S.H.; Schneider, J.A.; Pochet, N.; Krichevsky, A.M.; et al. Dissecting the role of non-coding RNAs in the accumulation of amyloid and tau neuropathologies in Alzheimer's disease. *Mol. Neurodegener.* **2017**, *12*, 51. [CrossRef] [PubMed]

9. Irier, H.A.; Jin, P. Dynamics of DNA methylation in aging and Alzheimer's disease. *DNA Cell Biol.* **2012**, *31* (Suppl. 1), S42–S48. [CrossRef] [PubMed]
10. Unnikrishnan, A.; Freeman, W.M.; Jackson, J.; Wren, J.D.; Porter, H.; Richardson, A. The role of DNA methylation in epigenetics of aging. *Pharmacol. Ther.* **2018**. [CrossRef] [PubMed]
11. Román, G.C. *MTHFR* gene mutations: A potential marker of late-onset Alzheimer's disease? *J. Alzheimer's Dis.* **2015**, *47*, 323–327. [CrossRef] [PubMed]
12. Wang, J.; Huff, A.M.; Spence, J.D.; Hegele, R.A. Single nucleotide polymorphism in *CTH* associated with variation in plasma homocysteine concentration. *Clin. Genet.* **2004**, *65*, 483–486. [CrossRef] [PubMed]
13. Sharma, R.P.; Gavin, D.P.; Grayson, D.R. CpG methylation in neurons: Message, memory, or mask? *Neuropsychopharmacology* **2010**, *35*, 2009–2020. [CrossRef] [PubMed]
14. Li, E.; Bestor, T.H.; Jaenisch, R. Targeted mutation of the DNA methyltransferase gene results in embryonic lethality. *Cell* **1992**, *69*, 915–926. [CrossRef]
15. Zhang, W.; Xu, J. DNA methyltransferases and their roles in tumorigenesis. *Biomark. Res.* **2017**, *5*, 1. [CrossRef] [PubMed]
16. Hutnick, L.K.; Golshani, P.; Namihira, M.; Xue, Z.; Matynia, A.; Yang, X.W.; Silva, A.J.; Schweizer, F.E.; Fan, G. DNA hypomethylation restricted to the murine forebrain induces cortical degeneration and impairs postnatal neuronal maturation. *Hum. Mol. Genet.* **2009**, *18*, 2875–2888. [CrossRef]
17. Grossi, E.; Stoccoro, A.; Tannorella, P.; Migliore, L.; Coppedè, F. Artificial neural networks link one-carbon metabolism to gene-promoter methylation in Alzheimer's disease. *J. Alzheimers Dis.* **2016**, *53*, 1517–1522. [CrossRef] [PubMed]
18. Jones, P.A.; Liang, G. Rethinking how DNA methylation patterns are maintained. *Nat. Rev. Genet.* **2009**, *10*, 805–811. [CrossRef] [PubMed]
19. Guan, J.Z.; Guan, W.P.; Maeda, T.; Makino, N. Analysis of telomere length and subtelomeric methylation of circulating leukocytes in women with Alzheimer's disease. *Aging Clin. Exp. Res.* **2013**, *25*, 17–23. [CrossRef]
20. Piaceri, I.; Raspanti, B.; Tedde, A.; Bagnoli, S.; Sorbi, S.; Nacmias, B. Epigenetic modifications in Alzheimer's disease: Cause or effect? *J. Alzheimers Dis.* **2015**, *43*, 1169–1173. [CrossRef] [PubMed]
21. West, R.L.; Lee, J.M.; Maroun, L.E. Hypomethylation of the amyloid precursor protein gene in the brain of an Alzheimer's disease patient. *J. Mol. Neurosci.* **1995**, *6*, 141–146. [CrossRef] [PubMed]
22. Tohgi, H.; Utsugisawa, K.; Nagane, Y.; Yoshimura, M.; Genda, Y.; Ukitsu, M. Reduction with age in methylcytosine in the promoter region -224 approximately -101 of the amyloid precursor protein gene in autopsy human cortex. *Brain Res. Mol. Brain Res.* **1999**, *70*, 288–292. [CrossRef]
23. Barrachina, M.; Ferrer, I. DNA methylation of Alzheimer disease and tauopathy-related genes in postmortem brain. *J. Neuropathol. Exp. Neurol.* **2009**, *68*, 880–891. [CrossRef] [PubMed]
24. Chouliaras, L.; Rutten, B.P.; Kenis, G.; Peerbooms, O.; Visser, P.J.; Verhey, F.; van Os, J.; Steinbusch, H.W.; van den Hove, D.L. Epigenetic regulation in the pathophysiology of Alzheimer's disease. *Prog. Neurobiol.* **2010**, *90*, 498–510. [CrossRef] [PubMed]
25. Bakulski, K.M.; Dolinoy, D.C.; Sartor, M.A.; Paulson, H.L.; Konen, J.R.; Lieberman, A.P.; Albin, R.L.; Hu, H.; Rozek, L.S. Genome-wide DNA methylation differences between late-onset Alzheimer's disease and cognitively normal controls in human frontal cortex. *J. Alzheimers Dis.* **2012**, *29*, 571–588. [CrossRef] [PubMed]
26. Bradley-Whitman, M.; Lovell, M.A. Epigenetic changes in the progression of Alzheimer's disease. *Mech. Ageing Dev.* **2013**, *134*, 486–495. [CrossRef] [PubMed]
27. Coppieters, N.; Dieriks, B.V.; Lill, C.; Faull, R.L.; Curtis, M.A.; Dragunow, M. Global changes in DNA methylation and hydroxymethylation in Alzheimer's disease human brain. *Neurobiol. Aging* **2014**, *35*, 1334–1344. [CrossRef] [PubMed]
28. Iwata, A.; Nagata, K.; Hatsuta, H.; Takuma, H.; Bundo, M.; Iwamoto, K.; Tamaoka, A.; Murayama, S.; Saido, T.; Tsuji, S. Altered CpG methylation in sporadic Alzheimer's disease is associated with APP and MAPT dysregulation. *Hum. Mol. Genet.* **2014**, *23*, 648–656. [CrossRef]
29. Humphries, C.E.; Kohli, M.A.; Nathanson, L.; Whitehead, P.; Beecham, G.; Martin, E.; Mash, D.C.; Pericak-Vance, M.A.; Gilbert, J. Integrated whole transcriptome and DNA methylation analysis identifies gene networks specific to late-onset Alzheimer's disease. *J. Alzheimers Dis.* **2015**, *44*, 977–987. [CrossRef]
30. Wang, S.C.; Oelze, B.; Schumacher, A. Age-specific epigenetic drift in late-onset Alzheimer's disease. *PLoS ONE* **2008**, *3*, e2698. [CrossRef]

31. Ellison, E.M.; Abner, E.L.; Lovell, M.A. Multiregional analysis of global 5-methylcytosine and 5-hydroxymethylcytosine throughout the progression of Alzheimer's disease. *J. Neurochem.* **2017**, *140*, 383–394. [CrossRef] [PubMed]
32. Chouliaras, L.; Mastroeni, D.; Delvaux, E.; Grover, A.; Kenis, G.; Hof, P.R.; Steinbusch, H.W.; Coleman, P.D.; Rutten, B.P.; van den Hove, D.L. Consistent decrease in global DNA methylation and hydroxymethylation in the hippocampus of Alzheimer's disease patients. *Neurobiol. Aging.* **2013**, *34*, 2091–2099. [CrossRef] [PubMed]
33. Hernández, H.G.; Sandoval-Hernández, A.G.; Garrido-Gil, P.; Labandeira-Garcia, J.L.; Zelaya, M.V.; Bayon, G.F.; Fernández, A.F.; Fraga, M.F.; Arboleda, G.; Arboleda, H. Alzheimer's disease DNA methylome of pyramidal layers in frontal cortex: Laser-assisted microdissection study. *Epigenomics* **2018**. [CrossRef] [PubMed]
34. Yu, L.; Chibnik, L.B.; Srivastava, G.P.; Pochet, N.; Yang, J.; Xu, J.; Kozubek, J.; Obholzer, N.; Leurgans, S.E.; Schneider, J.A.; et al. Association of brain DNA methylation in *SORL1, ABCA7, HLA-DRB5, SLC24A4*, and *BIN1* with pathological diagnosis of Alzheimer disease. *JAMA Neurol.* **2015**, *72*, 15–24. [CrossRef] [PubMed]
35. Lardenoije, R.; van den Hove, D.L.A.; Havermans, M.; van Casteren, A.; Le, K.X.; Palmour, R.; Lemere, C.A.; Rutten, B.P.F. Age-related epigenetic changes in hippocampal subregions of four animal models of Alzheimer's disease. *Mol. Cell. Neurosci.* **2018**, *86*, 1–15. [CrossRef] [PubMed]
36. OMIM®. Online Mendelian Inheritance in Man® Cystathionine Gamma-Lyase; CTH. Available online: http://www.omim.org/entry/607657 (accessed on 12 December 2018).
37. OMIM®. Online Mendelian Inheritance in Man® 5,10-Methylenetetrahydrofolate Reductase; MTHFR. Available online: http://www.omim.org/entry/607093 (accessed on 12 December 2018).
38. Linnebank, M.; Popp, J.; Smulders, Y.; Smith, D.; Semmler, A.; Farkas, M.; Kulic, L.; Cvetanovska, G.; Blom, H.; Stoffel-Wagner, B.; et al. S-adenosylmethionine is decreased in the cerebrospinal fluid of patients with Alzheimer's disease. *Neurodegener. Dis.* **2010**, *7*, 373–378. [CrossRef] [PubMed]
39. Kirsch, S.H.; Herrmann, W.; Obeid, R. Genetic defects in folate and cobalamin pathways affecting the brain. *Clin. Chem. Lab. Med.* **2013**, *51*, 139–155. [CrossRef] [PubMed]
40. Mitchell, E.S.; Conus, N.; Kaput, J. B vitamin polymorphisms and behavior: Evidence of associations with neurodevelopment, depression, schizophrenia, bipolar disorder and cognitive decline. *Neurosci. Biobehav. Rev.* **2014**, *47*, 307–320. [CrossRef]
41. Seripa, D.; Forno, G.D.; Matera, M.G.; Gravina, C.; Margaglione, M.; Palermo, M.T.; Wekstein, D.R.; Antuono, P.; Davis, D.G.; Daniele, A.; et al. Methylenetetrahydrofolate reductase, angiotensin converting enzyme gene polymorphisms in two genetically, and diagnostically distinct cohort of Alzheimer patients. *Neurobiol. Aging* **2003**, *24*, 933–939. [CrossRef]
42. Da Silva, V.C.; da Costa Ramos, F.J.; Malaquias Freitas, E.; de Brito-Marques, P.R.; de Holanda Cavalcanti, M.N.; D'Almeida, V.; Cabral-Filho, J.E.; Cartaxo Muniz, M.T. Alzheimer's disease in Brazilian elderly has a relation with homocysteine but not with MTHFR polymorphisms. *Arq. Neuro-Psiquiatr.* **2006**, *64*, 941–945. [CrossRef]
43. Nishiyama, M.; Kato, Y.; Hashimoto, M.; Yukawa, S.; Omori, K. Apolipoprotein E, methylenetetrahydrofolate reductase (MTHFR) mutation and the risk of senile dementia—An epidemiological study using the polymerase chain reaction (PCR) method. *Epidemiology* **2000**, *10*, 163–172. [CrossRef]
44. Ford, A.H.; Flicker, L.; Alfonso, H.; Hankey, G.J.; Norman, P.E.; van Bockxmeer, F.M.; Almeida, O.P. Plasma homocysteine and MTHFRC667T polymorphism as risk factors for incident dementia. *J. Neurol. Neurosurg. Psychiatry* **2012**, *83*, 70–75. [CrossRef] [PubMed]
45. De Lau, L.M.L.; van Meurs, J.B.; Uitterlinden, A.G.; Smith, A.D.; Refsum, H.; Johnston, C.; Breteler, M.M. Genetic variation in homocysteine metabolism, cognition, and white matter lesions. *Neurobiol. Aging* **2010**, *31*, 2020–2022. [CrossRef] [PubMed]
46. Mansouri, L.; Fekih-Mrissa, N.; Klai, S.; Mansour, M.; Gritli, N.; Mrissa, R. Association of methylenetetrahydrofolate reductase polymorphisms with susceptibility to Alzheimer's disease. *Clin. Neurol. Neurosurg.* **2013**, *115*, 1693–1696. [CrossRef] [PubMed]
47. Fraga, M.F.; Ballestar, E.; Paz, M.F.; Ropero, S.; Setien, F.; Ballestar, M.L.; Heine-Suñer, D.; Cigudosa, J.C.; Urioste, M.; Benitez, J.; et al. Epigenetic differences arise during the lifetime of monozygotic twins. *Proc. Natl. Acad. Sci. USA* **2005**, *102*, 10604–10609. [CrossRef]

48. Martin, G.M. Epigenetic drift in aging identical twins. *Proc. Natl. Acad. Sci. USA* **2005**, *102*, 10413–10414. [CrossRef]
49. Cook, R.H.; Schneck, S.A.; Clark, D.B. Twins with Alzheimer's disease. *Arch. Neurol.* **1981**, *38*, 300–301. [CrossRef]
50. Breitner, J.C.; Gatz, M.; Bergem, A.L.; Christian, J.C.; Mortimer, J.A.; McClearn, G.E.; Heston, L.L.; Welsh, K.A.; Anthony, J.C.; Folstein, M.F. Use of twin cohorts for research in Alzheimer's disease. *Neurology* **1993**, *43*, 261–267. [CrossRef]
51. Nee, L.E.; Lippa, C.F. Alzheimer's disease in 22 twin pairs—13-year follow-up: Hormonal, infectious and traumatic factors. *Dement. Geriatr. Cogn. Disord.* **1999**, *10*, 148–151. [CrossRef]
52. Coppedè, F. One-carbon metabolism and Alzheimer's disease: Focus on epigenetics. *Curr. Genom.* **2010**, *11*, 246–260. [CrossRef]
53. Spence, J.D.; Yi, Q.; Hankey, G.J. B vitamins in stroke prevention: Time to reconsider. *Lancet Neurol.* **2017**, *16*, 750–760. [CrossRef]
54. Smith, A.D.; Refsum, H. Homocysteine, B vitamins, and cognitive impairment. *Annu. Rev. Nutr.* **2016**, *36*, 211–239. [CrossRef] [PubMed]
55. Tucker, K.L.; Qiao, N.; Scott, T.; Rosenberg, I.; Spiro, A. High homocysteine and low B vitamins predict cognitive decline in aging men: The Veterans Affairs Normative Aging Study. *Am. J. Clin. Nutr.* **2005**, *82*, 627–635. [CrossRef] [PubMed]
56. Lipnicki, D.M.; Sachdev, P.S.; Crawford, J.; Reppermund, S.; Kochan, N.A.; Trollor, J.N.; Draper, B.; Slavin, M.J.; Kang, K.; Lux, O.; et al. Risk factors for late-life cognitive decline and variation with age and sex in the Sydney Memory and Ageing Study. *PLoS ONE* **2013**, *8*, e65841. [CrossRef] [PubMed]
57. Dufouil, C.; Alperovitch, A.; Ducros, V.; Tzourio, C. Homocysteine, white matter hyperintensities, and cognition in healthy elderly people. *Ann. Neurol.* **2003**, *53*, 214–221. [CrossRef] [PubMed]
58. McCaddon, A.; Hudson, P.; Davies, G.; Hughes, A.; Williams, J.H.; Wilkinson, C. Homocysteine and cognitive decline in healthy elderly. *Dement. Geriatr. Cogn. Disord.* **2001**, *12*, 309–313. [CrossRef] [PubMed]
59. Nurk, E.; Refsum, H.; Tell, G.S.; Engedal, K.; Vollset, S.E.; Ueland, P.M.; Nygaard, H.A.; Smith, A.D. Plasma total homocysteine and memory in the elderly: The Hordaland Homocysteine study. *Ann. Neurol.* **2005**, *58*, 847–857. [CrossRef] [PubMed]
60. Hooshmand, B.; Solomon, A.; Kåreholt, I.; Rusanen, M.; Hänninen, T.; Leiviskä, J.; Winblad, B.; Laatikainen, T.; Soininen, H.; Kivipelto, M. Associations between serum homocysteine, holotranscobalamin, folate and cognition in the elderly: A longitudinal study. *J. Intern. Med.* **2012**, *271*, 204–221. [CrossRef] [PubMed]
61. Clarke, R.; Birks, J.; Nexo, E.; Ueland, P.M.; Schneede, J.; Scott, J.; Molloy, A.; Evans, J.G. Low vitamin B-12 status and risk of cognitive decline in older adults. *Am. J. Clin. Nutr.* **2007**, *86*, 1384–1391. [CrossRef] [PubMed]
62. Hooshmand, B.; Mangialasche, F.; Kalpouzos, G.; Solomon, A.; Kåreholt, I.; Smith, A.D.; Refsum, H.; Wang, R.; Mühlmann, M.; Ertl-Wagner, B.; et al. Association of vitamin B12, folate, and sulfur amino acids with brain magnetic resonance imaging measures in older adults: A longitudinal population-based study. *JAMA Psychiatry* **2016**, *73*, 606–613. [CrossRef] [PubMed]
63. Seshadri, S.; Beiser, A.; Selhub, J.; Jacques, P.F.; Rosenberg, I.H.; D'Agostino, R.B.; Wilson, P.W.; Wolf, P.A. Plasma homocysteine as a risk factor for dementia and Alzheimer's disease. *N. Engl. J. Med.* **2002**, *346*, 476–483. [CrossRef] [PubMed]
64. Hooshmand, B.; Solomon, A.; Kåreholt, I.; Leiviskä, J.; Rusanen, M.; Ahtiluoto, S.; Winblad, B.; Laatikainen, T.; Soininen, H.; Kivipelto, M. Homocysteine and holotranscobalamin and the risk of Alzheimer disease: A longitudinal study. *Neurology* **2010**, *75*, 1408–1414. [CrossRef]
65. Faux, N.G.; Ellis, K.A.; Porter, L.; Fowler, C.J.; Laws, S.M.; Martins, R.N.; Pertile, K.K.; Rembach, A.; Rowe, C.C.; Rumble, R.L.; et al. Homocysteine, vitamin B12, and folic acid levels in Alzheimer's disease, mild cognitive impairment, and healthy elderly: Baseline characteristics in subjects of the Australian Imaging Biomarker Lifestyle study. *J. Alzheimers Dis.* **2011**, *27*, 909–922. [CrossRef] [PubMed]
66. Smith, A.D. The worldwide challenge of the dementias: A role for B vitamins and homocysteine? *Food Nutr. Bull.* **2008**, *29*, S143–S172. [CrossRef] [PubMed]
67. Smith, A.D.; Refsum, H.; Bottiglieri, T.; Fenech, M.; Hooshmand, B.; McCaddon, A.; Miller, J.W.; Rosenberg, I.H.; Obeid, R. Homocysteine and dementia: An international consensus statement. *J. Alzheimers Dis.* **2018**, *62*, 561–570. [CrossRef] [PubMed]

68. Minagawa, H.; Watanabe, A.; Akatsu, H.; Adachi, K.; Ohtsuka, C.; Terayama, Y.; Hosono, T.; Takahashi, S.; Wakita, H.; Jung, C.G.; et al. Homocysteine, another risk factor for Alzheimer disease, impairs apolipoprotein E3 function. *J. Biol. Chem.* **2010**, *285*, 38382–38388. [CrossRef] [PubMed]
69. Bhatia, P.; Singh, N. Homocysteine excess: Delineating the possible mechanism of neurotoxicity and depression. *Fundam. Clin. Pharmacol.* **2015**, *29*, 522–528. [CrossRef]
70. Lipton, S.A.; Kim, W.K.; Choi, Y.B.; Kumar, S.; D'Emilia, D.M.; Rayudu, P.V.; Arnelle, D.R.; Stamler, J.S. Neurotoxicity associated with dual actions of homocysteine at the N-methyl-D-aspartate receptor. *Proc. Natl. Acad. Sci. USA* **1997**, *94*, 5923–5928. [CrossRef]
71. Snowdon, D.A.; Tully, C.L.; Smith, C.D.; Riley, K.P.; Markesbery, W.R. Serum folate and the severity of atrophy of the neocortex in Alzheimer disease: Findings from the Nun study. *Am. J. Clin. Nutr.* **2000**, *71*, 993–998. [CrossRef] [PubMed]
72. Wang, H.; Odegaard, A.; Thyagarajan, B.; Hayes, J.; Cruz, K.S.; Derosiers, M.F.; Tyas, S.L.; Gross, M.D. Blood folate is associated with asymptomatic or partially symptomatic Alzheimer's disease in the Nun study. *J. Alzheimers Dis.* **2012**, *28*, 637–645. [CrossRef]
73. Blom, H.J.; Smulders, Y. Overview of homocysteine and folate metabolism. With special references to cardiovascular disease and neural tube defects. *J. Inherit. Metab. Dis.* **2011**, *34*, 75–81. [CrossRef] [PubMed]
74. Nazki, F.H.; Sameer, A.S.; Ganaie, B.A. Folate: Metabolism, genes, polymorphisms and the associated diseases. *Gene* **2014**, *533*, 11–20. [CrossRef] [PubMed]
75. Panossian, L.A.; Porter, V.R.; Valenzuela, H.F.; Zhu, X.; Reback, E.; Masterman, D.; Cummings, J.L.; Effros, R.B. Telomere shortening in T cells correlates with Alzheimer's disease status. *Neurobiol. Aging* **2003**, *24*, 77–84. [CrossRef]
76. Paul, L.; Cattaneo, M.; D'Angelo, A.; Sampietro, F.; Fermo, I.; Razzari, C.; Fontana, G.; Eugene, N.; Jacques, P.F.; Selhub, J. Telomere length in peripheral blood mononuclear cells is associated with folate status in men. *J. Nutr.* **2009**, *139*, 1273–1278. [CrossRef] [PubMed]
77. Friso, S.; Choi, S.-W.; Girelli, D.; Mason, J.B.; Dolnikowski, G.G.; Bagley, P.J.; Olivieri, O.; Jacques, P.F.; Rosenberg, I.H.; Corrocher, R.; et al. A common mutation in the 5,10-methylenetetrahydrofolate reductase gene affects genomic DNA methylation through an interaction with folate status. *Proc. Natl. Acad. Sci. USA* **2002**, *99*, 5606–5811. [CrossRef] [PubMed]
78. Blount, B.C.; Mack, M.M.; Wehr, C.M.; MacGregor, J.T.; Hiatt, R.A.; Wang, G.; Wickramasinghe, S.N.; Everson, R.B.; Ames, B.N. Folate deficiency causes uracil misincorporation into human DNA and chromosome breakage: Implications for cancer and neuronal damage. *Proc. Natl. Acad. Sci. USA* **1997**, *94*, 3290–3295. [CrossRef] [PubMed]
79. Troesch, B.; Weber, P.; Mohajeri, M. Potential links between impaired one-carbon metabolism due to polymorphisms, inadequate B-vitamin status, and the development of Alzheimer's disease. *Nutrients* **2016**, *8*, 803. [CrossRef]
80. Religa, D.; Styczynska, M.; Peplonska, B.; Gabryelewicz, T.; Pfeffer, A.; Chodakowska, M.; Luczywek, E.; Wasiak, B.; Stepien, K.; Golebiowski, M.; et al. Homocysteine, apolipoprotein E and methylenetetrahydrofolate reductase in Alzheimer's disease and mild cognitive impairment. *Dement. Geriatr. Cogn. Disord.* **2003**, *16*, 64–70. [CrossRef] [PubMed]
81. Smith, D.A.D.; Warren, M.J.; Refsum, H. Chapter Six—Vitamin B_{12}. *Adv. Food Nutr. Res.* **2018**, *83*, 215–279. [CrossRef] [PubMed]
82. Stabler, S.P. Vitamin B_{12} deficiency. *N. Engl. J. Med.* **2013**, *368*, 149–160. [CrossRef] [PubMed]
83. Valente, E.; Scott, J.M.; Ueland, P.-M.; Cunningham, C.; Casey, M.; Molloy, A.M. Diagnostic accuracy of holotranscobalamin, methylmalonic acid, serum cobalamin, and other indicators of tissue vitamin B_{12} status in the elderly. *Clin. Chem.* **2011**, *57*, 856–863. [CrossRef] [PubMed]
84. Cho, H.S.; Huang, L.K.; Lee, Y.T.; Chan, L.; Hong, C.T. Suboptimal baseline serum vitamin B_{12} is associated with cognitive decline in people with Alzheimer's disease undergoing cholinesterase inhibitor treatment. *Front. Neurol.* **2018**, *9*, 325. [CrossRef] [PubMed]
85. Garcia, A.; Haron, Y.; Evans, L.; Smith, M.; Freedman, M.; Román, G. Metabolic markers of cobalamin deficiency and cognitive function in normal older adults. *J. Am. Geriatr. Soc.* **2004**, *52*, 66–71. [CrossRef]
86. Garcia, A.; Zanibbi, K. Homocysteine and cognitive function in elderly people. *CMAJ* **2004**, *171*, 897–904. [CrossRef] [PubMed]

87. Román, G.C.; Ruiz, P.J. Neurologic complications of Sjögren syndrome. *MedLink Neurol.* **2010**, *11*, 1034.
88. Andrès, E.; Loukili, N.H.; Noel, E.; Kaltenbach, G.; Abdelgheni, M.B.; Perrin, A.E.; Noblet-Dick, M.; Maloisel, F.; Schlienger, J.L.; Blicklé, J.F. Vitamin B_{12} (cobalamin) deficiency in elderly patients. *CMAJ* **2004**, *171*, 251–259. [CrossRef] [PubMed]
89. Spence, D. Mechanisms of thrombogenesis in atrial fibrillation. *Lancet* **2009**, *373*, 1006. [CrossRef]
90. Wallin, A.; Román, G.C.; Esiri, M.; Kettunen, P.; Svensson, J.; Paraskevas, G.P.; Kapaki, E. Update on vascular cognitive impairment associated with subcortical small-vessel disease. *J. Alzheimers Dis.* **2018**, *62*, 1417–1441. [CrossRef] [PubMed]
91. Mohajeri, M.H.; Troesch, B.; Weber, P. Inadequate supply of vitamins and DHA in the elderly: Implications for brain aging and Alzheimer-type dementia. *Nutrition* **2015**, *31*, 261–275. [CrossRef]
92. Fuso, A.; Nicolia, V.; Cavallaro, R.A.; Ricceri, L.; D'Anselmi, F.; Coluccia, P.; Calamandrei, G.; Scarpa, S. B-vitamin deprivation induces hyperhomocysteinemia and brain S-adenosylhomocysteine, depletes brain S-adenosylmethionine, and enhances PS1 and BACE expression and amyloid-β deposition in mice. *Mol. Cell. Neurosci.* **2008**, *37*, 731–746. [CrossRef] [PubMed]
93. McCleery, J.; Abraham, R.P.; Denton, D.A.; Rutjes, A.W.; Chong, L.Y.; Al-Assaf, A.S.; Griffith, D.J.; Rafeeq, S.; Yaman, H.; Malik, M.A.; et al. Vitamin and mineral supplementation for preventing dementia or delaying cognitive decline in people with mild cognitive impairment. *Cochrane Database Syst. Rev.* **2018**, *11*, CD011905. [CrossRef]
94. Smith, A.D.; Smith, S.M.; de Jager, C.A.; Whitbread, P.; Johnston, C.; Agacinski, G.; Oulhaj, A.; Bradley, K.M.; Jacoby, R.; Refsum, H. Homocysteine-lowering by B vitamins slows the rate of accelerated brain atrophy in mild cognitive impairment. A randomized controlled trial. *PLoS ONE* **2010**, *5*, e12244. [CrossRef] [PubMed]
95. Jager, C.A.; Oulhaj, A.; Jacoby, R.; Refsum, H.; Smith, A.D. Cognitive and clinical outcomes of homocysteine-lowering B-vitamin treatment in mild cognitive impairment: A randomized controlled trial. *Int. J. Geriatr. Psychiatry* **2012**, *27*, 592–600. [CrossRef] [PubMed]
96. Douauda, G.; Refsum, H.; de Jager, C.A.; Jacoby, R.; Nichols, T.E.; Smith, S.M.; Smith, A.D. Preventing Alzheimer's disease-related gray matter atrophy by B-vitamin treatment. *PNAS Proc. Natl. Acad. Sci. USA* **2013**, *110*, 9523–9528. [CrossRef] [PubMed]
97. Sharma, A.; Gerbarg, P.; Bottiglieri, T.; Massoumi, L.; Carpenter, L.L.; Lavretsky, H.; Muskin, P.R.; Brown, R.P.; Mischoulon, D. As Work Group of the American Psychiatric Association Council on Research S-Adenosylmethionine (SAMe) for Neuropsychiatric Disorders: A Clinician-Oriented Review of Research. *J. Clin. Psychiatry* **2017**, *78*, e656–e667. [CrossRef] [PubMed]
98. Dayon, L.; Guiraud, S.P.; Corthésy, J.; Da Silva, L.; Migliavacca, E.; Tautvydaitė, D.; Oikonomidi, A.; Moullet, B.; Henry, H.; Métairon, S.; et al. One-carbon metabolism, cognitive impairment and CSF measures of Alzheimer pathology: Homocysteine and beyond. *Alzheimers. Res. Ther.* **2017**, *9*, 43. [CrossRef]
99. Galizia, I.; Oldani, L.; Macritchie, K.; Amari, E.; Dougall, D.; Jones, T.N.; Lam, R.W.; Massei, G.J.; Yatham, L.N.; Young, A.H. S-adenosyl methionine (SAMe) for depression in adults. *Cochrane Database Syst. Rev.* **2016**. [CrossRef]

2

New Insights into the Molecular Bases of Familial Alzheimer's Disease

Valeria D'Argenio [1,2,*] **and Daniela Sarnataro** [3,*]

[1] CEINGE-Biotecnologie Avanzate scarl, via G. Salvatore 486, 80145 Naples, Italy
[2] Department of Human Sciences and Quality of Life Promotion, San Raffaele Open University, via di val Cannuta 247, 00166 Rome, Italy
[3] Department of Molecular Medicine and Medical Biotechnology, Federico II University, via S. Pansini 5, 80131 Naples, Italy
* Correspondence: dargenio@ceinge.unina.it (V.D.); daniela.sarnataro@unina.it (D.S.)

Abstract: Like several neurodegenerative disorders, such as Prion and Parkinson diseases, Alzheimer's disease (AD) is characterized by spreading mechanism of aggregated proteins in the brain in a typical "prion-like" manner. Recent genetic studies have identified in four genes associated with inherited AD (amyloid precursor protein-*APP*, Presenilin-1, Presenilin-2 and Apolipoprotein E), rare mutations which cause dysregulation of APP processing and alterations of folding of the derived amyloid beta peptide (Aβ). Accumulation and aggregation of Aβ in the brain can trigger a series of intracellular events, including hyperphosphorylation of tau protein, leading to the pathological features of AD. However, mutations in these four genes account for a small of the total genetic risk for familial AD (FAD). Genome-wide association studies have recently led to the identification of additional AD candidate genes. Here, we review an update of well-established, highly penetrant FAD-causing genes with correlation to the protein misfolding pathway, and novel emerging candidate FAD genes, as well as inherited risk factors. Knowledge of these genes and of their correlated biochemical cascade will provide several potential targets for treatment of AD and aging-related disorders.

Keywords: Alzheimer's disease; *APP* mutations; *APOE* alleles; *PSEN1*; *PSEN2*; germline mutations; late onset AD; early onset AD; familial AD; genetics of AD

---

1. Introduction

Alzheimer's disease (AD) is responsible for about 60–70% of cases of dementia, equivalent to an estimated population of 40–50 million persons worldwide. This more than doubled from 1990 to 2016 [1]. Typically, AD is featured by a progressive neurodegeneration that lead to a gradual loss of memory and alterations affecting other cognitive functions, such as spatial cognition, reasoning, word-finding, judgment and problem-solving [2]. Aging is the most important AD risk factor and, even if it may occur at any age, more often AD appears in older individuals (later than 65 years of age) [3,4]. However, early onset AD cases, characterized by the occurrence of clinical signs between 30 and 65 years old, have been also reported [3,4]. Even if atypical phenotypes have been described, clinical and pathological features seem to be the same between early and late onset AD, so that it may be difficult to distinguish these 2 groups [4]. Interestingly, while late onset AD is usually sporadic and doesn't show any segregation within the families, it has been highlighted that early onset AD is featured by a high recurrence rate within the affected families, thus suggesting the presence of inherited forms of AD [3].

In particular, it has been estimated that 15–25% of total AD accounts for familial Alzheimer's disease (FAD) (Figure 1) [5].

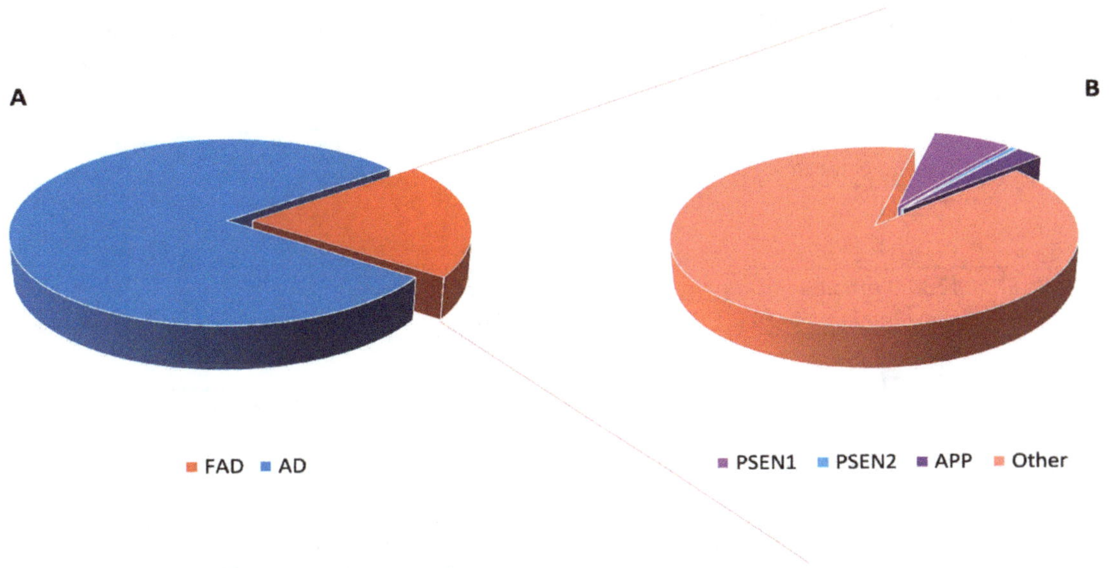

Figure 1. Prevalence and genetic causes of familial Alzheimer's disease (FAD). FAD represents only a small fraction (about 20%) of all Alzheimer's disease (AD) cases (**A**). In addition, within FAD, mutations the amyloid precursor protein (*APP*), presenilin 1 (*PSEN1*) or presenilin 2 (*PSEN2*) genes account for a small proportion of cases, underlying that the molecular bases of the larger fraction still remain to be unveiled (**B**).

In this category, it is included the autosomal dominant Alzheimer's disease (ADAD), associated to the presence of known causative gene mutations, mainly in the amyloid precursor protein (*APP*), presenilin 1 (*PSEN1*) or presenilin 2 (*PSEN2*) genes, that have been described as highly penetrant, disease-causing FAD genes [3–5]. However, mutations in these genes are able to explain just a small percentage of all FAD cases, suggesting the existence of other, inherited, disease-predisposing genes [4]. Since FAD typically shows a sequential, clinical progression from pre-dementia to dementia stage, thus it is crucial to recognize and diagnose it before symptoms onset in order to begin treatments as soon as possible [6,7]. As a consequence, a better understanding of FAD molecular bases, i.e., the identification of the causative genes, may ameliorate the management and the clinical outcome of these patients and of their families.

Recent advances in genomics, i.e., the availability of highly performing next generation sequencing (NGS)-based methods to accurately analyze single genes [8,9] or a subset of genes of interest [10–12], up to the whole exome [13,14] or the whole genome [13,14], has prompted the study of the molecular bases of human diseases and is a promising tool to discover novel FAD-related genes [4].

Here, we will review the current knowledge regarding the genetic etiology of FAD. In particular, we will focus first on well-established, highly penetrant, FAD-causing genes. In this context, the relationship between mutations affecting AD-related genes and proteins' trafficking, folding and aggregation properties will be highlighted, with special attention to APP. Next, novel, emerging and candidate FAD genes, as well as inherited risk factors will be also discussed, suggesting that enlarged genetic testing may be useful in FAD families in order to improve the identification and management of the at-risk subjects.

2. Methods

Indexed articles in English were searched in PubMed using the following keywords: "Alzheimer's disease molecular bases", "Alzheimer's disease mutations", "Alzheimer's disease germline mutations", "Alzheimer's disease genes", "inherited Alzheimer's disease", "familial Alzheimer's disease",

"*APP* mutations", "*PSEN1* mutations", "*PSEN2* mutations" and "novel Alzheimer's disease genes". In the attempt to focus on the most recent and updated papers on these topics, we fixed the time within 2010 and 2020 as temporal window; however, a manual search for oldest references mentioned in the found articles was also carried out. Papers in the search results reporting somatic mutations or describing genetic risk factors related to sporadic, late onset AD were not included since are out of the topic of the present review (Figure 2).

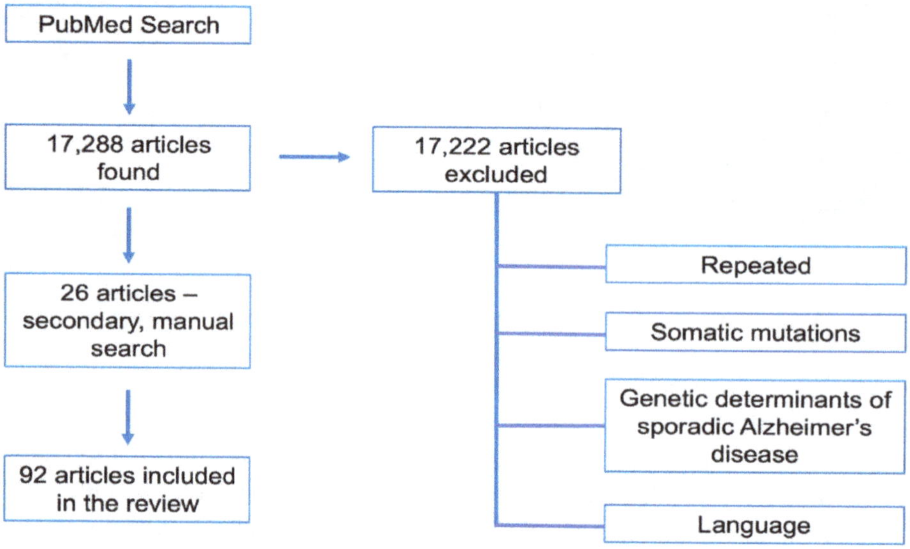

Figure 2. Flow-diagram summarizing the steps for the selection of the articles reviewed herein.

3. Highly Penetrant Familial Alzheimer Disease-Causing Genes

Genetic analysis of large FAD families allowed the discovery of the three well established and high-penetrant genes related to this disease, namely, *APP*, *PSEN1* and *PSEN2* (Figure 3).

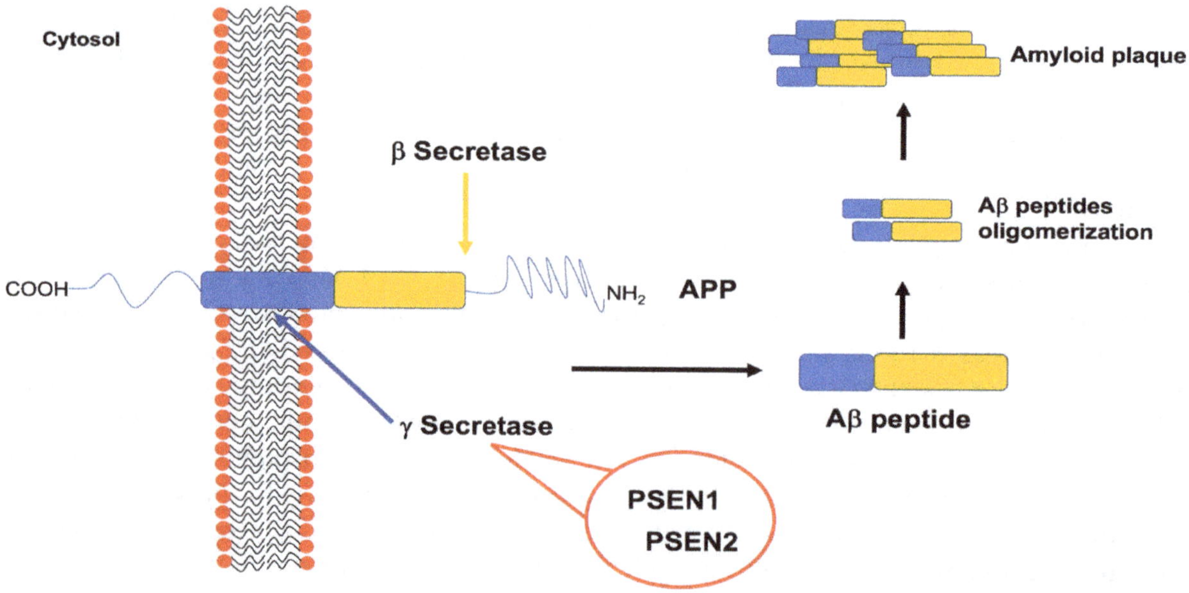

Figure 3. Amyloid precursor protein (APP) structure and amyloid beta (Aβ) peptide production. The cleavage of APP by specific secretases is required to produce the Aβ peptide. One of these secretases, namely the γ secretase, is a multimeric complex involving also presenilin 1 (PSEN1) and presenilin 2 (PSEN2). Mutations affecting *APP*, as well as *PSEN1* or *PSEN2* genes, have been associated to familial Alzheimer's disease (FAD) because of their ability to increase Aβ peptides production and, consequently, their aggregation up to amyloid plaques formation.

The amyloid precursor protein gene (*APP*, OMIM #104760, chromosome 21q21.3) encodes for an integral type 1 membrane glycoprotein that is almost ubiquitously expressed. APP is sequentially processed for proteolytic cleavage to produce amyloid β (Aβ), by β- and γ-secretases (the latter composed by PSEN1, PSEN2, Nicastrin and Aph-1). Because APP processing by γ-secretase is not restricted to a single site, it gives rise to different Aβ species, $A\beta_{42}$ being more prone to aggregate [15].

Recently it has become evident that the AD-typical Aβ assemblies are able to adopt alternative conformations and become self-propagating, like prions [16–19].

To date, 32 pathogenic mutations in *APP* were reported within or flanking the Aβ sequence (https://www.alzforum.org/mutations/app), being located mostly near the β- and γ-secretase sites [20]. As a consequence, *APP* mutations seem to be able to increase Aβ aggregation rate, thus causing FAD (Figure 3) [21].

The p.K670N and p.M671L Swedish AD-related pathogenic mutations are localized near to the γ-secretase site and lead to increased absolute levels of $A\beta_{42}$ (without changing $A\beta_{42}$ to $A\beta_{40}$ ratio) [22]. Interestingly, Del Prete et al., found that in a Swedish cell culture model of AD, APP and its catabolites are present in mitochondrial-ER associated membranes (MAMs) and β- and γ-secretases harbor APP processing activities in MAMs [23]. This finding is extremely interesting, considering the fact that the localization of APP and its enzymes plays a critical role in the Aβ generation and its signaling inside the cell [24]. The p.T714I, p.V715M, p.V715A, p.I716V, p.V717I and p.V717L *APP* mutations are all located in proximity of the γ-secretase site, affect the cleavage and, contrary to the double Swedish mutations, cause an increase of the $A\beta_{42}$ to $A\beta_{40}$ ratio and are able to influence the stability of APP C-terminal fragments [20,25]. Very recently, the p.I716T *APP* mutation [25], as well as the p.L723P featured by the local unfolding of the C-terminal turn [26], was described to affect the efficiency of the γ-secretase ε-cleavage and to induce a major $A\beta_{42}$ to $A\beta_{40}$ ratio. This effect is due to the additional H-bond between the T716 side chain and the transmembrane backbone, which can affect the cleavage domain dynamic [25].

Mutations within the Aβ sequence have been predicted not only to affect APP processing, thus regulating the amount of total Aβ production, but were also thought to affect the aggregation properties of the resulting Aβ peptide [25]. Indeed, the *APP* p.A692G, p.E693Q and p.D694N mutations, all located inside the Aβ sequence, have been described to have an increased aggregative ability and neurotoxicity respect to the wild type Aβ [21].

Although a common effect of these mutations is the dysregulation of the production of different Aβ forms of APP, a recent paper form Lumsden et al. proposed also a dysregulation of iron homeostasis as a common effect of mutations related to early onset AD [27].

Table 1 summarizes *APP* mutations, affecting protein stability, folding, processing, from the N- to the C-terminal.

Despite the above, it has been reported that *APP* dominant mutations account for about 16% of all ADAD [3]. Some years ago, 2 *APP* mutations, namely p.A673V and p.E693del, have been found to be able to cause FAD only in the homozygous status supporting the existence also of a recessive pattern of inheritance [28,29]. More recently, Conidi et al., described an Italian family carrying the *APP* p.A713T in homozygous status; surprisingly the clinical phenotype was not more severe respect to the heterozygous carriers [30]. This finding not only highlighted that the homozygosity for *APP* dominant mutations is not lethal, but also suggested that other, independently inherited genetic factors, may exert a protective effect and modify the clinical presentation of the disease.

Finally, in addition to single nucleotide variants and small insertion/deletions, dominantly inherited duplications of the *APP* locus have been also described and associated to AD [31–35]. In particular, small chromosomal duplications with different genomic coordinates, but all including the *APP* locus, have been described in some French FAD families [31,32]. Next, *APP* duplications were reported also in Finnish and Dutch FAD cases [33–35]. The clinical consequences of these duplications are not yet clearly defined and also their frequency as FAD cause is variable in the different studies [31–35]. Totally, 25 duplications have been identified so far and, respect to missense mutations, these duplications seem to have a reduced penetrance and a variable age of onset [36].

Table 1. Amyloid precursor protein (*APP*) pathogenic mutations and their effects at protein level.

Mutation and Protein Region	Protein Stability/Folding/Processing	Reference
N-terminal		
p.K670N/p.M671L	Leads to increased absolute levels of $A\beta_{42}$, doesn't alter $A\beta_{42}/A\beta_{40}$ ratio Present in MAMs	Kumar-Singh_2009 [22] Del Prete_2017 [23]
Amyloid-beta domain		
p.A692G p.E693Q p.E693K p.E693G p.D694N	Potent aggregative	Murakami_2002 [21]
p.A713T p.T714I	Increase $A\beta_{42}/A\beta_{40}$ ratio, affect stability of *APP* CTFs	Kumar-Singh_2009 [22]
Transmembrane/C-terminal		
p.V715M p.I716V p.V717L	Increase $A\beta_{42}/A\beta_{40}$ ratio, affect stability of *APP* CTFs	De Jonghe_2001 [20]
Pp.I716T	Increases $A\beta_{42}/A\beta_{40}$ ratio reducing the efficiency of the γ-secretase ε-cleavage	Götz_2019 [25]
p.L723P	Causes unfolding of C-terminal turn of *APP* TM domain helix	Bocharov_2019 [26]

Interestingly, Jonsson et al., identified a rare *APP* variant in the Icelandic population showing a protective effect [37]. Finally, a number of variants of unknown clinical significance have been also detected and further functional tests are required to establish their pathogenicity.

The presenilin 1 (*PSEN1*, OMIM #104311, chromosome 14q24.3) encodes for a protein that is a subunit of γ-secretase, i.e., one of the 2 enzymes responsible for APP proteolytic cleavage. As a consequence, mutations in *PSEN1*, impairing the activity of γ-secretase complex, may lead to the production of more aggregation-prone forms of the $A\beta$ peptide, that is a typical hallmark of AD, thus inducing the disease development (Figure 3) [3,4].

PSEN1 is the most common gene related to FAD. To date, 221 *PSEN1* pathogenic mutations have been described, accounting for up to 70% of ADAD cases (http://www.alzforum.org/mutations). These mutations can be both single nucleotide variants and small insertions/deletions; in addition, a deletion able to cause *PSEN1* exon 9 skipping, has been also described [38]. Typically, FAD onset in *PSEN1* mutations carriers ranges from 30 to 50 years, the mutations showing an autosomal dominant inheritance and almost always a complete penetrance [39]. Interestingly, *de novo* mutations, featured by a very early age of onset (before 30 years) have been also described [40–42].

As in the case of *APP*, Kosik et al., described a Colombian family carrying the *PSEN1* mutation p.E280A in homozygous status; also, in this case, the severity of the disease was not influenced by the homozygosity of the mutation [43].

The presenilin 2 (*PSEN2*, OMIM #600759, chromosome 1q31-q42) gene has a genetic structure very similar to *PSEN1*, sharing a sequence homology of 67% [3]. It encodes for another component of the γ-secretase complex; thus, its impairment, due to pathogenic mutations, is able to increase the $A\beta_{42}/A\beta_{40}$ ratio too (Figure 3).

To date, 19 different *PSEN2* pathogenic mutations have been reported (http://www.alzforum.org/mutations). As for *PSEN1*, these pathogenic mutations are scattered along the entire gene sequence with a higher frequency in the transmembrane domains [44,45]. The ADAD age of onset ranges from 40 to 70 years in *PSEN2* mutations carriers, the penetrance of these mutations being still controversial to assess, due to the few numbers of families reported to date and showing also a so wide age-range of onset [39].

It has been estimated that totally, *APP*, *PSEN1* and *PSEN2* mutations account only for about 5–10% of all FAD (Figure 1) [46,47]. Within the FAD, considering only the ADAD forms the contribution of these genes is highly heterogeneous based on the population studied, 23% up to 88% of patients remaining without a genetic diagnosis [47,48]. Since the clinical features of FAD can be variable, the diagnosis is often difficult and delayed, underlying the importance of identifying other molecular alterations responsible for the currently unexplained FAD cases.

4. Apolipoprotein E ε4 Risk Allele and Familial Alzheimer Disease

The apolipoprotein E gene (*APOE*, OMIM #107741, chromosome 19q13.2) encodes a glycoprotein involved in the mobilization of peripheral cholesterol, also during neuronal growth and regeneration [49,50]. Three APOE isoforms are known, namely ApoE2, ApoE3 and ApoE4, differing at level of 2 aminoacidic residues (the 112 and 158) and coded by 3 alleles, i.e., ε2, ε3 and ε4, whose frequency varies among different populations [3].

To date, an association between the ε4 allele and the sporadic, late-onset AD has been reported [3,4]. In particular, it has been assessed an increased risk up to 3-fold in the heterozygous carriers and up to 15-fold in the homozygous [51]. Interestingly, the ε2 allele has been reported as a protective factor, reducing the AD risk and also positively impacting longevity [52]. These different features have been related to ta different binding affinity of the encoded proteins for the Aβ peptide; in particular, ApoE4 shows the highest affinity leading to the creation of monofibrils that are able to produce dense precipitates [3]. However, it is important to underline that the ε4 allele is not a cause but an AD risk factor; thus, other genetic or environmental factors are required for disease development. A working model, attempting to explain the relationship between ApoE and Alzheimer's disease, has been proposed (Figure 4) [53].

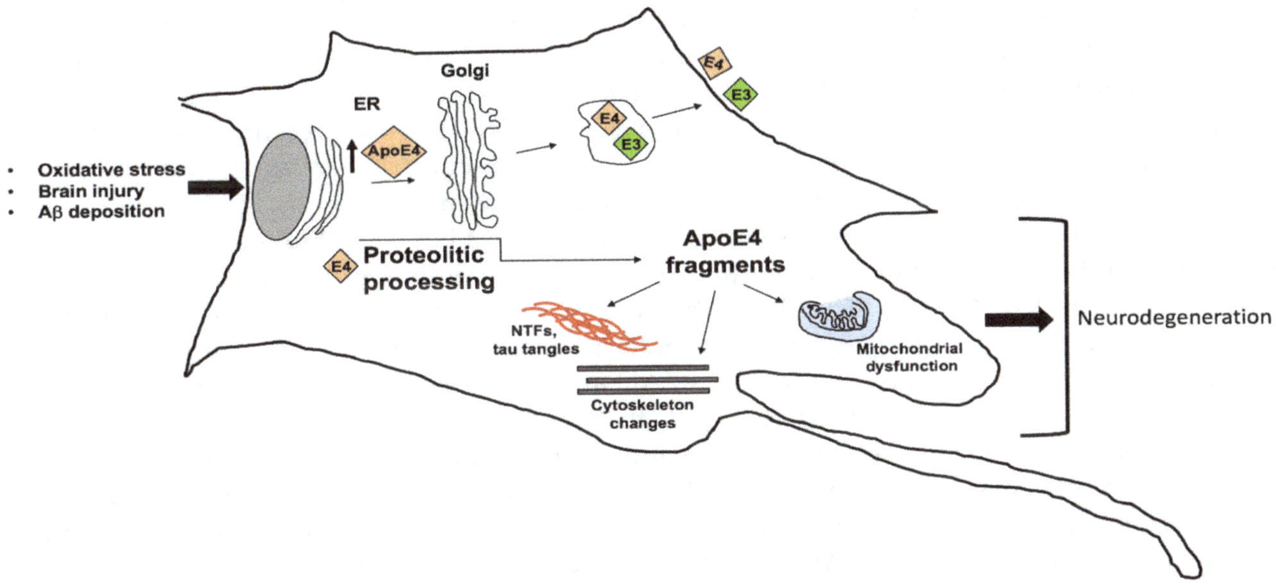

Figure 4. Working model for Apolipoprotein E4 (ApoE4) contribution to Alzheimer's disease (AD) development. Different stimuli can induce ApoE4 and ApoE3 overexpression, with E4 contribution to neurodegeneration in AD. ApoE4, undergoing to proteolytic cleavage, can generate different fragments which can contribute to mitochondrial dysfunction, cytoskeletal disorganization, neurofibrillary tangles and, consequently to neurodegeneration.

In particular, ApoE4, unlike ApoE3, contributes to AD by interacting with different factors through various pathways. In response to oxidative stress, aging, brain damage or Aβ deposition, neurons synthesize increasing amount of ApoE, that in turn undergoes proteolytic processing generating fragments which cause mitochondrial dysfunction, cytoskeletal changes, NFT (neurofibrillary tangles) formation, leading to neurodegeneration.

Interestingly, it has been shown that the *APOE* ε4 allele is able to increase also the risk for early onset AD in presence of familiarity for the disease [54]. In particular, in the ε4 homozygous carriers the risk was independent from other genetic factors, while in the heterozygous no, suggesting that it may act as disease phenotype-modifier in presence of other genetic mutations [4]. However, Genin et al., reported for *APOE* ε4 allele an AD risk comparable to that of other genetic factors [55]. Some studies, evaluating the effects of the *APOE* genotype on AD clinical features in families carrying pathogenic mutations in *APP*, *PSEN1* or *PSEN2* genes, showed that the ε4 allele is associated to an earlier age of onset in the mutations' carriers, while the carriers of the ε2 allele had a later onset [56–58]. Nevertheless, it is important to underline that the significance of *APOE* testing in clinical practice is still under debate and it has been recently reviewed to not significantly impact diagnostic and prognostic evaluations [59]. Indeed, being a risk factor, the *APOE* ε4 allele is common in the general population, i.e., also in healthy individual without a positive family history of AD. Further large longitudinal studies are required to assess the contribution of *APOE* to AD risk and its possible use in clinical routine settings.

5. Novel, Emerging and Candidate Genes Associated to Familial Alzheimer Disease

Mutations in *APP*, *PSEN1* and *PSEN2* genes, as well as the *APOE* ε4 risk allele, explain only a small percentage of all FAD cases, suggesting that other genes may play a role. In the last years, NGS based studies, through the analysis of large pedigrees, are allowing the detection of novel genes potentially related to FAD.

Guerreiro et al., analyzing a Turkish FAD family, identified a pathogenic mutation in the *NOTCH3* gene [60]. Interestingly, the same mutation was previously associated with a dementia disorder similar to AD and the proband belongs to a consanguineous family with a complex history of neurological disorders [60]. *NOTCH3* (OMIM# 600276, chromosome 19p13.12) encodes a transmembrane receptor involved in cellular signaling and embryonic development. More than 130 mutations have been reported in this gene and related to the rare syndrome cerebral arteriopathy autosomal dominant with subcortical infarcts and leukoencephalopathy; a role also in FAD has been recently proposed [61].

The finding of a shared gene between degenerative and vascular dementias suggests the presence of a similar neurovascular unit dysfunction. Accordingly, a consensus paper by Bordet et al., based on the observation that most of patients currently seem to be affected by mixed forms, proposed that also therapeutic strategies should be common [62]. Indeed, therapeutic approaches should be oriented towards an integrated strategy, including antioxidants, anti-inflammatory, modulation of proteins aggregation and neuronal plasticity. Since in older patients, vascular cognitive impairment (VCI) leading to vascular dementia is often mixed to AD and VCI is rarely "pure", a disease modifying strategy seems to be justified [62]. It is noteworthy that a mitochondrial dysfunction may play a role in this context as an additional cause of cognitive impairment, either of vascular, degenerative or both natures [63]. In particular, a reduction of respiratory chain complex I activity, related to mitochondrial dysfunction, has been reported in a group of patients with vascular dementia and several mitochondrial mechanisms have been invoked in Aβ-related cerebrovascular degeneration [63].

Pottier et al., carried out the WES of 29 probands from FAD families resulted negative for mutations in the 3 main FAD genes and found 7 mutations in the *SORL1* gene [64]. In particular, one of these mutations, i.e., the p.G511R, has been shown to be able to reduce the ability of the protein to bind the Aβ peptide, thus inducing its accumulation [65]. The sortilin-related receptor (*SORL1*, OMIM# 602005, chromosome 11q24.1) encodes for a mosaic protein that is the receptor of neuronal ApoE. Accordingly, *SORL-1* mutations have been described in 2 families with early onset AD. In particular, the *SORL-1* variants where shown to be able to weaken the interaction with APP, interfering with APP trafficking and altering the Aβ levels [66]. Other studies have confirmed the role of *SORL1* mutations in FAD and also in late onset AD [67,68]. Li et al., have recently reported the case of a patient with early onset AD and cognitive impairment, carrying a heterozygous mutation in the *SORL1* gene [69]. Taken together, these items of evidence suggest that *SORL1* mutations may be involved in FAD, its contribution being probably underestimated, and that this gene should be tested in the affected families in addition to *APP*, *PSEN1* and *PSEN2* genes. Indeed, the analysis of *SORL1* in larger cohorts of patients may allow to better clarify its contribution to FAD.

Interestingly, genome-wide association studies identified about 30 additional risk factors/alleles for late onset AD [70,71]. Among these, variants affecting *CLU* (*APOJ*) or *CR1* (complement component 3b/4b receptor 1), being involved in the clearance of Aβ have been associated to AD [72] and heterozygous missense mutations in *TREM2* (triggering receptor myeloid 2 cells) have been described to increase by 3-fold the risk of AD [73]. It has been proposed that these genes may be responsible also for FAD cases.

In particular, an increased frequency of *CLU* gene rare coding mutations has been highlighted in AD patients, predominantly affecting the β chain of the protein [74]. Clusterin (*CLU*, OMIM# 185430, chromosome 8p21.1) encodes a protein involved in synapsis turnover. Most of the CLU variants described so far are able to promote CLU degradation, thus reducing its activity [75].

Two NGS-based studies identified a rare variant (p.Arg47His) in *TREM2* gene [73,76] *TREM2* (OMIM# 605086, chromosome 6p21.1) encodes a type I transmembrane protein belonging to the immunoglobulin receptor superfamily and involved in immune responses activation. Interestingly, TREM2 has been found to be able to bind ApoE, thus increasing the phagocytosis of ApoE-bound apoptotic neurons [77]. Some *TREM2* variants may increase AD risk by reducing the affinity for ApoE, and thus decreasing Aβ peptide clearance. Additionally, it has been showed that *TREM2* mutations in its extracellular domain impair protein maturation and its phagocytic activity [78,79]. The *TREM2* p.Arg47His variant has been reported in different population as associated to AD, including some cases of FAD [73,76,80–82]. The role of other *TREM2* variants is still poorly understood.

Three independent studies identified loss-of-function mutations in the *ABCA7* gene in AD patients [83–85]. The ATP-binding cassette, subfamily A, member 7 (*ABCA7*, OMIM# 605414, chromosome 19p13.3) encodes a transporter protein able to move lipids across the membranes. It has been reported that the inhibition of ABCA7 expression is able to increase β secretase cleavage of APP, thus increasing the production of Aβ peptide [86]. In particular, Cuyvers et al., identified an *ABCA7* frameshift mutation as a founder mutation in a Belgian population, since it was detected in several FAD families showing a dominant pattern of inheritance [83].

Vardarajan et al., by sequencing 76 AD-related loci, identified a rare missense mutation in the *EPHA1* gene (p.P460L) segregating within a large Caribbean FAD family [85]. The Ephrin receptor (*EPHA1*, OMIM # 179610, chromosome 7q34-q35) encodes a tyrosine kinase receptor implicated in neuronal development.

The main features of novel FAD candidate genes are summarized in Table 2.

Table 2. Novel candidate genes and inherited risk factors associated to familial Alzheimer's disease (FAD).

Gene Name (Acronym)	Proposed Function in FAD	References
Apolipoprotein E (*APOE*)	Contribution of ApoE4 to mitochondrial dysfunction, cytoskeletal disorganization and neurofibrillary tangles	Huang_2006 [53]
Neurogenic Locus Notch Homolog Protein 3 (*NOTCH3*)	Cellular signaling impairment	Patel_2019 [61]
Sortilin-related receptor (*SORL1*)	Interference with APP trafficking and alteration of the Aβ levels	Cuccaro_2016 [66]
Complement component 3b/4b receptor 1 (*CR1*)	Aβ peptide clearance reduction	Shen 2016 [72]
Clusterin (*CLU*)	Synapsis turnover reduction	Bettens_2015 [75]
Triggering Receptor Expressed on Myeloid Cells 2 (*TREM2*)	Aβ peptide clearance reduction	Bailey_2015 [77] Lue_2015 [78] Kleinberger_2014 [79]
The ATP-binding cassette, subfamily a, member 7 (*ABCA7*)	Aβ peptide production increase	Satoh_2015 [86]
Ephrin receptor (*EPHA1*)	Alteration of neuronal development	Vardarajan_2016 [85]

It is noticeable that the same genes identified as risk factors for sporadic and late onset AD, harbor also rare variants segregating with FAD. Even if data in this field are still inconclusive since they are often based on isolated findings, however they suggest that some familial cases may be due the combination of rare variants and other risk factors. Recent NGS-based screening including FAD cases, identified established risk alleles with moderate penetrance and one or more variants of uncertain significance, thus suggesting the hypothesis, in presence of no mutations in the 3 main FAD genes, of a polygenic inheritance [87,88]. The use of NGS-based methods for the analysis of large genomic regions in several patients simultaneously may provide further insights to improve the diagnosis of disorders featured by high genetic and phenotypic variability, such as AD. However, the interpretation of NGS data, due to the large number of variants of unknown significance, is often challenging and inconclusive in clinical settings [14,89].

6. Conclusions

AD incidence is showing an increasing trend worldwide, so its early and accurate diagnosis has become mandatory. Indeed, the earlier the diagnosis is made, the sooner the treatments may begin, the latter being an important prognostic factor to ameliorate patients' clinical outcome. It is becoming evident that within the "AD" definition are included different entities, whose correct identification may be important to drive treatments choices. While most of AD cases are sporadic, featured by late onset and by the presence of polygenic risk factors, a small percentage of AD is familial, often featured by early age of onset and related to the presence of rare, pathogenic mutations segregating within the affected families. To date, 3 main genes (*APP*, *PSEN1* and *PSEN2*) have been related to autosomal dominant FAD, accounting just for a small percentage of cases. Novel candidate genes are being identified. Larger studies on large group of patients are required to better address their contribution to the disease and discover other potential candidates. This will allow a better prognostic classification of the patients and a better management of the probands and of their families, by the identification of the -at risk individuals. These genetic data, together with novel clues coming from other "omics" [90–92], will allow also the development of novel and even more personalized therapies for AD and FAD treatment.

Author Contributions: V.D. and D.S.: conceptualization; writing—original draft preparation; writing—review and editing. All authors have read and agreed to the published version of the manuscript.

References

1. Collaborators GBDD. Global, regional, and national burden of Alzheimer's disease and other dementias, 1990–2016: A systematic analysis for the Global Burden of Disease Study 2016. *Lancet Neurol.* **2019**, *181*, 88–106.
2. McKhann, G.M.; Knopman, D.S.; Chertkow, H.; Hyman, B.T.; Jack, C.R., Jr.; Kawas, C.H.; Klunk, W.E.; Koroshetz, W.J.; Manly, J.J.; Mayeux, R.; et al. The diagnosis of dementia due to Alzheimer's disease: Recommendations from the National Institute on Aging-Alzheimer's Association workgroups on diagnostic guidelines for Alzheimer's disease. *Alzheimers Dement.* **2011**, *7*, 263–269. [CrossRef]
3. Guerreiro, R.J.; Gustafson, D.R.; Hardy, J. The genetic architecture of Alzheimer's disease: Beyond APP, PSENs and APOE. *Neurobiol. Aging* **2012**, *33*, 437–456. [CrossRef]
4. Cacace, R.; Sleegers, K.; Van Broeckhoven, C. Molecular genetics of early-onset Alzheimer's disease revisited. *Alzheimers Dement.* **2016**, *12*, 733–748. [CrossRef]
5. Goldman, J.S.; Hahn, S.E.; Catania, J.W.; LaRusse-Eckert, S.; Butson, M.B.; Rumbaugh, M.; Strecker, M.N.; Roberts, J.S.; Burke, W.; Mayeux, R.; et al. American College of Medical Genetics and the National Society of Genetic Counselors. Genetic counseling and testing for Alzheimer disease: Joint practice guidelines of the American College of Medical Genetics and the National Society of Genetic Counselors. *Genet. Med.* **2011**, *136*, 597–605. [CrossRef]
6. Reiman, E.M.; Langbaum, J.B.; Tariot, P.N.; Lopera, F.; Bateman, R.J.; Morris, J.C.; Sperling, R.A.; Aisen, P.S.; Roses, A.D.; Welsh-Bohmer, K.A.; et al. CAP-advancing the evaluation of preclinical Alzheimer disease treatments. *Nat. Rev. Neurol.* **2016**, *121*, 56–61. [CrossRef]
7. Tariot, P.N.; Lopera, F.; Langbaum, J.B.; Thomas, R.G.; Hendrix, S.; Schneider, L.S.; Rios-Romenets, S.; Giraldo, M.; Acosta, N.; Tobon, C.; et al. The Alzheimer's Prevention Initiative Autosomal-Dominant Alzheimer's Disease Trial: A study of crenezumab versus placebo in preclinical PSEN1 E280A mutation

carriers to evaluate efficacy and safety in the treatment of autosomal-dominant Alzheimer's disease, including a placebo-treated noncarrier cohort. *Alzheimers Dement. (N. Y.)* **2018**, *4*, 150–160.

8. Bergougnoux, A.; D'Argenio, V.; Sollfrank, S.; Verneau, F.; Telese, A.; Postiglione, I.; Lackner, K.J.; Claustres, M.; Castaldo, G.; Rossman, H.; et al. Multicenter validation study for the certification of a CFTR gene scanning method using next generation sequencing technology. *Clin. Chem. Lab. Med.* **2018**, *56*, 1046–1053. [CrossRef]
9. D'Argenio, V.; Esposito, M.V.; Telese, A.; Precone, V.; Starnone, F.; Nunziato, M.; Cantiello, P.; Iorio, M.; Evangelista, E.; D'Aiuto, M.; et al. The molecular analysis of BRCA1 and BRCA2: Next-generation sequencing supersedes conventional approaches. *Clin. Chim. Acta* **2015**, *446*, 221–225. [CrossRef]
10. D'Argenio, V.; Frisso, G.; Precone, V.; Boccia, A.; Fienga, A.; Pacileo, G.; Limongelli, G.; Paolella, G.; Calabrò, R.; Salvatore, F. DNA sequence capture and next-generation sequencing for the molecular diagnosis of genetic cardiomyopathies. *J. Mol. Diagn.* **2014**, *16*, 32–44. [CrossRef]
11. Cariati, F.; D'Argenio, V.; Tomaiuolo, R. The evolving role of genetic tests in reproductive medicine. *J. Transl. Med.* **2019**, *17*, 267. [CrossRef]
12. Nunziato, M.; Esposito, M.V.; Starnone, F.; Diroma, M.A.; Calabrese, A.; Del Monaco, V.; Buono, P.; Frasci, G.; Botti, G.; D'Aiuto, M.; et al. A multi-gene panel beyond BRCA1/BRCA2 to identify new breast cancer-predisposing mutations by a picodroplet PCR followed by a next-generation sequencing strategy: A pilot study. *Anal. Chim. Acta* **2019**, *1046*, 154–162. [CrossRef]
13. Precone, V.; Del Monaco, V.; Esposito, M.V.; De Palma, F.D.; Ruocco, A.; Salvatore, F.; D'Argenio, V. Cracking the code of human diseases using next-generation sequencing: Applications, challenges, and perspectives. *Biomed. Res. Int.* **2015**, 161648. [CrossRef]
14. D'Argenio, V. The high-throughput analyses era: are we ready for the data struggle? *High. Throughput* **2018**, *7*, 8. [CrossRef]
15. Belinova, I.; Karran, E.; De Strooper, B. The toxic Ab oligomer and Alzheimer's disease: An emperor in need of clothes. *Nat. Neurosci.* **2012**, *15*, 349–357.
16. Goedert, M.; Clavaguera, F.; Tolnay, M. The propagation of prion-like protein inclusions in neurodegenerative diseases. *Trends Neurosci.* **2010**, *33*, 317–325. [CrossRef]
17. Jucker, M.; Walker, L.C. Self-propagation of pathogenic protein aggregates in neurodegenerative diseases. *Nature* **2013**, *501*, 45–51. [CrossRef]
18. Sarnataro, D.; Pepe, A.; Zurzolo, C. Cell biology of prion protein. *Prog. Mol. Biol. Transl. Sci.* **2017**, *150*, 57–82.
19. Sarnataro, D. Attempt to untangle the prion-like misfolding mechanism for neurodegenerative diseases. *Int. J. Mol. Sci.* **2018**, *19*, 3081. [CrossRef]
20. De Jonghe, C.; Esselens, C.; Kumar-Singh, S.; Craessaerts, K.; Serneela, S.; Checler, F.; Annaert, W.; Van Broeckhoven, C.; De Strooper, B. Pathogenic APP mutations near the γ-secretase cleavage site differentially affect Aβ secretion and APP C-terminal fragment stability. *Hum. Mol. Gen.* **2001**, *16*, 1665–1671. [CrossRef]
21. Murakami, K.; Irie, K.; Morimoto, A.; Ohigashi, H.; Shindo, M.; Nagao, M.; Shimizu, T.; Shirasawa, T. Synthesis, aggregation, neurotoxicity, and secondary structure of various Aβ1-42 mutants of familial Alzheimer's disease at positions 21–23. *Biochem. Biophys. Res. Commun.* **2002**, *294*, 5–10. [CrossRef]
22. Kumar-Singh, S. Hereditary and sporadic forms of Aβ-cerebrovascular amyloidosis and relevant transgenic mouse models. *Int. J. Mol. Sci.* **2009**, *10*, 1872–1895. [CrossRef] [PubMed]
23. Del Prete, D.; Suski, J.M.; Oulès, B.; Debayle, D.; Gay, A.S.; Lacas-Gervais, S.; Bussiere, R.; Bauer, C.; Pinton, P.; Paterlini-Bréchot, P.; et al. Localization and processing of the Amyloid-β protein precursor in mitochondria-associated membranes. *J. Alzheimers Dis.* **2017**, *55*, 1549–1570. [CrossRef] [PubMed]
24. Bhattacharya, A.; Limone, A.; Napolitano, F.; Cerchia, C.; Parisi, S.; Minopoli, G.; Montuori, N.; Lavecchia, A.; Sarnataro, D. APP maturation and intracellular localization are controlled by a specific inhibitor of 37/67 kDa laminin-1 receptor in neuronal cells. *Int. J. Mol. Sci.* **2020**, *21*, 1738. [CrossRef] [PubMed]
25. Götz, A.; Hogel, P.; Silber, M.; Chaitoglou, I.; Luy, B.; Muhle-Goll, C.; Scharnagl, C.; Langosch, D. Increased H-bond stability relates to altered e-cleavage efficiency and Ab levels in the I45T familial Alzheimer's disease mutant of APP. *Sci. Rep.* **2019**, *9*, 5321. [CrossRef]
26. Bocharov, E.V.; Nadezhdin, K.D.; Urban, A.S.; Volynsky, P.E.; Pavlov, K.V.; Efremov, R.G.; Arseniev, A.S.; Bocharova, O.V. Familial L723P mutation can shift the distribution between the alternative APP transmembrane domain cleavage cascades by local unfolding of the E-cleavage site suggesting a straightforward mechanism of Alzheimer's disease pathogenesis. *ACS Chem. Biol.* **2019**, *4*, 1573–1582. [CrossRef]

27. Lumsden, A.L.; Rogers, J.T.; Majd, S.; Newman, M.; Sutherland, G.T.; Verdile, G.; Lardelli, M. Dysregulation of neuronal iron homeostasis as an alternative unifying effect of mutations causing familial Alzheimer's disease. *Front. Neurosci.* **2018**, *12*, 533. [CrossRef]
28. Di Fede, G.; Catania, M.; Morbin, M.; Rossi, G.; Suardi, S.; Mazzoleni, G.; Merlin, M.; Giovagnoli, A.R.; Prioni, S.; Erbetta, A.; et al. A recessive mutation in the APP gene with dominant-negative effect on amyloidogenesis. *Science* **2009**, *323*, 1473–1477. [CrossRef]
29. Tomiyama, T.; Nagata, T.; Shimada, H.; Teraoka, R.; Fukushima, A.; Kanemitsu, H.; Takuma, H.; Kuwano, R.; Imagawa, M.; Ataka, S.; et al. A new amyloid beta variant favoring oligomerization in Alzheimer'stype dementia. *Ann. Neurol.* **2008**, *63*, 377–387. [CrossRef]
30. Conidi, M.E.; Bernardi, L.; Puccio, G.; Smirne, N.; Muraca, M.G.; Curcio, S.A.; Colao, R.; Piscopo, P.; Gallo, M.; Anfossi, M.; et al. Homozygous carriers of APP A713T mutation in an autosomal dominant Alzheimer disease family. *Neurology* **2015**, *84*, 2266–2273. [CrossRef]
31. Cabrejo, L.; Guyant-Marechal, L.; Laquerriere, A.; Vercelletto, M.; De la Fourniere, F.; Thomas-Anterion, C.; Verny, C.; Letournel, F.; Pasquier, F.; Vital, A.; et al. Phenotype associated with APP duplication in five families. *Brain* **2006**, *129*, 2966–2976. [CrossRef] [PubMed]
32. Rovelet-Lecrux, A.; Hannequin, D.; Raux, G.; Le Meur, N.; Laquerriere, A.; Vital, A.; Dumanchin, C.; Feuillette, S.; Brice, A.; Vercelletto, M.; et al. APP locus duplication causes autosomal dominant early-onset Alzheimer disease with cerebral amyloid angiopathy. *Nat. Genet.* **2006**, *38*, 24–26. [CrossRef] [PubMed]
33. Remes, A.M.; Finnila, S.; Mononen, H.; Tuominen, H.; Takalo, R.; Herva, R.; Majamaa, K. Hereditary dementia with intracerebral hemorrhages and cerebral amyloid angiopathy. *Neurology* **2004**, *63*, 234–240. [CrossRef] [PubMed]
34. Rovelet-Lecrux, A.; Frebourg, T.; Tuominen, H.; Majamaa, K.; Campion, D.; Remes, A.M. APP locus duplication in a Finnish family with dementia and intracerebral haemorrhage. *J. Neurol. Neurosurg. Psychiatry* **2007**, *78*, 1158–1159. [CrossRef] [PubMed]
35. Sleegers, K.; Brouwers, N.; Gijselinck, I.; Theuns, J.; Goossens, D.; Wauters, J.; Del-Favero, J.; Cruts, M.; van Duijn, C.M.; Van Broeckhoven, C. APP duplication is sufficient to cause early onset Alzheimer's dementia with cerebral amyloid angiopathy. *Brain* **2006**, *129*, 2977–2983. [CrossRef] [PubMed]
36. Hooli, B.V.; Mohapatra, G.; Mattheisen, M.; Parrado, A.R.; Roehr, J.T.; Shen, Y.; Gusella, J.F.; Moir, R.; Saunders, A.J.; Lange, C.; et al. Role of common and rare APP DNA sequence variants in Alzheimer disease. *Neurology* **2012**, *78*, 1250–1257. [CrossRef]
37. Jonsson, T.; Atwal, J.K.; Steinberg, S.; Snaedal, J.; Jonsson, P.V.; Bjornsson, S.; Stefansson, H.; Sulem, P.; Gudbjartsson, D.; Maloney, J.; et al. A mutation in APP protects against Alzheimer's disease and age-related cognitive decline. *Nature* **2012**, *488*, 96–99. [CrossRef]
38. Cruts, M.; Theuns, J.; Van Broeckhoven, C. Locus-specific mutation databases for neurodegenerative brain diseases. *Hum. Mutat.* **2012**, *33*, 1340–1344. [CrossRef]
39. Pilotto, A.; Padovani, A.; Borroni, B. Clinical, biological, and imaging features of monogenic Alzheimer's Disease. *Biomed. Res. Int.* **2013**, 689591. [CrossRef]
40. Portet, F.; Dauvilliers, Y.; Campion, D.; Raux, G.; Hauw, J.J.; Lyon-Caen, O.; Camu, W.; Touchon, J. Very early onset AD with a de novo mutation in the presenilin 1 gene (Met 233 Leu). *Neurology* **2003**, *61*, 1136–1137. [CrossRef]
41. Golan, M.P.; Styczynska, M.; Jozwiak, K.; Walecki, J.; Maruszak, A.; Pniewski, J.; Lugiewicz, R.; Filipek, S.; Zekanowski, C.; Barcikowska, M. Early-onset Alzheimer's disease with a de novo mutation in the presenilin 1 gene. *Exp. Neurol.* **2007**, *208*, 264–268. [CrossRef] [PubMed]
42. Lanoiselèe, H.M.; Nicolas, G.; Wallon, D.; Rovelet-Lecrux, A.; Lacour, M.; Rousseau, S.; Richard, A.C.; Pasquier, F.; Rollin-Sillaire, A.; Martinaud, O.; et al. Collaborators of the CNR-MAJ project. APP, PSEN1, and PSEN2 mutations in early-onset Alzheimer disease: A genetic screening study of familial and sporadic cases. *PLoS Med.* **2017**, *14*, e1002270. [CrossRef] [PubMed]
43. Kosik, K.S.; Munoz, C.; Lopez, L.; Arcila, M.L.; Garcia, G.; Madrigal, L.; Moreno, S.; Ríos Romenets, S.; Lopez, H.; Gutierrez, M.; et al. Homozygosity of the autosomal dominant Alzheimer disease presenilin 1 E280A mutation. *Neurology* **2015**, *84*, 206–208. [CrossRef]
44. Hardy, J.; Crook, R. Presenilin mutations line up along transmembrane alpha-helices. *Neurosci. Lett.* **2001**, *306*, 203–205. [CrossRef]
45. Guerreiro, R.J.; Beck, J.; Gibbs, J.R.; Santana, I.; Rossor, M.N.; Schott, J.M.; Nalls, M.A.; Ribeiro, H.; Santiago, B.;

Fox, N.C.; et al. Genetic Variability in CLU and Its Association with Alzheimer's Disease. *PLoS ONE* **2010**, *5*, e9510. [CrossRef]

46. Brouwers, N.; Sleegers, K.; Van Broeckhoven, C. Molecular genetics of Alzheimer's disease: An update. *Ann. Med.* **2008**, *40*, 562–583. [CrossRef]
47. Wingo, T.S.; Lah, J.J.; Levey, A.I.; Cutler, D.J. Autosomal recessive causes likely in early-onset Alzheimer disease. *Arch. Neurol.* **2012**, *69*, 59–64. [CrossRef]
48. Jarmolowicz, A.I.; Chen, H.Y.; Panegyres, P.K. The Patterns of Inheritance in Early-Onset Dementia: Alzheimer's Disease and Frontotemporal Dementia. *Am. J. Alzheimers Dis. Other Dement.* **2014**, *30*, 299–306. [CrossRef]
49. Mahley, R.W. Apolipoprotein E: Cholesterol transport protein with expanding role in cell biology. *Science* **1988**, *240*, 622–630. [CrossRef]
50. Mahley, R.W.; Rall, S.C., Jr. Apolipoprotein E: Far more than a lipid transport protein. *Annu Rev. Genomics Hum. Genet.* **2000**, *1*, 507–537. [CrossRef]
51. Ashford, J.W. APOE genotype effects on Alzheimer's disease onset and epidemiology. *J. Mol. Neurosci.* **2004**, *23*, 157–165. [CrossRef]
52. Corder, E.H.; Saunders, A.M.; Risch, N.J.; Strittmatter, W.J.; Schmechel, D.E.; Gaskell, P.C., Jr.; Rimmler, J.B.; Locke, P.A.; Conneally, P.M.; Schmader, K.E. Protective effect of apolipoprotein E type 2 allele for late onset Alzheimer disease. *Nat. Genet.* **1994**, *7*, 180–184. [CrossRef]
53. Huang, Y. Apolipoprotein E and Alzheimer disease. *Neurology* **2006**, *66*, S79–S85. [CrossRef] [PubMed]
54. Van Duijn, C.M.; de Knijff, P.; Cruts, M.; Wehnert, A.; Havekes, L.M.; Hofman, A.; Van Broeckhoven, C. Apolipoprotein E4 allele in a population-based study of early-onset Alzheimer's disease. *Nat. Genet.* **1994**, *7*, 74–78. [CrossRef] [PubMed]
55. Genin, E.; Hannequin, D.; Wallon, D.; Sleegers, K.; Hiltunen, M.; Combarros, O.; Bullido, M.J.; Engelborghs, S.; De Deyn, P.; Berr, C.; et al. APOE and Alzheimer disease: A major gene with semi-dominant inheritance. *Mol. Psychiatry* **2011**, *16*, 903–907. [CrossRef] [PubMed]
56. Sorbi, S.; Nacmias, B.; Forleo, P.; Piacentini, S.; Latorraca, S.; Amaducci, L. Epistatic effect of APP717 mutation and apolipoprotein E genotype in familial Alzheimer's disease. *Ann. Neurol.* **1995**, *38*, 124–127. [CrossRef] [PubMed]
57. Pastor, P.; Roe, C.M.; Villegas, A.; Bedoya, G.; Chakraverty, S.; Garcia, G.; Bedoya, G.; Chakraverty, S.; García, G.; Tirado, V.; et al. Apolipoprotein Eepsilon4 modifies Alzheimer's disease onset in an E280A PS1 kindred. *Ann. Neurol.* **2003**, *54*, 163–169. [CrossRef]
58. Wijsman, E.M.; Daw, E.W.; Yu, X.; Steinbart, E.J.; Nochlin, D.; Bird, T.D.; Schellenberg, G.D. APOE and other loci affect age-at-onset in Alzheimer's disease families with PS2 mutation. *Am. J. Med. Genet. Part B Neuropsychiatr. Genet.* **2005**, *132*, 14–20. [CrossRef]
59. Petersen, R.C. Mild Cognitive Impairment. *Continuum (Minneap Minn)* **2016**, *22*, 404–418. [CrossRef]
60. Guerreiro, R.J.; Lohmann, E.; Kinsella, E.; Bras, J.M.; Luu, N.; Gurunlian, N.; Dursun, B.; Bilgic, B.; Santana, I.; Hanagasi, H.; et al. Exome sequencing reveals an unexpected genetic cause of disease: NOTCH3 mutation in a Turkish family with Alzheimer's disease. *Neurobiol. Aging* **2012**, *33*, 1008–1023. [CrossRef]
61. Patel, D.; Mez, J.; Vardarajan, B.N.; Staley, L.; Chung, J.; Zhang, X.; Farrell, J.J.; Rynkiewicz, M.J.; Cannon-Albright, L.A.; Teerlink, C.C.; et al. Alzheimer's Disease Sequencing Project. Association of Rare Coding Mutations with Alzheimer Disease and Other Dementias Among Adults of European Ancestry. *JAMA Netw. Open* **2019**, *2*, 191350. [CrossRef] [PubMed]
62. Bordet, R.; Ihl, R.; Korczyn, A.D.; Lanza, G.; Jansa, J.; Hoerr, R.; Guekht, A. Towards the concept of disease-modifier in post-stroke or vascular cognitive impairment: A consensus report. *BMC Med.* **2017**, *15*, 107. [CrossRef] [PubMed]
63. Lanza, G.; Cantone, M.; Musso, S.; Borgione, E.; Scuderi, C.; Ferri, R. Early-onset subcortical ischemic vascular dementia in an adult with mtDNA mutation 3316G>A. *J. Neurol.* **2018**, *265*, 968–969. [CrossRef] [PubMed]
64. Pottier, C.; Hannequin, D.; Coutant, S.; Rovelet-Lecrux, A.; Wallon, D.; Rousseau, S.; Legallic, S.; Paquet, C.; Bombois, S.; Pariente, J.; et al. PHRC GMAJ Collaborators. High frequency of potentially pathogenic SORL1 mutations in autosomal dominant early-onset Alzheimer disease. *Mol. Psychiatry* **2012**, *17*, 875–879. [CrossRef]

65. Caglayan, S.; Takagi-Niidome, S.; Liao, F.; Carlo, A.S.; Schmidt, V.; Burgert, T.; Kitago, Y.; Füchtbauer, E.M.; Füchtbauer, A.; Holtzman, D.M.; et al. Lysosomal sorting of amyloid-beta by the SORLA receptor is impaired by a familial Alzheimer's disease mutation. *Sci. Transl. Med.* **2014**, *6*, 223. [CrossRef]
66. Cuccaro, M.L.; Camey, R.M.; Zhang, Y.; Bohm, C.; Kunkle, B.W.; Vardarajan, B.N.; Whitehead, P.L.; Cukier, H.N.; Mayeux, R.; George-Hyslop, P.; et al. SORL1 mutations in early- and late-onset Alzheimer disease. *Neurol. Genet.* **2016**, *2*, e116.
67. Nicolas, G.; Charbonnier, C.; Wallon, D.; Quenez, O.; Bellenguez, C.; Grenier-Boley, B.; Rousseau, S.; Richard, A.C.; Rovelet-Lecrux, A.; Le Guennec, K.; et al. CNR-MAJ collaborators. SORL1 rare variants: A major risk factor for familial early-onset Alzheimer's disease. *Mol. Psychiatry* **2016**, *21*, 831–836. [CrossRef]
68. Vardarajan, B.N.; Zhang, Y.; Lee, J.H.; Cheng, R.; Bohm, C.; Ghani, M.; Cheng, R.; Bohm, C.; Ghani, M.; Reitz, C.; et al. Coding mutations in SORL1 and Alzheimer disease. *Ann. Neurol.* **2015**, *77*, 215–227. [CrossRef]
69. Li, X.; Xiong, Z.; Liu, Y.; Yuan, Y.; Deng, J.; Xiang, W.; Li, Z. Case report of first—Episode psychotic symptoms in a patient with early-onset Alzheimer's disease. *BMC Psychiatry* **2020**, *20*, 128. [CrossRef]
70. Cuyvers, E.; Sleegers, K. Genetic variations underlying Alzheimer's disease: Evidence from genome-wide association studies and beyond. *Lancet Neurol.* **2016**, *15*, 857–868. [CrossRef]
71. Shen, L.; Jia, J. An overview of Genome-Wide Association Studies in Alzheimer's Disease. *Neurosci. Bull.* **2016**, *32*, 183–190. [CrossRef] [PubMed]
72. Lambert, J.C.; Heath, S.; Even, G.; Campion, D.; Sleegers, K.; Hiltunen, M.; Combarros, O.; Zelenika, D.; Bullido, M.J.; Tavernier, B.; et al. Genome-wide association study identifies variants at CLU and CR1 associated with Alzheimer's disease. *Nat. Gen.* **2009**, *41*, 1094–1099. [CrossRef] [PubMed]
73. Jonsson, T.; Stefansson, H.; Steinberg, S.; Jonsdottir, I.; Jonsson, P.V.; Snaedal, J.; Bjornsson, S.; Huttenlocher, J.; Levey, A.I.; Lah, J.J.; et al. Variant of TREM2 associated with the risk of Alzheimer's disease. *N. Engl. J. Med.* **2013**, *368*, 107–116. [CrossRef] [PubMed]
74. Bettens, K.; Brouwers, N.; Engelborghs, S.; Lambert, J.C.; Rogaeva, E.; Vandenberghe, R.; Le Bastard, N.; Pasquier, F.; Vermeulen, S.; Van Dongen, J.; et al. Both common variations and rare non-synonymous substitutions and small insertion/deletions in CLU are associated with increased Alzheimer risk. *Mol. Neurodegener.* **2012**, *7*, 3. [CrossRef] [PubMed]
75. Bettens, K.; Vermeulen, S.; Van Cauwenberghe, C.; Heeman, B.; Asselbergh, B.; Robberecht, C.; Engelborghs, S.; Vandenbulcke, M.; Vandenberghe, R.; De Deyn, P.P.; et al. Reduced secreted clusterin as a mechanism for Alzheimer-associated CLU mutations. *Mol. Neurodegener.* **2015**, *10*, 30. [CrossRef]
76. Guerreiro, R.; Wojtas, A.; Bras, J.; Carrasquillo, M.; Rogaeva, E.; Majounie, E.; Cruchaga, C.; Sassi, C.; Kauwe, J.S.; Younkin, S.; et al. Alzheimer Genetic Analysis Group. TREM2 variants in Alzheimer's disease. *Engl. J. Med.* **2013**, *368*, 117–127. [CrossRef]
77. Bailey, C.C.; DeVaux, L.B.; Farzan, M. The triggering receptor expressed on myeloid cells 2 binds apolipoprotein E. *J. Biol. Chem.* **2015**, *290*, 26033–26042. [CrossRef]
78. Lue, L.F.; Schmitz, C.; Walker, D.G. What happens to microglial TREM2 in Alzheimer's disease: Immunoregulatory turned into immunopathogenic? *Neuroscience* **2015**, *302*, 138–150. [CrossRef] [PubMed]
79. Kleinberger, G.; Yamanishi, Y.; Suarez-Calvet, M.; Czirr, E.; Lohmann, E.; Cuyvers, E.; Struyfs, H.; Pettkus, N.; Wenninger-Weinzierl, A.; Mazaheri, F.; et al. TREM2 mutations implicated in neurodegeneration impair cell surface transport and phagocytosis. *Sci. Transl. Med.* **2014**, *6*, 243ra86. [CrossRef] [PubMed]
80. Cuyvers, E.; Bettens, K.; Philtjens, S.; Van Langenhove, T.; Gijselinck, I.; van der Zee, J.; Engelborghs, S.; Vandenbulcke, M.; Van Dongen, J.; Geerts, N.; et al. BELNEU consortium. Investigating the role of rare heterozygous TREM2 variants in Alzheimer's disease and frontotemporal dementia. *Neurobiol. Aging* **2014**, *35*, 726–729. [CrossRef] [PubMed]
81. Pottier, C.; Wallon, D.; Rousseau, S.; Rovelet-Lecrux, A.; Richard, A.C.; Rollin-Sillaire, A.; Frebourg, T.; Campion, D.; Hannequin, D. TREM2 R47H variant as a risk factor for early-onset Alzheimer's disease. *J. Alzheimers Dis.* **2013**, *35*, 45–49. [CrossRef] [PubMed]
82. Cruchaga, C.; Karch, C.M.; Jin, S.C.; Benitez, B.A.; Cai, Y.; Guerreiro, R.; Harari, O.; Norton, J.; Budde, J.; Bertelsen, S.; et al. Rare coding variants in the phospholipase D3 gene confer risk for Alzheimer's disease. *Nature* **2014**, *505*, 550–554. [CrossRef] [PubMed]
83. Cuyvers, E.; De Roeck, A.; Van den Bossche, T.; Van Cauwenberghe, C.; Bettens, K.; Vermeulen, S.; Mattheijssens, M.; Peeters, K.; Engelborghs, S.; Vandenbulcke, M.; et al. Mutations in 74 ABCA7 in a Belgian

cohort of Alzheimer's disease patients: A targeted resequencing study. *Lancet Neurol.* **2015**, *14*, 814–822. [CrossRef]
84. Steinberg, S.; Stefansson, H.; Jonsson, T.; Johannsdottir, H.; Ingason, A.; Helgason, H.; Sulem, P.; Magnusson, O.T.; Gudjonsson, S.A.; Unnsteinsdottir, U.; et al. Loss-of-function variants in ABCA7 confer risk of Alzheimer's disease. *Nat. Genet.* **2015**, *47*, 445–447. [CrossRef]
85. Vardarajan, B.N.; Ghani, M.; Kahn, A.; Sheikh, S.; Sato, C.; Barral, S.; Lee, J.H.; Cheng, R.; Reitz, C.; Lantigua, R.; et al. Rare coding mutations identified by sequencing of Alzheimer disease genome-wide 76 association studies loci. *Ann. Neurol.* **2015**, *78*, 487–498. [CrossRef] [PubMed]
86. Satoh, K.; Abe-Dohmae, S.; Yokoyama, S.; St George-Hyslop, P.; Fraser, P.E. ATP-binding cassette transporter A7 (ABCA7) loss of function alters Alzheimer amyloid processing. *J. Biol. Chem.* **2015**, *290*, 24152–24165. [CrossRef]
87. Bonvicini, C.; Scassellati, C.; Benussi, L.; Di Maria, E.; Maj, C.; Ciani, M.; Fostinelli, S.; Mega, A.; Bocchetta, M.; Lanzi, G.; et al. Next Generation Sequencing Analysis in Early Onset Dementia Patients. *J. Alzheimers Dis.* **2019**, *67*, 243–256. [CrossRef]
88. Cochran, J.N.; McKinley, E.C.; Cochran, M.; Amaral, M.D.; Moyers, B.A.; Lasseigne, B.N.; Gray, D.E.; Lawlor, J.M.J.; Prokop, J.W.; Geier, E.G.; et al. Genome sequencing for early-onset or atypical dementia: High diagnostic yield and frequent observation of multiple contributory alleles. *Cold Spring Harb. Mol. Case Stud.* **2019**, *5*, a003491. [CrossRef] [PubMed]
89. Cali, F.; Cantone, M.; Cosentino, F., II; Lanza, G.; Ruggeri, G.; Chiavetta, V.; Salluzzo, R.; Ragalmuto, A.; Vinci, M.; Ferri, R. Interpreting Genetic Variants: Hints from a Family Cluster of Parkinson's Disease. *J. Parkinsons Dis.* **2019**, *9*, 203–206. [CrossRef] [PubMed]
90. Qazi, T.J.; Quan, Z.; Mir, A.; Qing, H. Epigenetics in Alzheimer's Disease: Perspective of DNA Methylation. *Mol. Neurobiol.* **2018**, *55*, 1026–1044. [CrossRef]
91. D'Argenio, V.; Sarnataro, D. Microbiome influence in the pathogenesis of prion and Alzheimer's Diseases. *Int. J. Mol. Sci.* **2019**, *20*, 4704. [CrossRef] [PubMed]
92. Lee, S.Y.; Song, M.Y.; Kim, D.; Park, C.; Park, D.K.; Kim, D.G.; Yoo, J.S.; Kim, Y.H. A Proteotranscriptomic-based computational drug-repositioning method for Alzheimer's Disease. *Front. Pharmacol.* **2020**, *10*, 1653. [CrossRef] [PubMed]

3

The Brain Metabolic Correlates of the Main Indices of Neuropsychological Assessment in Alzheimer's Disease

Agostino Chiaravalloti [1,2], Maria Ricci [1,*], Daniele Di Biagio [3], Luca Filippi [4], Alessandro Martorana [5,6] and Orazio Schillaci [1,2]

1 Department of Biomedicine and Prevention, University Tor Vergata, 00133 Rome, Italy; agostino.chiaravalloti@uniroma2.it (A.C.); orazio.schillaci@uniroma2.it (O.S.)
2 IRCCS Neuromed, 86077 Pozzilli, Italy
3 UOC Nuclear Medicine, Policlinico Tor Vergata, 00133 Rome, Italy; danieledibiagio@gmail.com
4 UOC Nuclear Medicine, Santa Maria Goretti Hospital, 04100 Latina, Italy; lucfil@hotmail.com
5 UOSD Centro Demenze Policlinico Tor Vergata, 00133 Rome, Italy; martorana@med.uniroma2.it
6 Department of System Medicine, University Tor Vergata, 00133 Rome, Italy
* Correspondence: maria.ricci28@gmail.com
† This paper is a revised version of our paper published as conference paper in the 29th European Association of Nuclear Medicine congress.

Abstract: Background: The study aimed to investigate the relationships between F-18 fluorodeoxyglucose (18F)FDG uptake and neuropsychological assessment in Alzheimer's disease (AD). Methods: We evaluated 116 subjects with AD according to the NINCDS-ADRDA criteria. All the subjects underwent a brain PET/CT with (18F)FDG, cerebrospinal fluid (CSF) assay, mini-mental state examination (MMSE) and further neuropsychological tests: Rey auditory verbal learning test, immediate recall (RAVLT immediate); Rey auditory verbal learning test, delayed recall (RAVLT, delayed); Rey complex figure test, copy (RCFT, copy); Rey complex figure test, delayed recall (RCFT, delayed); Raven's colored progressive matrices (RCPM); phonological word fluency test (PWF) and Stroop test. We performed the statistical analysis by using statistical parametric mapping (SPM12; Wellcome Department of Cognitive Neurology, London, UK). Results: A significant relationship has been reported between (18F)FDG uptake and RAVLT immediate test in Brodmann area (BA)37 and BA22 and with RCFT, copy in BA40, and BA7. We did not find any significant relationships with other tests. Conclusion: In the AD population, brain (18F)FDG uptake is moderately related to the neuropsychological assessment, suggesting a limited impact on statistical data analysis of glucose brain metabolism.

Keywords: Alzheimer's disease; PET/CT; (18F)FDG; neuropsychological assessment

---

1. Introduction

Subjective memory deficit, together with evidence of memory decline and cognitive impairment during the past months or few years, are key features for Alzheimer's disease (AD) already at the prodromal (or mild cognitive impairment; MCI) stage [1]. Although cognitive tests are frequently used as outcome measures in clinical trials, there are a number of limitations associated with their use [2].

Neurodegenerative AD-related changes are known to accumulate progressively 15 to 20 years before dementia, and even years before the detection of clinical deficits [3]. Cognitive decline in AD, generally assessed by neuropsychological battery [4], is postulated as consequential from neurological pathology as portrayed by biomarkers [5], but the specificity of these associations is still a matter of debate [6]. Particularly, the correspondence between the neuropsychological assessment and standard neuroimaging biomarkers remains incomplete, and the relationship between neuropsychological performance and individual variation in clinical AD neuroimaging markers is likely to be both convergent and unique [5,7]. Although it is tempting to presume neurological substrates causing poor performance at a common neuropsychological assessment, the substrates underlying the cognitive process may be reorganized in the diseased brain of patients with MCI, possibly due to neurodegenerative changes or functional compensation. It is important to understand how these biomarkers, interact to influence cognitive change to isolate the combination of pathologies that contribute most to decline, in order to inform the clinical utility and validation of cognitive tests [5] and the neuroimaging correlates to test performance.

In particular, data concerning the relationship between glucose metabolism and common neuropsychological assessment are poor, even if the results of the neuropsychological tests may be considered as statistical parameters in research papers that include brain data analysis, by using computer-aided metrics such as statistical parametric mapping (SPM) [8,9].

The present study aimed to evaluate the brain metabolic correlates of the main indices of neuropsychological assessment by studying their relationships to cortical and subcortical F-18 fluorodeoxyglucose (18F)FDG uptake in a cohort of subjects with AD. Moreover, this paper aimed to evaluate the impact of neuropsychological assessment as parameters in SPM brain data analysis. For this purpose, all the subjects underwent a brain PET/CT scan using (18F)FDG, a complete neuropsychological assessment that included mini-mental state examination (MMSE). Moreover, the following indices of neuropsychological assessment were determined in the AD population: Rey auditory verbal learning test, immediate recall (RAVLT immediate); Rey auditory verbal learning test, delayed recall (RAVLT, delayed); Rey complex figure test, copy (RCFT, copy); Rey complex figure test, delayed recall (RCFT, delayed); Raven colored progressive matrices (RCPM); phonological word fluency test (PWF) and Stroop test. A cerebrospinal fluid (CSF) assay for amyloid, total tau, and phosphorylated tau was performed in all patients.

An initial version of this paper was presented as a conference paper at the 29th European Association of Nuclear Medicine Congress.

2. Materials and Methods

We evaluated 116 subjects with a new clinical diagnosis of AD (males = 66; females = 50) according to the NINCDS-ADRDA criteria [10]. The mean age was 71.4 ± 6 years old. A complete clinical investigation was performed in all patients, including medical history, mini-mental state examination (MMSE), a complete blood screening (including routine exams, thyroid hormones, and level of B12). Moreover, in all patients, a neurologist examination, neuropsychological examination, a complete neuropsychiatric evaluation, and neuroimaging consisting of magnetic resonance imaging (1.5 T MRI) was performed. Exclusion criteria were the following: isolated deficits and/or unmodified MMSE (<25/30) on revisit (6, 12, and 18 months follow-up), clinically manifest acute stroke in the last 6 months (Hachinsky scale >4, and radiological evidence of subcortical lesions), as described in previous papers [11–13]. None of the patients enrolled had pyramidal and/or extrapyramidal signs reported at the neurological examination. At the time of enrollment, in the 30 days before participating in this study, none of the patients had been treated with drugs that might have modulated cerebral cortex excitability, including antidepressants, neuroactive drugs (i.e., benzodiazepines, antiepileptic drugs or neuroleptics), or cholinesterase inhibitors. The study was performed according to the Declaration of Helsinki and approved by the local ethics committee of the Tor Vergata University in Rome. All participants or their legal guardians gave the written informed consent after receiving an extensive disclosure of the study. A cognitive profile consistent with mild dementia (according to neuropsychological evaluation, including the MMSE) has been described in all AD patients.

In order to improve the diagnostic accuracy of the AD patients, a lumbar puncture and CSF sampling was performed in all patients. The first 12 mL of CSF was collected in a polypropylene tube, then directly transported to the local laboratory for centrifugation at 2000× *g* at +4 °C for 10 min. The supernatant was pipetted off, gently stirred and mixed to avoid potential gradient effects, and aliquoted in 1 mL portions in polypropylene tubes that were stored at −80 °C pending biochemical analyses, without being thawed and re-frozen. Then, CSF total Tau (T-Tau) and phosphorylated Tau (Thr181, p-Tau) concentration was evaluated using a sandwich ELISA (Innotest hTAU-Ag, Innogenetics, Gent, Belgium). CSF Aβ1–42 levels were determined using a sandwich ELISA (Innotest® ß- amyloid (1–42), Innogenetics, Gent, Belgium), specifically elaborated to measure Aβ containing both the first and 42nd amino acid, as described in previous papers [11–15].

All the subjects underwent a brain PET/CT scan using (18F)FDG, mini-mental state examination (MMSE). Several indices of neuropsychological assessment were explored: Rey auditory verbal learning test, immediate recall (RAVLT immediate); Rey auditory verbal learning test, delayed recall (RAVLT, delayed); Rey complex figure test, copy (RCFT, copy); Rey complex figure test, delayed recall (RCFT, delayed); Raven's colored progressive matrices (RCPM); phonological word fluency Test (PWF) and Stroop test. The relationship between brain uptake of (18F)FDG and CSF biomarkers were analyzed using statistical parametric mapping (SPM12; Wellcome Department of Cognitive Neurology, London, UK) implemented in Matlab R2018a using sex, age, and CSF biomarkers as covariates.

2.1. PET/CT Scanning

The PET/CT system Discovery VCT (GE Medical Systems, Tennessee, TN, USA) has been used to assess (18F)FDG brain distribution in all patients using a 3D-mode standard technique in a 256 × 256 matrix. Reconstruction was performed using the 3-dimensional reconstruction method of ordered-subsets expectation maximization (OSEM) with 20 subsets and with 4 iterations. The system combines a high-speed ultra 16-detector-row (912 detectors per row) CT unit and a PET scanner with 10,080 bismuth germanate crystals in 24 rings (axial full width at half-maximum 1 cm radius, 5.2 mm in 3D mode, an axial field of view 157 mm). A low-amperage CT scan of the head for attenuation correction (40 mA; 120 Kv) was performed before PET image acquisition. All subjects fasted for at least 5 h before intravenous injection of (18F)FDG ; the serum glucose level was up to 95 mg/mL in all of them. All the subjects were injected intravenously with 185–210 MBq of (18F)FDG and hydrated with 500 mL of saline (0.9% sodium chloride). The scan started 30 min after the injection in all the subjects according to standard guidelines, as described in previous papers [13,16,17].

2.2. Statistical Analysis

Differences in brain (18F)FDG uptake were analyzed using statistical parametric mapping (SPM12, Wellcome Department of Cognitive Neurology, London, UK) implemented in Matlab R2018a (Mathworks, Natick, Massachusetts, USA). PET data were subjected to affine and nonlinear spatial normalization into the MNI space. Then, the spatially set of images was smoothed with an 8 mm isotropic Gaussian filter to blur individual variations in gyral anatomy and to increase the signal-to-noise ratio. Images were globally normalized using proportional scaling to remove confounding effects to global CBF changes, with a threshold masking of 0.8. The statistical parametric maps were transformed into a normal distribution unit. Correction of SPM coordinates to match the Talairach coordinates was achieved by the subroutine implemented by Matthew Brett (http://www.mrc-cbu.cam.ac.uk/Imaging). Brodmann areas (BA) were then identified at a range of 0 to 3 mm from the corrected Talairach coordinates of the SPM output isocentres, after importing them by Talairach client (http://www.talairach.org/index.html). A statistical height threshold was equal to or lower than $p < 0.001$ at both clusters, and voxel-level was accepted as significant. We considered significant a cluster extension of more than 125 (5 × 5 × 5 voxels, i.e., 11 × 11 × 11 mm) contiguous voxels, based on the calculation of the partial volume effect resulting from the spatial resolution of the PET camera (about the double of full width at half maximum), as described in previous papers of the same research group [13].The resulting SPM data was correlated to each index of neuropsychological assessment, in order to study their relationships to cortical and subcortical (18F)FDG uptake.

3. Results

The values of CSF amyloid, total tau, and phosphorylated tau were respectively 363.6 ± 162, 689 ± 338.1, and 92.4 ± 70.7 pg/mL. A general overview of the patient population is reported in Table 1. Most of the cases were sporadic, but in about 15% of enrolled patients, there was a family link.

Table 1. A general overview of age, mini-mental state examination (MMSE), and Cerebral spinal fluid (CSF) parameters in the whole population.

Whole Population (n = 116)	Mean ± SD (Range)
Age (years)	71.4 ± 6 (48–82)
MMSE	20.3 ± 4.9 (9–30)
Amyloid (pg/mL)	363.6 ± 162 (70–913)
T-Tau (pg/mL)	689 ± 338.1 (173–1749)
P-Tau (pg/mL)	92.4 ± 70.7 (34–661)

Neuropsychological assessment resulted in 22.6 ± 8.6 for RAVLT, immediate; 71.4 ± 5,9 for RAVLT, delayed; 18.2 ± 10.4 for RCFT, copy; 7.6 ± 6 for RCFT, delayed; 18.8 ± 9 (RCPM); 22.2 ± 10.1 for PWF and 44.6 ± 36.2 for Stroop test (Table 2).

Table 2. A general overview of Neuropsychological tests results in the whole population: Rey auditory verbal learning test, immediate recall (RAVLT immediate); Rey auditory verbal learning test, delayed recall (RAVLT, delayed); Rey complex figure test, copy (RCFT, copy); Rey complex figure test, delayed recall (RCFT, delayed); Raven's colored progressive matrices (RCPM); phonological word fluency test (PWF) and Stroop test.

Neuropsychological Test	Mean ± SD (Range)
RAVLT immediate	22.6 ± 8.6 (0–43)
RAVLT delayed	71.4 ± 5.9 (48–82)
RCFT copy	18.2 ± 10.4 (0–36)
RCFT delayed	7.6 ± 6 (0–26)
RCPM	18.8 ± 9 (0–36)
PWF	22.2 ± 10.1 (0–55)
Stroop Test	44.6 ± 36.2 (0–162)

A positive correlation was reported in the statistical analysis between the PET data and performance in RAVLT immediate. We found a significant relationship between (18F)FDG uptake and performance in RAVLT immediate in a large portion of the left temporal lobe, in a cluster of 1141 voxels that included left temporal middle and superior gyrus, as shown in Figure 1 and Table 3 (positive correlation in Brodmann area 37 and Brodmann area 22).

Furthermore, a significant correlation was described between the PET data and performance in RCFT, copy. We found a significant positive relationship between (18F)FDG uptake and performance in RCFT, copy in a cluster of 1177 voxels that included left parietal inferior lobule and precuneus, and in a cluster of 804 voxels that include right parietal superior and inferior lobules (left and right BA40 and left and right BA7), as reported in Figure 2 and Table 4. We did not find any significant relationships between (18F)FDG uptake and other tests performed.

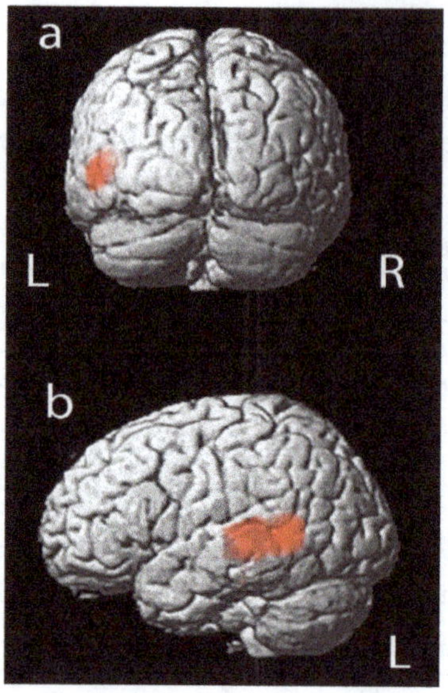

Figure 1. 3D rendering of the results of statistical parametric mapping analyses between (18F)FDG uptake and performance in RAVLT immediate that shows a positive correlation in a large portion of the left temporal lobe (Brodmann area 37 and Brodmann area BA22): (**a**) posterior view; (**b**) left lateral view.

Table 3. A general overview of statistical parametric mapping analyses that detected a positive correlation in Brodmann area (BA) 37 and Brodmann area 22 of FDG uptake and performance in RAVL immediate test. The Brodmann areas were then identified at a range of 0 to 3 mm from the corrected Talairach coordinates of the SPM output isocentres. A statistical height threshold was equal to or lower than $p < 0.001$ at both clusters, and voxel-level was accepted as significant. We considered as significant a cluster extension of more than 125 contiguous voxels.

Analysis	Cluster Level					Voxel Level	
Positive Correlation	p(FWE-corr)	q(FDRcorr)	Extent	Cortical Region	Z Score of Maximum	Talairach Coordinates	Cortical Region
	0.003	0.007	1141	Left temporal, middle temporal gyrus	4.55	−48, −52, 4	BA 37
				Left temporal, middle temporal gyrus	3.68	−54, −36, 8	BA 22
				Left temporal, superior temporal gyrus	3.60	−56, −28, 6	BA 22

Table 4. A general overview of statistical parametric mapping analyses that detected a positive correlation in left and right Brodmann area (BA) 7 and left and right Brodmann area 40 of FDG uptake and performance in RCFT, copy test. The Brodmann areas were then identified at a range of 0 to 3 mm from the corrected Talairach coordinates of the SPM output isocentres. A statistical height threshold was equal to or lower than $p < 0.001$ at both clusters, and voxel-level was accepted as significant. We considered as significant a cluster extension of more than 125 contiguous voxels.

Analysis	Cluster Level					Voxel Level	
Positive Correlation	p(FWE-corr)	q(FDRcorr)	Extent	Cortical Region	Z Score of Maximum	Talairach Coordinates	Cortical Region
	0.002	0.005	1177	Left parietal, inferior parietal lobule	4.84	−34, −50, 36	BA 40
				left parietal, precuneus	4.25	−24, −76, 42	BA 7
				left parietal, precuneus	4.08	−16, −74, 48	BA 7
	0.011	0.013	804	Right parietal, superior parietal lobule	4.52	34, −56, 48	BA 7
				right parietal, superior parietal lobule	3.90	28, −66, 48	BA 7
				right parietal, inferior parietal lobule	3.70	42, −40, 42	BA 40

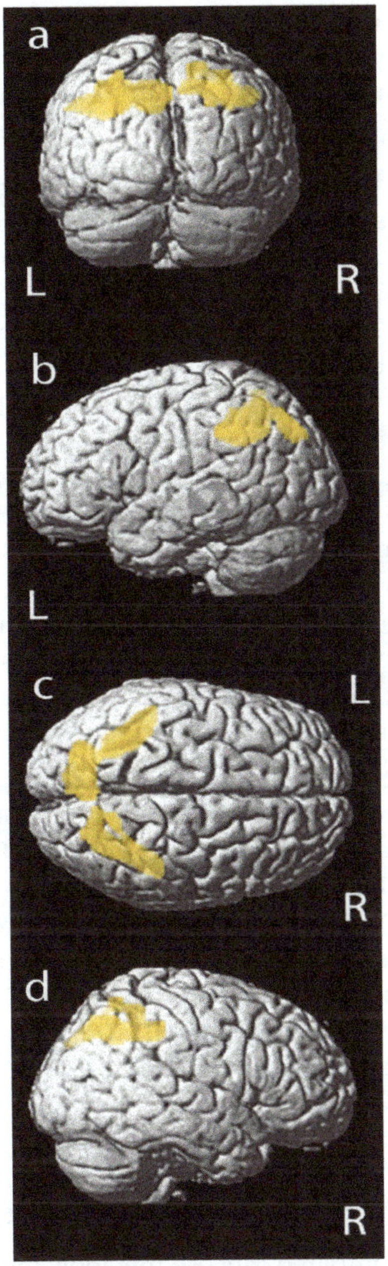

Figure 2. 3D rendering of the results of statistical parametric mapping analyses between (18F)FDG uptake and performance in RCFT copy that shows a positive correlation in left and right Brodmann area 40 and left and right Brodmann area 7: (**a**) posterior view; (**b**) left lateral view; (**c**) superior view; (**d**) right lateral view.

4. Discussion

Cognitive performance is an important outcome measure in AD diagnosis and progression. Nevertheless, the symptomatic significance of improvement or decline in clinical tests has not been well established, making it difficult to set a standard for what is meant by meaningful improvement [6]. Cognitive decline in AD is generally assessed by a neuropsychological battery [4]. An optimal outcome measure would reflect clinically-significant patient function, provide reliable measurements with minimal variability, and track a physiologically relevant disease process. However, the cognitive assessment also has several limitations, such as a large inter and intraindividual variability and floor and ceiling effects [2].

The neuropsychological test results may be considered as statistical parameters in research papers that include brain data analysis by using computer-aided metrics, such as statistical parametric mapping (SPM) [8]. For each cognitive measure, difference scores were entered into a regression analysis in SPM as the independent variable [9] or as a covariate.

The goal of the present study was to examine the brain metabolic correlates of the main indices of neuropsychological assessment tests in order to evaluate their impact on SPM brain data analysis.

We found a significant relationship between (18F)FDG uptake and performance in RAVLT immediate in a large portion of the left temporal lobe (positive correlation in BA37 and BA22) and with RCFT, copy (positive correlation in left and right BA40 and left and right BA7). We did not find any significant relationships with other tests.

A previous paper evaluated the brain metabolic correlates of the main indices of RAVLT, showing a significant correlation between the delayed recall score and metabolism in the posterior cingulate gyrus of both hemispheres and left precuneus, as well as between a score of long-term percent retention and metabolism in the left posterior cingulate gyrus, precuneus, and orbitofrontal areas. No correlation was found between immediate or total recall scores and glucose metabolism [1]. Nevertheless, the sample analyzed was a group of 54 elderly subjects with memory complaints. Therefore these differences, with our results, may be both due to the different sized sample and to the worse clinical conditions of our patients (elderly subjects with memory complaints vs. clinically diagnosed AD) with subsequent cortical hypometabolism according to the AD pattern. Neurological substrates underlying the tests widely used, such as delayed recall and executive function, were explored in MCI, whereas it was only partially explored in diagnosed AD.

A paper concerning MCI performances on delayed recall and executive function suggested that hypometabolism in the right medial temporal cortex, right prefrontal cortex, left superior parietal cortex, and bilateral posterior cingulate reflect impairments in delayed recall, while hypometabolism in the right prefrontal cortex mirrors deficits in executive function in MCI [18]. The differences with our results may be due to differences in both the methods and in the stage of disease of the examined population. A further paper evaluated the relationships of FDG-PET metabolism with cognition in MCI: the composite score predicted variation in cortical metabolism, and TMT B was significantly correlated with PET metabolism. The results indicated that RAVLT and TMT B are sensitive to variation in AD neuroimaging markers in MCI but, contrary to our paper focused on SPM brain analysis; the Statistical Package for the Social Sciences (SPSS version 22.0) was used [5]. Even if both statistical analysis and enrolled populations are different from our methods, these findings partially support our results concerning the correlation of RAVLT test performance with FDG uptake in AD.

Furthermore, a previous study compared glucose metabolism and clinical measurements, reporting that baseline and longitudinal FDG-ROI measures are sensitive to poor performance at neuropsychological assessment and validate the cognitive and functional relevance of longitudinal changes in (18F)FDG measurement. Nevertheless, the indices used in this paper were The Functional Activities Questionnaire (FAQ) and Alzheimer's Disease Assessment Scale—cognitive subscale (ADAS-cog) [6].

The patients and methods applied in the literature are as heterogeneous as the results obtained. According to our results concerning diagnosed AD, glucose metabolism of the left temporal lobe correlated to RAVLT, whereas glucose metabolism of the bilateral parietal lobe correlated to RCFT, copy. We did not find any significant relationships with other tests. Therefore, cortical and subcortical glucose consumption appear moderately related to the neuropsychological assessment. Even if the clinical usefulness of neuropsychological assessment is well established, our results suggest a limited impact on the data analysis of brain metabolism in patients with AD. Therefore, we suggest using these parameters in the statistical analysis of neuroimaging biomarkers by dedicated software, especially FDG uptake, just in the particular analysis concerning specific clinical aspects. Generally, considering the heterogeneous data about the influence of neuropsychological assessment on PET data, the use of neuropsychological indices as a covariate or independent variables in SPM analysis can be avoided in these patients.

Author Contributions: A.C., conceptualization, data curation, writing, supervision; M.R., data curation, formal analysis, writing; D.D.B., data curation, formal analysis; L.F., data curation, formal analysis; A.M., supervision, validation; O.S., supervision, validation, writing. All authors have read and agreed to the published version of the manuscript.

Acknowledgments: The authors wish to thank Tiziana Martino (IRCCS Neuromed) for data collection. This study was supported by the PICASO project (grant no. 689209). An initial version of this paper has been presented as a conference paper at the 29th European Association of Nuclear Medicine congress https://link.springer.com/article/10.1007%2Fs00259-016-3484-4

References

1. Brugnolo, A.; Morbelli, S.; Arnaldi, D.; De Carli, F.; Accardo, J.; Bossert, I.; Dessi, B.; Famà, F.; Ferrara, M.; Girtler, N.; et al. Metabolic Correlates of Rey Auditory Verbal Learning Test in Elderly Subjects with Memory Complaints. *J. Alzheimer's Dis.* **2014**, *39*, 103–113. [CrossRef] [PubMed]
2. Visser, P.J. Role of cognitive testing in disease modifying AD trials. *J. Nutr. Heal. Aging* **2006**, *10*, 132–133.
3. Tomadesso, C.; De La Sayette, V.; De Flores, R.; Bourgeat, P.; Villemagne, V.L.; Egret, S.; Eustache, F.; Chételat, G. Neuropsychology and neuroimaging profiles of amyloid-positive versus amyloid-negative amnestic mild cognitive impairment patients. *Alzheimer's Dementia Diagn. Assess. Dis. Monit.* **2018**, *10*, 269–277. [CrossRef] [PubMed]
4. Carlesimo, G.A.; Fadda, L.; Sabbadini, M.; Caltagirone, C. Recency effect in Alzheimer's disease: A reappraisal. *Q. J. Exp. Psychol. A* **1996**, *49*, 315–325. [CrossRef] [PubMed]
5. Eliassen, C.F.; Reinvang, I.; Selnes, P.; Fladby, T.; Hessen, E. Convergent Results from Neuropsychology and from Neuroimaging in Patients with Mild Cognitive Impairment. *Dement. Geriatr. Cogn. Disord.* **2017**, *43*, 144–154. [CrossRef] [PubMed]
6. Landau, S.M.; Harvey, D.; Madison, C.M.; Koeppe, R.A.; Reiman, E.M.; Foster, N.L.; Weiner, M.W.; Jagust, W.J.; Initiative, T.A.D.N. Associations between cognitive, functional, and FDG-PET measures of decline in AD and MCI. *Neurobiol. Aging* **2009**, *32*, 1207–1218. [CrossRef] [PubMed]
7. Hedden, T.; Schultz, A.; Rieckmann, A.; Mormino, E.C.; Johnson, K.A.; Sperling, R.A.; Buckner, R.L. Multiple Brain Markers are Linked to Age-Related Variation in Cognition. *Cereb. Cortex* **2014**, *26*, 1388–1400. [CrossRef] [PubMed]
8. Chiaravalloti, A.; Fiorentini, A.; Francesco, U.; Martorana, A.; Koch, G.; Belli, L.; Torniolo, S.; Di Pietro, B.; Motta, C.; Schillaci, O. Is cerebral glucose metabolism related to blood–brain barrier dysfunction and intrathecal IgG synthesis in Alzheimer disease? *Medicine* **2016**, *95*, e4206. [CrossRef] [PubMed]
9. Racine, A.; Adluru, N.; Alexander, A.L.; Christian, B.T.; Okonkwo, O.C.; Oh, J.; Cleary, C.A.; Birdsill, A.; Hillmer, A.T.; Murali, D.; et al. Associations between white matter microstructure and amyloid burden in preclinical Alzheimer's disease: A multimodal imaging investigation. *NeuroImage Clin.* **2014**, *4*, 604–614. [CrossRef] [PubMed]
10. Dubois, B.; Feldman, H.H.; Jacova, C.; DeKosky, S.T.; Barberger-Gateau, P.; Cummings, J.; Delacourte, A.; Galasko, D.; Gauthier, S.; Jicha, G.; et al. Research criteria for the diagnosis of Alzheimer's disease: Revising the NINCDS-ADRDA criteria. *Lancet Neurol.* **2007**, *6*, 734–746. [CrossRef]
11. Chiaravalloti, A.; Barbagallo, G.; Martorana, A.; Castellano, A.E.; Ursini, F.; Schillaci, O. Brain metabolic patterns in patients with suspected non-alzheimer's pathophysiology (SNAP) and alzheimer's disease (AD): Is [(18)F] FDG a specific biomarker in these patients? *Eur. J. Nucl. Med. Mol. Imaging* **2019**, *46*, 1796–1805. [CrossRef] [PubMed]
12. Chiaravalloti, A.; Barbagallo, G.; Ricci, M.; Martorana, A.; Ursini, F.; Sannino, P.; Karalis, G.; Schillaci, O. Brain metabolic correlates of CSF Tau protein in a large cohort of Alzheimer's disease patients: A CSF and FDG PET study. *Brain Res.* **2018**, *1678*, 116–122. [CrossRef] [PubMed]
13. Ricci, M.; Chiaravalloti, A.; Martorana, A.; Koch, G.; De Lucia, V.; Barbagallo, G.; Schillaci, O. The role of epsilon phenotype in brain glucose consumption in Alzheimer's disease. *Ann. Nucl. Med.* **2020**, *34*, 254–262. [CrossRef] [PubMed]
14. Liguori, C.; Chiaravalloti, A.; Sancesario, G.; Stefani, A.; Sancesario, G.; Mercuri, N.B.; Schillaci, O.; Pierantozzi, M. Cerebrospinal fluid lactate levels and brain [18F]FDG PET hypometabolism within the default mode network in Alzheimer's disease. *Eur. J. Nucl. Med. Mol. Imaging* **2016**, *43*, 2040–2049. [CrossRef] [PubMed]

15. Chiaravalloti, A.; Martorana, A.; Koch, G.; Toniolo, S.; Di Biagio, D.; Di Pietro, B.; Schillaci, O. Functional correlates of t-Tau, p-Tau and Aβ1–42 amyloid cerebrospinal fluid levels in Alzheimer's disease. *Nucl. Med. Commun.* **2015**, *36*, 1. [CrossRef] [PubMed]
16. Chiaravalloti, A.; Pagani, M.; Cantonetti, M.; Di Pietro, B.; Tavolozza, M.; Travascio, L.; Di Biagio, D.; Danieli, R.; Schillaci, O. Brain metabolic changes in Hodgkin disease patients following diagnosis and during the disease course: An 18F-FDG PET/CT study. *Oncol. Lett.* **2014**, *9*, 685–690. [CrossRef] [PubMed]
17. Chiaravalloti, A.; Koch, G.; Toniolo, S.; Belli, L.; Di Lorenzo, F.; Gaudenzi, S.; Schillaci, O.; Bozzali, M.; Sancesario, G.; Martorana, A. Comparison between Early-Onset and Late-Onset Alzheimer's Disease Patients with Amnestic Presentation: CSF and (18)F-FDG PET Study. *Dement. Geriatr. Cogn. Disord. Extra* **2016**, *6*, 108–119. [CrossRef] [PubMed]
18. Nishi, H.; Sawamoto, N.; Namiki, C.; Yoshida, H.; Thuy, D.H.D.; Ishizu, K.; Hashikawa, K.; Fukuyama, H. Correlation between Cognitive Deficits and Glucose Hypometabolism in Mild Cognitive Impairment. *J. Neuroimaging* **2010**, *20*, 29–36. [CrossRef] [PubMed]

4

The "develOpment of metabolic and functional markers of Dementia IN Older people" (ODINO) Study: Rationale, Design and Methods

Anna Picca [1], Daniela Ronconi [2], Hélio J. Coelho-Junior [2], Riccardo Calvani [1], Federico Marini [3], Alessandra Biancolillo [4], Jacopo Gervasoni [1,2], Aniello Primiano [1,2], Cristina Pais [1], Eleonora Meloni [1], Domenico Fusco [1], Maria Rita Lo Monaco [1], Roberto Bernabei [1,2,*], Maria Camilla Cipriani [1], Emanuele Marzetti [1,2,*] and Rosa Liperoti [1,2]

1 Fondazione Policlinico Universitario "Agostino Gemelli" IRCCS, 00168 Rome, Italy; anna.picca@guest.policlinicogemelli.it (A.P.); riccardo.calvani@guest.policlinicogemelli.it (R.C.); jacopo.gervasoni@policlinicogemelli.it (J.G.); anielloprim@gmail.com (A.P.); cristina.pais@guest.policlinicogemelli.it (C.P.); meloni.eleonora@hotmail.it (E.M.); domenico.fusco@policlinicogemelli.it (D.F.); mariarita.lomonaco@policlinicogemelli.it (M.R.L.M.); mariacamilla.cipriani@policlinicogemelli.it (M.C.C.); rosa.liperoti@policlinicogemelli.it (R.L.)

2 Università Cattolica del Sacro Cuore, 00168 Rome, Italy; danielaronconi88@gmail.com (D.R.); coelhojunior@hotmail.com.br (H.J.C.-J.)

3 Department of Chemistry, Sapienza Università di Roma, 00185 Rome, Italy; federico.marini@uniroma1.it

4 Department of Physical and Chemical Sciences, Università degli Studi dell'Aquila, 67100 L'Aquila, Italy; alessandra.biancolillo@univaq.it

* Correspondence: roberto.bernabei@unicatt.it (R.B.); emanuele.marzetti@policlinicogemelli.it (E.M.)

Abstract: Mild cognitive impairment (MCI), also termed mild neurocognitive disorder, includes a heterogeneous group of conditions characterized by declines in one or more cognitive domains greater than that expected during "normal" aging but not severe enough to impair functional abilities. MCI has been associated with an increased risk of developing dementia and even considered an early stage of it. Therefore, noninvasively accessible biomarkers of MCI are highly sought after for early identification of the condition. Systemic inflammation, metabolic perturbations, and declining physical performance have been described in people with MCI. However, whether biological and functional parameters differ across MCI neuropsychological subtypes is presently debated. Likewise, the predictive value of existing biomarkers toward MCI conversion into dementia is unclear. The "develOpment of metabolic and functional markers of Dementia IN Older people" (ODINO) study was conceived as a multi-dimensional investigation in which multi-marker discovery will be coupled with innovative statistical approaches to characterize patterns of systemic inflammation, metabolic perturbations, and physical performance in older adults with MCI. The ultimate aim of ODINO is to identify potential biomarkers specific for MCI subtypes and predictive of MCI conversion into Alzheimer's disease or other forms of dementia over a three-year follow-up. Here, we describe the rationale, design, and methods of ODINO.

Keywords: aging; biomarkers; cytokines; cognitive decline; Alzheimer's disease; metabolomics; neuroinflammation; multivariate analysis; physical performance; person-tailored

1. Introduction

Mild cognitive impairment (MCI), also termed mild neurocognitive disorder according to the Diagnostic and Statistical Manual of Mental Disorders, Fifth Edition (DSM-5) [1], is a condition characterized by a decline in cognitive function that is greater than that expected for the individual's age and education level but not severe enough to compromise engagement in daily activities [2]. From a neuropsychological perspective, MCI involves reduced cognitive abilities (non-amnestic subtype) in one (single domain) or more (multiple domains) domains or a reduced ability to recall stored information (amnestic subtype) [3]. Other cognitive domains including language, visuospatial function, complex attention, and executive functions may also be affected [3]. Noticeably, people diagnosed with MCI, especially those with the amnestic subtype (aMCI), have a 10-fold increased risk of progression toward Alzheimer's disease (AD) or other forms of dementia [4]. Therefore, establishing whether MCI is indeed a prodromal stage of dementia and understanding the mechanisms of its progression are necessary for the early take-in-charge of affected individuals and for the implementation of preventive interventions [5,6]. To this aim, biomarkers capable of identifying persons with MCI, especially those at higher risk of developing AD or other forms of dementia, are highly sought after.

Signs of neuroinflammation (e.g., detection of inflammatory cytokines in the proximity of ß-amyloid deposits and neurofibrillary tangles), whole-body metabolic perturbations, and declining physical performance (e.g., slow gait speed, impaired performance on dual-task tests) have been documented in people with MCI [7,8]. However, the existence of specific patterns of biological and functional markers across MCI subtypes and their predictive value for the conversion of MCI into dementia are debated.

Multi-marker approaches covering different physiological domains are increasingly implemented for the appraisal of complex and dynamic conditions [9–11]. These approaches are conceptualized within the notion of allostatic load, that is the exposure of cells and biological systems to recurrent or chronic stressors inflicting cumulative damage [12]. Within this paradigm, biomarkers represent endophenotypes of physiological dysregulation that may support diagnosis, tracking, clinical and therapeutic decision-making, and verification of the efficacy of an intervention before it is clinically detectable. In this scenario, the quantification of specific parameters coupled with ad hoc multivariate statistical approaches may allow identifying patterns of biomarkers that can be applied at the individual level as a measure of departure from his/her "normal operating conditions" [13].

The "develOpment of metabolic and functional markers of Dementia IN Older people" (ODINO) study has been conceived as an innovative multi-dimensional investigation in which clinical, neuropsychological, functional, and biological parameters will be analyzed through ad hoc statistical analyses to provide a comprehensive characterization of MCI subtypes. Biological and functional markers will be tested for their ability to predict MCI conversion into AD and other forms of dementia over a three-year follow-up.

2. Materials and Methods

2.1. Study Design and Population

The protocol of this observational study was approved by the Ethics Committee of the Fondazione Policlinico Universitario "Agostino Gemelli" IRCCS (Rome, Italy) (protocol #230/19). A convenience sample of 120 participants will be enrolled in ODINO. The study will be carried out through a two-step analytical process: (1) collection of clinical data, evaluation of cognitive and physical performance, and analysis of biological markers to evaluate patterns of physical performance, systemic inflammation, and metabolic perturbations in older adults with MCI, and (2) a longitudinal three-year follow-up to obtain indications of biomarkers associated with the conversion of MCI into dementia.

Participant recruitment will take place at the Fondazione Policlinico Universitario "Agostino Gemelli" IRCCS under the coordination of the outpatient clinic of the Department of Geriatrics. Participants will be recruited by convenience and asked about their willingness to participate in the study. Candidates aged ≥65 and ≤85 years with a diagnosis of MCI according to the criteria of the National Institute on Aging-Alzheimer's Association [14] will be considered eligible for enrolment. After obtaining written informed consent, participants will be stratified in MCI subtypes (i.e., amnestic single domain, non-amnestic single domain, amnestic multi-domains, and non-amnestic multi-domains).

Exclusion criteria will be: active treatment for cancer or cancer diagnosis (except for non-melanoma skin cancer), severe knee or hip osteoarthritis limiting mobility, inflammatory diseases (e.g., rheumatoid arthritis, vasculitis, autoimmune disorders, inflammatory bowel disease), stroke with upper and/or lower extremity involvement, Parkinson's disease or other neurological disorders likely to interfere with physical function, major psychiatric illnesses, sleep disorders, heart failure New York Heart Association (NYHA) class III–IV, respiratory insufficiency requiring supplemental oxygen, and use of long-acting benzodiazepines or antipsychotic drugs. Temporary exclusion criteria will be acute illnesses (e.g., infections, re-exacerbation of chronic obstructive pulmonary disease), major surgery, and traumata.

Participant assessment will be carried out at the geriatric outpatient clinic of the Fondazione Policlinico Universitario "Agostino Gemelli" IRCCS during four visits at baseline and every 12 months over a three-year follow-up. The activities expected at each visit will be completed over three days within one week (Table 1).

Table 1. Visit schedule and related activities.

Activity	Visit 1 (Baseline)	V2 (12 Months)	V3 (24 Months)	V4 (36 Months)
Informed Consent	x			
Sociodemographic Characteristics	x	x	x	x
Medical History	x	x	x	x
Medication Inventory	x	x	x	x
CDR Scale	x	x	x	x
MMSE	x	x	x	x
RAVLT	x	x	x	x
Digit Span	x	x	x	x
Corsi Span	x	x	x	x
Visuospatial Abilities and Praxis	x	x	x	x
Language	x	x	x	x
Attention and Executive Functions	x	x	x	x
GDS-15	x	x	x	x
Anthropometry	x	x	x	x
Body Composition	x	x	x	x
Muscle Strength	x	x	x	x
TUG	x	x	x	x
SPPB	x	x	x	x
6MWT	x	x	x	x
ADL	x	x	x	x
IADL	x	x	x	x
7-Day Activity and EE Monitor	x	x	x	x
Blood Draw	x	x	x	x

The activities of each visit will be completed over three days within one week. Abbreviations: CDR, clinical dementia rating; MMSE, mini-mental state examination; RAVLT, Rey auditory verbal learning test; GDS-15, geriatric depression scale 15 items; TUG, timed-up-and-go; SPPB, short physical performance battery; 6MWT, six-min walking test; ADL, activities of daily living; IADL, instrumental activities of daily living; EE, energy expenditure.

2.2. *General Characteristics*

Information on age, sex, smoking habit, alcohol consumption, comorbid conditions, and medications will be recorded by an attending physician through a structured interview and careful review of medical records. Vital signs will also be assessed. Standard blood biochemistry will be carried out by the centralized diagnostic laboratory of the Fondazione Policlinico Universitario "Agostino Gemelli" IRCCS.

2.3. Neuropsychological Assessment and Cognitive Evaluation

Participants will receive a comprehensive neuropsychological assessment and cognitive evaluation by means of the clinical dementia rating (CDR) scale [15] and a battery of neuropsychological tests exploring global cognitive function (mini-mental state examination, MMSE) [16], verbal learning and episodic memory (Rey auditory verbal learning test, RAVLT) [17], verbal short-term memory and verbal working memory (digit span) [18], visuospatial short-term memory and visuospatial working memory (Corsi span) [19,20], visuospatial abilities and praxis (copying drawings; copying drawings with landmarks; Rey-Osterrieth complex figure copy) [21], language (phonological verbal fluency task, semantic verbal fluency task, nouns naming test, and verbs naming test) [22], and attention and executive functions (Stroop color word interference test, multiple features target cancellation test, MFTC) [23,24]. Mood will be assessed through the 15-item geriatric depression scale (GDS-15) [25].

2.4. Anthropometry and Body Composition

Body mass and height will be measured by means of a medical graded weight scale with a stadiometer. Body mass index (BMI) will be calculated as the ratio between body mass (kg) and the square of height (m^2).

A flexible and inextensible anthropometric tape will be used to measure waist circumference (WC), hip circumference (HC), and mid-arm circumference (MAC). The waist-to-hip ratio will be calculated. For these measurements, participants will be requested to wear light clothes and to stay in standing position, head held erect, eyes forward, with arms relaxed at the sides of the body, and feet kept together. WC will be taken at the mid-point between the last floating rib and the highest point of the iliac crest. HC will be measured at the highest point of the buttocks. MAC will be taken at the mid-point between the elbow and the deltoid muscle [26].

Bone mineral density and appendicular lean mass will be measured by dual X-ray absorptiometry (DXA) on a Hologic® Discovery A (Hologic, Inc., Bedford, MA, USA), as previously described [27].

2.5. Assessment of Muscle Strength, Physical Function, and Disability Status

Upper and lower-limb muscle strength will be measured by isometric handgrip strength (IHG) and isokinetic analysis, respectively. IHG will be measured using a Jamar handheld hydraulic dynamometer (Patterson Medical Products, Inc., Cincinnati, OH, USA) [28]. For the test, participants will remain seated on a standard chair with shoulders abducted, and the elbow flexed at 90° and near to the trunk, and the wrist in a neutral position (thumb up). The contralateral arm will remain relaxed under the thigh [29]. IHG will be measured during four s. Participants will be familiarized and warmed up before performing three maximal efforts with a one-min rest period. Encouragement to perform the test as quickly and forcefully as possible will be provided during the entire experiment. The maximal concentric isokinetic strength of knee extensors of the dominant side will be measured on a REV9000 isokinetic dynamometer (Technogym, Gambettola, Italy), as previously described [30]. Briefly, participants will be asked to produce their maximum force while extending the knee from 90° to 0° of flexion at 60°/s with a hip angle of 90°–100°. Two practice repetitions will be completed prior to three test repetitions. The maximal peak torque achieved will be used for the analysis.

The timed-up-and-go (TUG) test involves getting up from a chair, walking three meters around a marker placed on the floor, coming back to the same position, and sitting back on the chair. Participants will begin the test while wearing their regular footwear, with their back against the chair, arms resting on the chair's arms, and with the feet in contact with the ground. A researcher will instruct them to, on the word "go", get up and walk at a normal pace through the demarcation of three meters on the ground, turn, return to the chair, and sit down again. Timing will start when participants get up from the chair and will stop when their back touches the backrest of the chair again [31]. After completing the standard TUG test, participants will be asked to perform TUG combined with a verbal fluency task (i.e., naming as many animals as they can remember), with a motor task (i.e., carrying a full cup of water), and with both cognitive and motor tasks (i.e., performing the verbal fluency test while carrying a full cup of water) [32].

The short physical performance battery (SPPB) is composed of three subtasks: standing balance, usual gait speed, and the five-repetition chair-stand test [33]. For the standing balance test, participants will be asked to stand in three progressively more difficult positions for 10 s each: a side-by-side feet standing position, a semi-tandem position and a full-tandem position. Gait speed will be measured over a four m course at the person's usual pace. The faster of two trials will be used for the analysis. For the five-repetition chair-stand test, participants will be asked to perform five repetitions of standing up and sitting down from a chair without using hands and the performance will be timed. Each of the three SPPB subtasks will be categorized into a five-level score, with zero representing the inability to do the test and four corresponding to the highest level of performance.

The six-min walk test will be performed according to the guidelines of the American Thoracic Society [34]. The test will be conducted indoors on a 30-m track. After remaining seated for 15 min, participants will be requested to walk on the track as fast as possible for six min. The test will be interrupted if participants show any sign of chest pain, intolerable dyspnea, leg cramps, staggering, diaphoresis, a pale or ashen appearance, or any other complaint. The distance walked (m) will be used for the analysis.

Disability status will be assessed through the activities of daily living (ADL) and instrumental ADL (IADL) scales [35,36].

2.6. *Measurement of Physical Activity Levels and Energy Expenditure*

Free-living physical activity levels and energy expenditure will be quantified through a SenseWear® armband (SWA, BodyMedia, Inc., Pittsburgh, PA, USA) over seven consecutive days. The SWA is a body monitor wearable on the back of the arm that enables the continuous monitoring of physical activity at low intensities and during unstructured or intermittent activities. The SWA utilizes a unique combination of sensors to measure the amount of heat being dissipated by the body as well as the skin and near-armband temperature. Measures of galvanic skin response to physical and emotional stimuli are also recorded. A two-axis accelerometer tracks the arm movements and provides information about the body position. Wireless transmission, communication, and wired data download are ensured by a radio and a data port. All information collected is integrated and processed by software using proprietary algorithms according to the participant's characteristics (sex, age, height, and weight) to provide minute-by-minute estimates of energy expenditure during different levels of physical activity [37].

2.7. *Collection of Blood Samples*

Blood will be drawn in the morning by venipuncture of the median cubital vein. For plasma separation, blood will be collected using tubes containing ethylenediaminetetraacetic acid (EDTA) and will subsequently be centrifuged at 1000× *g* for 15 min at 4 °C. For serum separation, blood samples will be collected in tubes without EDTA and will be kept at room temperature for 30 min to allow clotting. Afterward, samples will be centrifuged as described above. Aliquots will be prepared from the upper clear fraction (plasma or serum) and stored at −80 °C until analysis.

2.8. *Determination of Biomarkers of Inflammation and Neurodegeneration*

A biomarker panel has been designed based on previous investigations by our group in older populations, including older adults with neurodegenerative conditions [10,38–43]. Markers of systemic inflammation will be assayed as described elsewhere [40]. Briefly, a set of 27 pro- or anti-inflammatory mediators (e.g., cytokines, chemokines, and growth factors) will be measured in serum samples using the Bio-Plex Pro™ Human Cytokine 27-plex Assay kit (#M500KCAF0Y, Bio-Rad, Hercules, CA, USA)

(Table 2). Experiments will be run on a Bio-Plex® System with Luminex xMap Technology (Bio-Rad) and data will be acquired on the Bio-Plex Manager Software 6.1 (Bio-Rad) with instrument default settings. Outliers will be automatically removed by optimization of standard curves across all analytes and results will be obtained as concentration (pg/mL).

Table 2. Serum inflammatory biomolecules assayed by multiplex immunoassay.

Biomarker Class	Components of the Biomarker Panel
Cytokines	IFNγ, IL1β, IL1Ra, IL2, IL4, IL5, IL6, IL7, IL8, IL9, IL10, IL12, IL13, IL15, IL17, TNF-α
Chemokines	CCL5, CCL11, IP-10, MCP-1, MIP-1α, MIP-1β
Growth Factors	FGF-β, G-CSF, GM-CSF, PDGF-BB

Abbreviations: IFN, interferon; IL, interleukin; IL1Ra, interleukin 1 receptor agonist; TNF-α, tumor necrosis factor-alpha; CCL, C-C motif chemokine ligand; IP: interferon-induced protein; MCP-1: monocyte chemoattractant protein 1; MIP: macrophage inflammatory protein; FGF, fibroblast growth factor; G-CSF, granulocyte colony-stimulating factor; GM-CSF, granulocyte macrophage colony-stimulating factor; PDGF-BB, platelet-derived growth factor BB.

Traditional and automated enzyme-linked immunosorbent assays will be run to quantify serum levels of amyloid beta (aa1-42) (#DAB142, R&D Systems, Minneapolis, MN, USA), neurofilament light polypeptide (#SPCKB-PS-002448-000190, R&D Systems), Tau (#NBP2-62749, Novus Biologicals, Littleton, CO, USA), and Tau [p Ser739] (#NBP2-66711, Novus Biologicals) proteins according to the manufacturer's instructions.

2.9. *Measurement of Plasma Fatty Acid Concentrations*

A panel of 14 fatty acids that were previously associated with AD [44] will be measured in plasma by a gas chromatography-electron ionization-mass spectrometry (GC-EI-MS) validated methodology (Eureka One Lab Division Kit, code GC75010; Ancona, Italy) according to the manufacturer's instructions (Table 3).

Table 3. Plasma fatty acids assayed by gas chromatography-electron ionization-mass spectrometry.

Fatty Acid	Fragments
Tetradecanoic acid	74.1; 87.0; 143.0
Hexadecanoic acid	227.0; 270.0
Cis-9-hexadecenoic acid	55.0; 81.0; 96.0; 237.0
Heptadecanoic acid (internal standard)	74.1; 87.0; 284.0
Octadecanoic acid	75.0; 255.0; 298.0
Cis-9-octadecenoic acid	81.1; 96.0; 264.0
Trans-9-octadecenoic acid	81.1; 96.0; 264.0
All cis 9,12-octadecadienoic acid	67.0; 81.1; 95.0
Trans-9,trans-12-octadecadienoic acid	67.0; 81.1; 95.0
All cis 9,12,15 octadecatrienoic acid	67.0; 79.1; 93.0; 95.0
All cis 6,9,12 octadecatrienoic acid	67.0; 79.1; 93.0; 95.0
All cis 8,11,14 eicosatrienoic acid	67.0; 79.1; 93.0
All cis 5,8,11,14 eicosatetraenic acid	67.0; 79.1; 91.0
All cis 5,8,11,14,17 eicosapentaenoic acid	67.0; 79.1; 91.0; 105.0

Following extraction and washing, samples will be treated with a derivatizing solution for 15 min at 100 °C, diluted and directly injected into the GC-MS. GC-MS analyses will be performed on a Trace GC Ultra (Thermo Fisher Scientific, Waltham, MA, USA) equipped with Durabond HP-88 column, 100 m × 0.25 mm × 0.2 μm film thickness (Agilent Technologies, Santa Clara, CA, USA), and connected to an ISQ mass spectrometer (Thermo Fisher Scientific). One μL of the sample will be injected in split mode (1:10 ratio), with injector temperature set at 250 °C. Helium will be used as carrier gas and the flow-rate will be maintained constant at 1 mL/min. The initial oven temperature of 100 °C will be held for 1 min, then raised to 220 °C at 10 °C/min, and maintained for 4 min. Afterward, the oven temperature will be increased up to 240 °C at 10 °C/min and held for 10 min. The mass transfer line will be maintained at 270 °C and the ion source at 200 °C. Analyses will be performed in the selected ion monitoring (SIM) mode. Ions monitored in the analysis are shown in Table 3. The analytical process will be monitored using fatty acid controls (code GC75019, level 1 and level 2) manufactured by Eureka One Lab Division.

2.10. *Measurement of Serum Concentrations of Amino Acids and Derivatives*

The serum concentration of a panel of 37 amino acids and derivatives will be determined by ultraperformance liquid chromatography/MS (UPLC/MS), as described elsewhere [9]. The panel has been chosen based on previous work by our group in older populations [9,41,45,46] and will include: 1-methylhistidine, 3-methylhistidine, 4-hydroxyproline, α-aminobutyric acid, β-alanine, β-aminobutyric acid, γ-aminobutyric acid, alanine, aminoadipic acid, anserine, arginine, asparagine, aspartic acid, carnosine, citrulline, cystathionine, cystine, ethanolamine, glutamic acid, glycine, histidine, isoleucine, leucine, lysine, methionine, ornithine, phenylalanine, phosphoethanolamine, phosphoserine, proline, sarcosine, serine, taurine, threonine, tryptophan, tyrosine, and valine.

Briefly, 50 μL of the sample will be added to 100 μL 10% (w/v) sulfosalicylic acid containing an internal standard mix (50 μM) (Cambridge Isotope Laboratories, Inc., Tewksbury, MA, USA). The mixture will be centrifuged at 1000× *g* for 15 min. Seventy μL of borate buffer and 20 μL of AccQ Tag reagents (Waters Corporation, Milford, MA, USA) will be added to 10 μL of the obtained supernatant and heated at 55 °C for 10 min. Next, samples will be loaded onto a CORTECS UPLC C18 column 1.6 μm, 2.1 mm × 150 mm (Waters Corporation) for chromatographic separation (ACQUITY H-Class, Waters Corporation). Elution will be accomplished at 500 μL/min flow-rate with a linear gradient (9 min) from 99:1 to 1:99 water 0.1% formic acid/acetonitrile 0.1% formic acid. Finally, analytes will be detected on an ACQUITY QDa single quadrupole mass spectrometer equipped with an electrospray source operating in positive mode (Waters Corporation). Amino acid controls manufactured by the MCA laboratory of the Queen Beatrix Hospital (Winterswijk, The Netherlands) will be used to monitor the analytic process.

2.11. *Statistical Analysis*

Since no studies have explored the multi-marker profile of MCI chosen in ODINO, no power analysis could be run for sample size calculation. Based on the number of older persons diagnosed with MCI at our center, we estimate that 120 participants will be enrolled over one year. The rate of losses to follow-up over three years is expected to be 20%, leaving a total of 100 cases from whom all variables of interest will be collected. Participants will be censored at the end of follow-up, at the date of conversion to dementia, or at the date of death, as applicable.

Descriptive statistics will be run for all variables. After ascertainment of data distribution, comparisons of variables of interest among MCI subtypes will be performed via analysis of variance (ANOVA) or Kruskal –Wallis H for continuous variables, as appropriate. Categorical variables will be compared through χ^2 statistics. Survival analyses (Kaplan–Meier and Cox regression) will be used to investigate the impact of clinical variables on conversion to dementia. Descriptive statistics will be performed using SAS version 9.2 (SAS Institute Inc., Cary, NC, USA).

In the cross-sectional stage of the study, to characterize MCI subtypes, different classification strategies will be enacted. First, a purely discriminant approach will be adopted. In discriminant classification, data are used to build a predictive model aiming at assigning each individual to one specific group (in this case, any of the MCI subtypes). To this aim, a classification strategy based on partial least squares discriminant analysis (PLS-DA) will be adopted [47]. PLS-DA offers the advantage of processing datasets containing a high number of variables even if they are highly correlated with one another. The analysis of the whole dataset, which encompasses multi-block data, will be performed through the recently developed sequential and orthogonalized covariance selection (SO-CovSel) [48]. The method, which allows a highly parsimonious variable selection, was used by our group for the identification of a gut microbial, inflammatory and metabolic fingerprint in older adults with physical frailty & sarcopenia [41].

To rule out the possibility of chance correlations and to estimate the reliability of predictive models, a thorough validation process by means of double cross-validation (DCV) and permutation tests will be operated. DCV consists of two nested loops of cross-validation; the external loop is used to unbiasedly estimate the predictive ability of the model parameters that are optimized on the basis of the internal loop. The classification ability of the optimal model is then expressed by means of various figures of merit, such as the number of misclassifications (NMC), the area under the receiver operating characteristic (AUROC) curve, and the discriminant Q2 (DQ2), the distributions of which under the null hypothesis are estimated via permutation tests [49]. This allows the establishment of the statistical significance of the observed discrimination. A detailed description of PLS-DA, SO-CovSel, and DCV procedures may be found elsewhere [9,41,43].

Classification will be repeated with a modeling approach based on soft independent modeling of class analogies (SIMCA) [50], in order to assess the degrees of similarity among MCI subtypes. Modeling approaches use data to define which experimental profiles are to be expected from individuals belonging to a particular category (i.e., the so-called model space). Accordingly, a class model allows the prediction of how likely it is for an individual to belong to a class or not, on the basis of the measurements considered. Since each category (MCI subtype) will be modeled independently from the others, the results of this analytical stage will provide information on the effectiveness of the characterization of different MCI subtypes. The analysis will also indicate how likely it is for specific subtypes of participants to be confounded with one another. A SIMCA model was recently built by our group to verify the accuracy of the classification of older adults with Parkinson's disease based on extracellular vesicle cargo [43].

In the longitudinal phase of the study, multilevel ANOVA (MANOVA) coupled with simultaneous component analysis (SCA) or with PLS-DA will be used to characterize the time dynamics of participants over the follow-up [51]. MANOVA may be considered to be equivalent to multivariate ANOVA for repeated measurements. In such a configuration, SCA, which under the constraints of MANOVA is identical to principal component analysis, or PLS-DA allows applying the method to data matrices containing a high number of possibly correlated variables. The statistical significance of MANOVA will be assessed non-parametrically by permutation tests. Multivariate statistics will be conducted using functions written in-house and run under the Matlab environment (The Mathworks, Natick, MA, USA).

3. Discussion

The possibility that MCI, at least in some variants, may be a prodromal stage of dementia has ignited a great deal of research primarily aimed at testing possible strategies to impede MCI progression [52]. However, the clinical heterogeneity of MCI and its multifactorial pathogenesis have been major hurdles in identifying meaningful biomarkers and devising effective interventions.

Different cognitive domains may be affected in MCI, which has allowed the clinical identification of various subtypes. In the aMCI, memory loss is predominant and shows a higher risk for further conversion to AD [53]. Non-amnestic MCI subtypes are characterized by impairments in cognitive domains other than memory and have a greater propensity to convert into other forms of dementia, such as diffuse Lewy body dementia and vascular dementia [53]. Both aMCI and naMCI variants can be further categorized into single- and multi-domain subtypes, depending on the number of cognitive domains affected. The distinction between aMCI and naMCI is not only based on neuropsychological parameters, but is sustained by specific brain structural characteristics, primarily involving the hippocampus, the cortical thickness, and the entorhinal cortex [54–57].

The development of biomarkers able to capture complex phenomena, such as MCI and dementia, are highly sought after. Several investigations have been conducted to evaluate candidate biomarkers for MCI. However, these studies investigated differences between MCI and healthy controls, whereas none of them explored distinct features across MCI subtypes [58,59].

The development of cost-effective omics platforms enabling the simultaneous analysis of a vast repertoire of biological mediators in biofluids has shown great value in providing a comprehensive read-out of the environmental and clinical disturbances affecting cell homeostasis in different settings [11]. Metabolomics analyses of the cerebrospinal fluid (CSF) allowed differentiating MCI from dementia in older people, a task in which traditional biomarkers of AD such as Aβ42 failed [60]. Core CSF biomarkers including total (T-Tau) and phosphorylated Tau (P-Tau) protein, Aβ42, and neurofilament light polypeptide have been strongly associated with AD, such that their clinical implementation for diagnostic purposes has been suggested [61]. However, biomarkers specific for MCI are still missing.

Recent advances in lipidomics suggest that fatty acid dysmetabolism and imbalance in fatty acid lipidome are involved in the initiation and progression of several neurodegenerative diseases, including AD [62]. Indeed, fatty acid β-oxidation and its byproducts impact immune cell function, thereby possibly contributing to neuroinflammation [62]. However, no studies have yet addressed whether specific lipid markers distinguish aMCI and naMCI and predict their conversion into dementia. Furthermore, an investigation involving eight prospective cohorts with over 20,000 participants found an inverse association between serum concentrations of branch-chained amino acids and incident AD [63]. Similar to lipids, it is presently unclear whether specific patterns of circulating amid acids are selectively associated with MCI subtypes.

Inflammatory cytokines, including interleukin (IL) 1β, IL6 and tumor necrosis factor-alpha (TNF-α), are involved in local inflammation triggered by amyloid plaque deposition and may induce neurotoxicity when produced chronically, favoring the generation of Aβ peptides [64]. Therefore, a role for these cytokines in inter- and intracellular signaling in microglia and astrocytes has been hypothesized in AD [65]. Interestingly, peripheral inflammatory markers associated with MCI are distinct from those found in patients with AD [66]. Though, no conclusive data are presently available.

Since markers pertaining to a single domain (e.g., inflammatory rather than metabolic) may fail at capturing the intertwined relationship between local and systemic changes, we decided to combine metabolomics analysis and immunoassays to characterize the metabolic and inflammatory profile of older adults with MCI. A biomarker panel has been designed based on previous investigations by our group in older populations, including older adults with neurodegenerative conditions [10,38–43]. This approach was also guided by the recent advances made in the field of geroscience [67]. To gain insights into the etiology of the MCI subtypes, the panel also includes the analysis of circulating levels of T-Tau and P-Tau protein, Aβ42, and neurofilament light polypeptide [61].

Other lines of evidence indicate that specific impairments in physical performance are associated with MCI. In particular, people with aMCI show significant decreases in gait speed and increases in stride time and time variability when changing from a single- to a dual-task [68,69]. Notably, poor gait performance, particularly under dual-tasking, has been proposed as a motor signature of aMCI [8]. It is noteworthy that the co-occurrence of cognitive complaints and slow gait, a condition referred to as motoric cognitive risk syndrome, identifies individuals at especially high risk to progress to dementia [70,71]. Along similar lines, low muscle strength of upper and lower extremities has shown to increase the risk of MCI progression into AD [72]. The neurophysiologic substratum of reduced physical performance in MCI has its roots in the existence of neuronal networks involved in both cognition and lower extremity function. Indeed, atrophy and amyloid deposition in a network encompassing the dorsolateral prefrontal cortex, cingulate gyrus, parietal association areas, basal ganglia, and medial temporal lobes (particularly the hippocampus) are thought to mediate the relationship between cognitive function and physical performance [73]. Thus, individuals who exhibit both cognitive and motor deficits may have greater underlying brain damage [71]. This implies that the simultaneous analysis of cognitive and physical function may help identify a subset of MCI persons at greater risk of conversion to dementia [71,74]. The observation that low muscle mass is commonly observed in conjunction with cognitive impairment [75,76] suggests that the inclusion of body composition analysis might further refine the identification of people more likely to progress from MCI to dementia. Indeed, muscle loss and cognitive dysfunction share a number of predisposing factors, including inflammation, oxidative stress, insulin resistance, and an inactive lifestyle [76]. With regard to the latter, studies have shown that engagement in regular physical activity is negatively associated with the risk of developing dementia [77–79]. Furthermore, findings from a systematic review and meta-analyses indicated that an increase of 500 kcal or 10 MET-h per week was associated with a 10% decrease in the risk of dementia [79].

4. Conclusions

The ODINO study was conceived as an innovative multi-dimensional investigation aimed at exploring biological and physical performance signatures of MCI subtypes. Measures of inflammatory metabolic markers and physical performance will be integrated through advanced multivariate statistical analyses to gain insights into the heterogeneity of MCI subtypes and their risk to progress toward dementia. The results obtained from the ODINO study and their comparison with those collected from a thoroughly characterized cohort of non-MCI older adults with similar age and sociodemographic characteristics [9–11] may enable discerning pathways involved in "physiologic" age-related cognitive decline from those implicated in the progression of MCI to early dementia. This knowledge will, therefore, pave the way for the clinical implementation of composite biomarkers of MCI. Our results will also allow the possible identification of therapeutic targets amenable for person-tailored interventions that may hold people with MCI back from the doorstep of dementia.

Author Contributions: Conceptualization, A.P. (Anna Picca), D.F., M.C.C., M.R.L.M., R.C., and R.L.; methodology, A.P. (Anna Picca), A.P. (Aniello Primiano), H.J.C.-J., and J.G.; software, F.M. and R.L.; validation, R.C. and R.L.; development of the data analysis plan, A.B. and F.M.; investigation, C.P., D.R., E.M. (Eleonora Meloni); resources, F.M. and R.B.; writing—original draft preparation, A.P. (Anna Picca), E.M. (Emanuele Marzetti) and R.C.; writing—review and editing, F.M., J.G., and R.L.; supervision, E.M. (Emanuele Marzetti), D.F., M.C.C., M.R.L.M., and R.B.; funding acquisition, R.B. All authors have read and agreed to the published version of the manuscript.

References

1. American Psychiatric Association. *Diagnostic and Statistical Manual of Mental Disorders*, 5th ed.; American Psychiatric Association: Washington, DC, USA, 2013; ISBN 0-89042-555-8.
2. Petersen, R.C.; Smith, G.E.; Waring, S.C.; Ivnik, R.J.; Kokmen, E.; Tangelos, E.G. Aging, Memory, and Mild Cognitive Impairment. *Int. Psychogeriatr.* **1997**, *9*, 65–69. [CrossRef] [PubMed]
3. Sachdev, P.S.; Blacker, D.; Blazer, D.G.; Ganguli, M.; Jeste, D.V.; Paulsen, J.S.; Petersen, R.C. Classifying neurocognitive disorders: The DSM-5 approach. *Nat. Rev. Neurol.* **2014**, *10*, 634–642. [CrossRef] [PubMed]
4. Petersen, R.C. Mild cognitive impairment as a clinical entity. *J. Intern. Med.* **2004**, *256*, 183–194. [CrossRef] [PubMed]
5. Morris, J.C.; Storandt, M.; Miller, J.P.; McKeel, D.W.; Price, J.L.; Rubin, E.H.; Berg, L. Mild cognitive impairment represents early-stage Alzheimer disease. *Arch. Neurol.* **2001**, *58*, 397–405. [CrossRef]
6. Levey, A.; Lah, J.; Goldstein, F.; Steenland, K.; Bliwise, D. Mild cognitive impairment: An opportunity to identify patients at high risk for progression to Alzheimer's disease. *Clin. Ther.* **2006**, *28*, 991–1001. [CrossRef]
7. Chi, G.C.; Fitzpatrick, A.L.; Sharma, M.; Jenny, N.S.; Lopez, O.L.; DeKosky, S.T. Inflammatory Biomarkers Predict Domain-Specific Cognitive Decline in Older Adults. *J. Gerontol. A Biol. Sci. Med. Sci.* **2017**, *72*, 796–803. [CrossRef]

8. Montero-Odasso, M.; Oteng-Amoako, A.; Speechley, M.; Gopaul, K.; Beauchet, O.; Annweiler, C.; Muir-Hunter, S.W. The motor signature of mild cognitive impairment: Results from the gait and brain study. *J. Gerontol. Ser. A Biol. Sci. Med. Sci.* **2014**, *69*, 1415–1421. [CrossRef] [PubMed]
9. Calvani, R.; Picca, A.; Marini, F.; Biancolillo, A.; Gervasoni, J.; Persichilli, S.; Primiano, A.; Coelho-Junior, H.J.; Bossola, M.; Urbani, A.; et al. Distinct Pattern of Circulating Amino Acids Characterizes Older Persons with Physical Frailty and Sarcopenia: Results from the BIOSPHERE Study. *Nutrients* **2018**, *10*, 1691. [CrossRef]
10. Marzetti, E.; Picca, A.; Marini, F.; Biancolillo, A.; Coelho-Junior, H.J.; Gervasoni, J.; Bossola, M.; Cesari, M.; Onder, G.; Landi, F.; et al. Inflammatory signatures in older persons with physical frailty and sarcopenia: The frailty "cytokinome" at its core. *Exp. Gerontol.* **2019**, *122*, 129–138. [CrossRef]
11. Picca, A.; Coelho-Junior, H.J.; Cesari, M.; Marini, F.; Miccheli, A.; Gervasoni, J.; Bossola, M.; Landi, F.; Bernabei, R.; Marzetti, E.; et al. The metabolomics side of frailty: Toward personalized medicine for the aged. *Exp. Gerontol.* **2019**, *126*, 110692. [CrossRef]
12. Seeman, T.E.; McEwen, B.S.; Rowe, J.W.; Singer, B.H. Allostatic load as a marker of cumulative biological risk: MacArthur studies of successful aging. *Proc. Natl. Acad. Sci. USA* **2001**, *98*, 4770–4775. [CrossRef]
13. Calvani, R.; Marini, F.; Cesari, M.; Tosato, M.; Anker, S.D.; von Haehling, S.; Miller, R.R.; Bernabei, R.; Landi, F.; Marzetti, E. SPRINTT consortium Biomarkers for physical frailty and sarcopenia: State of the science and future developments. *J. Cachexia Sarcopenia Muscle* **2015**, *6*, 278–286. [CrossRef] [PubMed]
14. Albert, M.S.; DeKosky, S.T.; Dickson, D.; Dubois, B.; Feldman, H.H.; Fox, N.C.; Gamst, A.; Holtzman, D.M.; Jagust, W.J.; Petersen, R.C.; et al. The diagnosis of mild cognitive impairment due to Alzheimer's disease: Recommendations from the National Institute on Aging-Alzheimer's Association workgroups on diagnostic guidelines for Alzheimer's disease. *Alzheimer's Dement.* **2011**, *7*, 270–279. [CrossRef] [PubMed]
15. Hughes, C.P.; Berg, L.; Danziger, W.L.; Coben, L.A.; Martin, R.L. A new clinical scale for the staging of dementia. *Br. J. Psychiatry* **1982**, *140*, 566–572. [CrossRef] [PubMed]
16. Folstein, M.F.; Folstein, S.E.; McHugh, P.R. "Mini-mental state". A practical method for grading the cognitive state of patients for the clinician. *J. Psychiatr. Res.* **1975**, *12*, 189–198. [CrossRef]
17. Carlesimo, G.A.; Caltagirone, C.; Gainotti, G. The Mental Deterioration Battery: Normative data, diagnostic reliability and qualitative analyses of cognitive impairment. The Group for the Standardization of the Mental Deterioration Battery. *Eur. Neurol.* **1996**, *36*, 378–384. [CrossRef]
18. Wechsler, D. A Standardized Memory Scale for Clinical Use. *J. Psychol. Interdiscip. Appl.* **1945**, *19*, 87–95. [CrossRef]
19. Berch, D.B.; Krikorian, R.; Huha, E.M. The Corsi block-tapping task: Methodological and theoretical considerations. *Brain Cogn.* **1998**, *38*, 317–338. [CrossRef]
20. Busch, R.M.; Farrell, K.; Lisdahl-Medina, K.; Krikorian, R. Corsi Block-Tapping task performance as a function of path configuration. *J. Clin. Exp. Neuropsychol.* **2005**, *27*, 127–134. [CrossRef]
21. Shin, M.-S.; Park, S.-Y.; Park, S.-R.; Seol, S.-H.; Kwon, J.S. Clinical and empirical applications of the Rey-Osterrieth Complex Figure Test. *Nat. Protoc.* **2006**, *1*, 892–899. [CrossRef]
22. Zarino, B.; Crespi, M.; Launi, M.; Casarotti, A. A new standardization of semantic verbal fluency test. *Neurol. Sci.* **2014**, *35*, 1405–1411. [CrossRef] [PubMed]
23. Scarpina, F.; Tagini, S. The Stroop Color and Word Test. *Front. Psychol.* **2017**, *8*, 557. [CrossRef] [PubMed]
24. Marra, C.; Gainotti, G.; Scaricamazza, E.; Piccininni, C.; Ferraccioli, M.; Quaranta, D. The Multiple Features Target Cancellation (MFTC): An attentional visual conjunction search test. Normative values for the Italian population. *Neurol. Sci.* **2013**, *34*, 173–180. [CrossRef] [PubMed]
25. Yesavage, J.A.; Sheikh, J.I. 9/Geriatric Depression Scale (GDS). *Clin. Gerontol.* **1986**, *5*, 165–173. [CrossRef]
26. Landi, F.; Russo, A.; Liperoti, R.; Pahor, M.; Tosato, M.; Capoluongo, E.; Bernabei, R.O.G. Midarm muscle circumference, physical performance and mortality: Results from the aging and longevity study in the Sirente geographic area (ilSIRENTE study). *Clin. Nutr.* **2010**, *29*, 441–447. [CrossRef]
27. Marzetti, E.; Cesari, M.; Calvani, R.; Msihid, J.; Tosato, M.; Rodriguez-Mañas, L.; Lattanzio, F.; Cherubini, A.; Bejuit, R.; Di Bari, M.; et al. The "Sarcopenia and Physical fRailty IN older people: Multi-componenT Treatment strategies" (SPRINTT) randomized controlled trial: Case finding, screening and characteristics of eligible participants. *Exp. Gerontol.* **2018**, *113*, 48–57. [CrossRef]
28. Mathiowetz, V.; Wiemer, D.M.; Federman, S.M. Grip and pinch strength: Norms for 6- to 19-year-olds. *Am. J. Occup. Ther. Off. Publ. Am. Occup. Ther. Assoc.* **1986**, *40*, 705–711. [CrossRef]

29. Landi, F.; Calvani, R.; Tosato, M.; Martone, A.M.; Picca, A.; Ortolani, E.; Savera, G.; Salini, S.; Ramaschi, M.; Bernabei, R.; et al. Animal-Derived Protein Consumption Is Associated with Muscle Mass and Strength in Community-Dwellers: Results from the Milan EXPO Survey. *J. Nutr. Health Aging* **2017**, *21*, 1050–1056. [CrossRef]
30. Marzetti, E.; Lees, H.A.; Manini, T.M.; Buford, T.W.; Aranda, J.M.; Calvani, R.; Capuani, G.; Marsiske, M.; Lott, D.J.; Vandenborne, K.; et al. Skeletal muscle apoptotic signaling predicts thigh muscle volume and gait speed in community-dwelling older persons: An exploratory study. *PLoS ONE* **2012**, *7*, e32829. [CrossRef]
31. Richardson, S. The Timed "Up & Go": A Test of Basic Functional Mobility for Frail Elderly Persons. *J. Am. Geriatr. Soc.* **1991**, *39*, 142–148. [CrossRef]
32. de Melo Borges, S.; Radanovic, M.; Forlenza, O.V. Functional mobility in a divided attention task in older adults with cognitive impairment. *J. Mot. Behav.* **2015**, *47*, 378–385. [CrossRef] [PubMed]
33. Guralnik, J.M.; Simonsick, E.M.; Ferrucci, L.; Glynn, R.J.; Berkman, L.F.; Blazer, D.G.; Scherr, P.A.; Wallace, R.B. A short physical performance battery assessing lower extremity function: Association with self-reported disability and prediction of mortality and nursing home admission. *J. Gerontol.* **1994**, *49*, M85–M94. [CrossRef] [PubMed]
34. Crapo, R.O.; Casaburi, R.; Coates, A.L.; Enright, P.L.; MacIntyre, N.R.; McKay, R.T.; Johnson, D.; Wanger, J.S.; Zeballos, R.J.; Bittner, V.; et al. ATS statement: Guidelines for the six-minute walk test. *Am. J. Respir. Crit. Care Med.* **2002**, *166*, 111–117.
35. Katz, S. Assessing self-maintenance: Activities of daily living, mobility, and instrumental activities of daily living. *J. Am. Geriatr. Soc.* **1983**, *31*, 721–727. [CrossRef]
36. Lawton, M.P.; Brody, E.M. Assessment of older people: Self-maintaining and instrumental activities of daily living. *Gerontologist* **1969**, *9*, 179–186. [CrossRef]
37. Almeida, G.J.M.; Wasko, M.C.M.; Jeong, K.; Moore, C.G.; Piva, S.R. Physical activity measured by the SenseWear Armband in women with rheumatoid arthritis. *Phys. Ther.* **2011**, *91*, 1367–1376. [CrossRef]
38. Ponziani, F.R.; Bhoori, S.; Castelli, C.; Putignani, L.; Rivoltini, L.; Del Chierico, F.; Sanguinetti, M.; Morelli, D.; Paroni Sterbini, F.; Petito, V.; et al. Hepatocellular carcinoma is associated with gut microbiota profile and inflammation in nonalcoholic fatty liver disease. *Hepatology* **2019**, *69*, 107–120. [CrossRef]
39. Picca, A.; Guerra, F.; Calvani, R.; Bucci, C.; Lo Monaco, M.R.; Bentivoglio, A.R.; Landi, F.; Bernabei, R.; Marzetti, E. Mitochondrial-derived vesicles as candidate biomarkers in parkinson's disease: Rationale, Design and Methods of the EXosomes in PArkiNson Disease (EXPAND) Study. *Int. J. Mol. Sci.* **2019**, *20*, 2373. [CrossRef]
40. Ponziani, F.R.; Putignani, L.; Paroni Sterbini, F.; Petito, V.; Picca, A.; Del Chierico, F.; Reddel, S.; Calvani, R.; Marzetti, E.; Sanguinetti, M.; et al. Influence of hepatitis C virus eradication with direct-acting antivirals on the gut microbiota in patients with cirrhosis. *Aliment. Pharmacol. Ther.* **2018**, *48*, 1301–1311. [CrossRef]
41. Picca, A.; Ponziani, F.R.; Calvani, R.; Marini, F.; Biancolillo, A.; Coelho-Junior, H.J.; Gervasoni, J.; Primiano, A.; Putignani, L.; Del Chierico, F.; et al. Gut microbial, inflammatory and metabolic signatures in older people with physical frailty and sarcopenia: Results from the BIOSPHERE Study. *Nutrients* **2019**, *12*, 65. [CrossRef]
42. Addolorato, G.; Ponziani, F.R.; Dionisi, T.; Mosoni, C.; Vassallo, G.A.; Sestito, L.; Petito, V.; Picca, A.; Marzetti, E.; Tarli, C.; et al. Gut microbiota compositional and functional fingerprint in patients with alcohol use disorder and alcohol-associated liver disease. *Liver Int.* **2020**, *40*, 878–888. [CrossRef] [PubMed]
43. Picca, A.; Guerra, F.; Calvani, R.; Marini, F.; Biancolillo, A.; Landi, G.; Beli, R.; Landi, F.; Bernabei, R.; Bentivoglio, A.R.; et al. Mitochondrial Signatures in Circulating Extracellular Vesicles of Older Adults with Parkinson's Disease: Results from the EXosomes in PArkiNson's Disease (EXPAND) Study. *J. Clin. Med.* **2020**, *9*, 504. [CrossRef] [PubMed]
44. Cunnane, S.C.; Schneider, J.A.; Tangney, C.; Tremblay-Mercier, J.; Fortier, M.; Bennett, D.A.; Morris, M.C. Plasma and brain fatty acid profiles in mild cognitive impairment and Alzheimer's disease. *J. Alzheimer's. Dis.* **2012**, *29*, 691–697. [CrossRef] [PubMed]
45. Picca, A.; Calvani, R.; Landi, G.; Marini, F.; Biancolillo, A.; Gervasoni, J.; Persichilli, S.; Primiano, A.; Urbani, A.; Bossola, M.; et al. Circulating amino acid signature in older people with Parkinson's disease: A metabolic complement to the EXosomes in PArkiNson Disease (EXPAND) study. *Exp. Gerontol.* **2019**, *128*, 110766. [CrossRef] [PubMed]

46. Calvani, R.; Rodriguez-Mañas, L.; Picca, A.; Marini, F.; Biancolillo, A.; Laosa, O.; Pedraza, L.; Gervasoni, J.; Primiano, A.; Conta, G.; et al. Identification of a Circulating Amino Acid Signature in Frail Older Persons with Type 2 Diabetes Mellitus: Results from the Metabofrail Study. *Nutrients* **2020**, *12*, 199. [CrossRef] [PubMed]
47. Ståhle, L.; Wold, S. Partial least squares analysis with cross-validation for the two-class problem: A Monte Carlo study. *J. Chemom.* **1987**, *1*, 185–196. [CrossRef]
48. Biancolillo, A.; Marini, F.; Roger, J.M. SO-CovSel: A novel method for variable selection in a multiblock framework. *J. Chemom.* **2020**, *34*, e3120. [CrossRef]
49. Westerhuis, J.A.; Hoefsloot, H.C.J.; Smit, S.; Vis, D.J.; Smilde, A.K.; van Velzen, E.J.J.; van Duijnhoven, J.P.M.; van Dorsten, F.A. Assessment of PLSDA cross validation. *Metabolomics* **2008**, *4*, 81–89. [CrossRef]
50. Wold, S.; Sjöström, M. SIMCA: A Method for Analyzing Chemical Data in Terms of Similarity and Analogy. In *Chemometrics, Theory and Application*; Kowalski, B.R., Ed.; American Chemical Society: Washington, DC, USA, 1977; Volume 52, pp. 243–282. ISBN 9780841203792.
51. Westerhuis, J.A.; van Velzen, E.J.J.; Hoefsloot, H.C.J.; Smilde, A.K. Multivariate paired data analysis: Multilevel PLSDA versus OPLSDA. *Metabolomics* **2010**, *6*, 119–128. [CrossRef]
52. Rosenberg, P.B.; Lyketsos, C. Mild cognitive impairment: Searching for the prodrome of Alzheimer's disease. *World Psychiatry* **2008**, *7*, 72–78. [CrossRef]
53. Grundman, M.; Petersen, R.C.; Ferris, S.H.; Thomas, R.G.; Aisen, P.S.; Bennett, D.A.; Foster, N.L.; Jack, C.R.; Galasko, D.R.; Doody, R.; et al. Alzheimer's Disease Cooperative Study. Mild cognitive impairment can be distinguished from Alzheimer disease and normal aging for clinical trials. *Arch. Neurol.* **2004**, *61*, 59–66. [CrossRef] [PubMed]
54. Csukly, G.; Sirály, E.; Fodor, Z.; Horváth, A.; Salacz, P.; Hidasi, Z.; Csibri, É.; Rudas, G.; Szabó, Á. The Differentiation of Amnestic Type MCI from the Non-Amnestic Types by Structural MRI. *Front. Aging Neurosci.* **2016**, *8*, 52. [CrossRef] [PubMed]
55. Mosconi, L.; Perani, D.; Sorbi, S.; Herholz, K.; Nacmias, B.; Holthoff, V.; Salmon, E.; Baron, J.C.; De Cristofaro, M.T.R.; Padovani, A.; et al. MCI conversion to dementia and the APOE genotype: A prediction study with FDG-PET. *Neurology* **2004**, *63*, 2332–2340. [CrossRef] [PubMed]
56. Jack, C.R.; Petersen, R.C.; Xu, Y.C.; O'Brien, P.C.; Smith, G.E.; Ivnik, R.J.; Boeve, B.F.; Waring, S.C.; Tangalos, E.G.; Kokmen, E. Prediction of AD with MRI-based hippocampal volume in mild cognitive impairment. *Neurology* **1999**, *52*, 1397–1403. [CrossRef]
57. deToledo-Morrell, L.; Stoub, T.R.; Bulgakova, M.; Wilson, R.S.; Bennett, D.A.; Leurgans, S.; Wuu, J.; Turner, D.A. MRI-derived entorhinal volume is a good predictor of conversion from MCI to AD. *Neurobiol. Aging* **2004**, *25*, 1197–1203. [CrossRef]
58. Wang, W.; Cheng, X.; Lu, J.; Wei, J.; Fu, G.; Zhu, F.; Jia, C.; Zhou, L.; Xie, H.; Zheng, S. Mitofusin-2 is a novel direct target of p53. *Biochem. Biophys. Res. Commun.* **2010**, *400*, 587–592. [CrossRef]
59. Serra, L.; Giulietti, G.; Cercignani, M.; Spanò, B.; Torso, M.; Castelli, D.; Perri, R.; Fadda, L.; Marra, C.; Caltagirone, C.; et al. Mild cognitive impairment: Same identity for different entities. *J. Alzheimer's. Dis.* **2013**, *33*, 1157–1165. [CrossRef]
60. Jääskeläinen, O.; Hall, A.; Tiainen, M.; van Gils, M.; Lötjönen, J.; Kangas, A.J.; Helisalmi, S.; Pikkarainen, M.; Hallikainen, M.; Koivisto, A.; et al. Metabolic Profiles Help Discriminate Mild Cognitive Impairment from Dementia Stage in Alzheimer's Disease. *J. Alzheimer's Dis.* **2020**, 1–10. [CrossRef]
61. Olsson, B.; Lautner, R.; Andreasson, U.; Öhrfelt, A.; Portelius, E.; Bjerke, M.; Hölttä, M.; Rosén, C.; Olsson, C.; Strobel, G.; et al. CSF and blood biomarkers for the diagnosis of Alzheimer's disease: A systematic review and meta-analysis. *Lancet Neurol.* **2016**, *15*, 673–684. [CrossRef]
62. Bogie, J.F.J.; Haidar, M.; Kooij, G.; Hendriks, J.J.A. Fatty acid metabolism in the progression and resolution of CNS disorders. *Adv. Drug Deliv. Rev.* **2020**. [CrossRef]
63. Tynkkynen, J.; Chouraki, V.; van der Lee, S.J.; Hernesniemi, J.; Yang, Q.; Li, S.; Beiser, A.; Larson, M.G.; Sääksjärvi, K.; Shipley, M.J.; et al. Association of branched-chain amino acids and other circulating metabolites with risk of incident dementia and Alzheimer's disease: A prospective study in eight cohorts. *Alzheimer's Dement.* **2018**, *14*, 723–733. [CrossRef] [PubMed]
64. Wang, W.Y.; Tan, M.S.; Yu, J.T.; Tan, L. Role of pro-inflammatory cytokines released from microglia in Alzheimer's disease. *Ann. Transl. Med.* **2015**, *3*, 136. [CrossRef] [PubMed]

65. Kim, S.-M.; Song, J.; Kim, S.; Han, C.; Park, M.H.; Koh, Y.; Jo, S.A.; Kim, Y.-Y. Identification of peripheral inflammatory markers between normal control and Alzheimer's disease. *BMC Neurol.* **2011**, *11*, 51. [CrossRef] [PubMed]
66. Bermejo, P.; Martín-Aragón, S.; Benedí, J.; Susín, C.; Felici, E.; Gil, P.; Ribera, J.M.; Villar, A.M. Differences of peripheral inflammatory markers between mild cognitive impairment and Alzheimer's disease. *Immunol. Lett.* **2008**, *117*, 198–202. [CrossRef]
67. Justice, J.N.; Ferrucci, L.; Newman, A.B.; Aroda, V.R.; Bahnson, J.L.; Divers, J.; Espeland, M.A.; Marcovina, S.; Pollak, M.N.; Kritchevsky, S.B.; et al. A framework for selection of blood-based biomarkers for geroscience-guided clinical trials: Report from the TAME Biomarkers Workgroup. *GeroScience* **2018**, *40*, 419–436. [CrossRef]
68. Muir, S.W.; Speechley, M.; Wells, J.; Borrie, M.; Gopaul, K.; Montero-Odasso, M. Gait assessment in mild cognitive impairment and Alzheimer's disease: The effect of dual-task challenges across the cognitive spectrum. *Gait Posture* **2012**, *35*, 96–100. [CrossRef]
69. Pedersen, M.M.; Holt, N.E.; Grande, L.; Kurlinski, L.A.; Beauchamp, M.K.; Kiely, D.K.; Petersen, J.; Leveille, S.; Bean, J.F. Mild cognitive impairment status and mobility performance: An analysis from the Boston RISE study. *J. Gerontol. A. Biol. Sci. Med. Sci.* **2014**, *69*, 1511–1518. [CrossRef]
70. Verghese, J.; Wang, C.; Lipton, R.B.; Holtzer, R. Motoric cognitive risk syndrome and the risk of dementia. *J. Gerontol. A Biol. Sci. Med. Sci.* **2013**, *68*, 412–418. [CrossRef]
71. Semba, R.D.; Tian, Q.; Carlson, M.C.; Xue, Q.L.; Ferrucci, L. Motoric cognitive risk syndrome: Integration of two early harbingers of dementia in older adults. *Ageing Res. Rev.* **2020**, *58*, 101022. [CrossRef]
72. Boyle, P.A.; Buchman, A.S.; Wilson, R.S.; Leurgans, S.E.; Bennett, D.A. Association of muscle strength with the risk of Alzheimer disease and the rate of cognitive decline in community-dwelling older persons. *Arch. Neurol.* **2009**, *66*, 1339–1344. [CrossRef]
73. Del Campo, N.; Payoux, P.; Djilali, A.; Delrieu, J.; Hoogendijk, E.O.; Rolland, Y.; Cesari, M.; Weiner, M.W.; Andrieu, S.; Vellas, B. MAPT/DSA Study Group Relationship of regional brain β-amyloid to gait speed. *Neurology* **2016**, *86*, 36–43. [CrossRef]
74. Tian, Q.; Resnick, S.M.; Mielke, M.M.; Yaffe, K.; Launer, L.J.; Jonsson, P.V.; Grande, G.; Welmer, A.-K.; Laukka, E.J.; Bandinelli, S.; et al. Association of Dual Decline in Memory and Gait Speed With Risk for Dementia Among Adults Older Than 60 Years: A Multicohort Individual-Level Meta-analysis. *JAMA Netw. Open* **2020**, *3*, e1921636. [CrossRef]
75. Nourhashémi, F.; Andrieu, S.; Gillette-Guyonnet, S.; Reynish, E.; Albarède, J.-L.; Grandjean, H.; Vellas, B. Is there a relationship between fat-free soft tissue mass and low cognitive function? Results from a study of 7105 women. *J. Am. Geriatr. Soc.* **2002**, *50*, 1796–1801. [CrossRef] [PubMed]
76. Cabett Cipolli, G.; Sanches Yassuda, M.; Aprahamian, I. Sarcopenia Is Associated with Cognitive Impairment in Older Adults: A Systematic Review and Meta-Analysis. *J. Nutr. Health Aging* **2019**, *23*, 525–531. [CrossRef] [PubMed]
77. Rovio, S.; Kåreholt, I.; Helkala, E.-L.; Viitanen, M.; Winblad, B.; Tuomilehto, J.; Soininen, H.; Nissinen, A.; Kivipelto, M. Leisure-time physical activity at midlife and the risk of dementia and Alzheimer's disease. *Lancet Neurol.* **2005**, *4*, 705–711. [CrossRef]
78. Scarmeas, N.; Luchsinger, J.A.; Schupf, N.; Brickman, A.M.; Cosentino, S.; Tang, M.X.; Stern, Y. Physical activity, diet, and risk of Alzheimer disease. *JAMA* **2009**, *302*, 627–637. [CrossRef]
79. Xu, W.; Wang, H.F.; Wan, Y.; Tan, C.-C.; Yu, J.-T.; Tan, L. Leisure time physical activity and dementia risk: A dose-response meta-analysis of prospective studies. *BMJ Open* **2017**, *7*, e014706. [CrossRef]

5

Obesity and Diabetes Mediated Chronic Inflammation: A Potential Biomarker in Alzheimer's Disease

Md Shahjalal Hossain Khan and Vijay Hegde *

Obesity and Metabolic Health Laboratory, Department of Nutritional Sciences, Texas Tech University, Lubbock, TX 79409, USA; Md-Shahjalal.Khan@ttu.edu

* Correspondence: vijay.hegde@ttu.edu

Abstract: Alzheimer's disease (AD) is the sixth leading cause of death and is correlated with obesity, which is the second leading cause of preventable diseases in the United States. Obesity, diabetes, and AD share several common features, and inflammation emerges as the central link. High-calorie intake, elevated free fatty acids, and impaired endocrine function leads to insulin resistance and systemic inflammation. Systemic inflammation triggers neuro-inflammation, which eventually hinders the metabolic and regulatory function of the brain mitochondria leading to neuronal damage and subsequent AD-related cognitive decline. As an early event in the pathogenesis of AD, chronic inflammation could be considered as a potential biomarker in the treatment strategies for AD.

Keywords: obesity; diabetes; inflammation; Alzheimer's disease; Amyloid Beta; Tau; biomarker; mitochondrial dysfunction

---

1. Introduction

Alzheimer's disease (AD) is a progressive and irreversible brain disorder that begins well before the clinical symptoms appear. The actual symptoms may appear only after several years of changes in the brain due to damage or destruction of brain cells (neurons) in the area involved in cognitive function such as memory, thinking, and learning [1]. AD slowly abolishes brain function and hinders thinking ability. AD is recognized as a common cause of an estimated 60–80% of cases of dementia [2]. The early clinical symptoms of AD have been described as difficulty in conversations and depression and is followed by disorientation, confusion, impaired communication, behavioral changes, and, eventually, trouble in speaking and walking. At the critical stage, consequences are fatal and the patients are bed-bound and need special attention such as round-the-clock care [3].

AD prevalence is escalating rapidly worldwide especially among the population aged 65 years and older. In the United States, it has been reported that, in 2019, an estimated 5.8 million Americans were living with AD-related dementia and, among them, 81% were aged 75 or older and 200,000 individuals were under 65 years of age [3]. The numbers have been projected to grow from the current 55 million to 88 million [3], approximately doubling by 2050 [4]. This alone depicts the magnitude of the burden of AD on health care and the overall society in the future. Considering disability-adjusted life years (DALYs) as a primary measure of disease burden, in the United States, AD has risen from the 12th most burdensome disease in 1990 to the 6th most burdensome disease in 2016 [5]. It has been estimated that, in 2019, the healthcare burden will be around $290 million [3]. Collectively, the above statistics indicate that AD does not only affect morbidity or mortality, but AD is also affecting the socio-economic and healthcare burden in the USA. There have been numerous studies elucidating the pathogenesis, molecular and clinical mechanisms, the association of diabetes and metabolic syndromes, and consequences in a broader range. Yet no single or combined treatment has shown to have satisfactory levels of efficiency to delay or prevent AD pathogenesis.

In this review, we will focus on a much narrower context of AD pathogenesis considering inflammation as the central mechanistic link among obesity, diabetes, and AD-related dementia. In obesity, the elevated circulating free fatty acids (FFA) attributes to inflammation, initiated by Toll-like receptors (TLR-4) and release of pro-inflammatory cytokines, which is also associated with insulin resistance and diabetes [6,7] via nuclear factor-kappa B (NF-*k*B) mediated inflammation that might mediate the intracellular signaling impairments [8]. In the brain, pro-inflammatory cytokines activated by microglia can induce oxidative stress and compromised antioxidant defense [9]. Collectively, they contribute to impaired insulin signaling, synapses loss, reduced mitochondrial axonal transport [10], mitochondrial fragmentation, dynamics, and eventual dysfunction [11]. Mitochondrial dysfunction has been considered as an early event for AD pathogenesis and is also associated with a metabolic syndrome including obesity, diabetes, insulin resistance, and cardiovascular diseases [8]. Thus, it is possible that mitochondrial dysfunction has an evident role in the initiation and development of the metabolic disorder, and it is worthy to investigate to what extent inflammation and mitochondrial health affect the progression of AD.

2. Pathogenesis of AD

The characteristic features of AD involve two major fundamental processes: extracellular beta amyloid (Aβ) deposition and intracellular tau protein hyper accumulation. Aβ is insoluble and is a major component for senile plaques. Insoluble tau is the major component of neurofibrillary tangles (NFT) [12]. Aβ is a 36 to 43 amino acid peptide, which is a part of the large transmembrane protein, Amyloid Precursor Protein (APP), and derived from cleavage of APP by β- and γ–secretase enzymes. Defective clearance of Aβ during the cleaving process of APP results in the accumulation of insoluble Aβ [13]. Initially, the Aβ monomer polymerizes into soluble oligomers and then into larger insoluble fragments like Aβ42 that can precipitate as amyloid fibrils [14]. On the other hand, tau is a protein associated with the microtubule and helps in modulating the axonal microtubule stability [15]. In an AD patient's brain, the tau protein gets hyper-phosphorylated and causes the protein to lose microtubule-binding ability and dissociate from the microtubules, which can progressively disrupt the transport structure and result in starvation of neurons and, ultimately, neuronal cell death [16]. Deposition of neuronal bodies and processing of insoluble phosphorylated tau protein into paired helical filaments can cause neurofibrillary degeneration. These deposits interfere with the spacing between microtubules and hinder the axonal terminals and dendrite nutrient transport [17].

3. Obesity, Diabetes, and AD

Obesity is a chronic and multifactorial disease characterized by excessive body fat accumulation. It is considered a risk factor for many diseases and disorders including hypertension, type 2 diabetes mellitus, coronary heart disease, and AD [18]. Adipose tissue possesses endocrine function secreting adipokines, inflammatory cytokines, and other bioactive mediators that influence energy homeostasis in metabolically active organs like adipose tissue, liver, pancreas, and even brain [19]. During a positive energy balance, adipocyte size and proliferation increases result in the expansion of adipose tissue to accommodate the excess energy, which leads to an increase in adipose tissue mass. This is followed by adipose tissue dysfunction promoting chronic low-grade inflammation [20], elevated oxidative stress [21,22], and altered mitochondrial dysfunction [23–25]. Although how obesity contributes to the mitochondrial dysfunction is still not clear, it is postulated that the induced inflammation and metabolic alteration implicated by impaired insulin function could be a possible factor [26,27].

Altered glucose homeostasis due to hyperinsulinemia and insulin resistance in diabetes is also one of the most prominent features of obesity. Obesity and a high fat diet (HFD) can induce insulin resistance, which, subsequently, impairs insulin signaling in the periphery as well as in the brain [28]. It is well-established that insulin has a significant role in the central nervous system (CNS) [29–33].

In the brain, insulin along with insulin growth factors (IGF) modulate neuronal growth, differentiation, survival, migration, metabolism, protein synthesis, gene expression, synapse formation, and synaptic plasticity [34]. Moreover, insulin regulates myelin production and oligodendrocyte maintenance [34]. Defective insulin signaling is also associated with impaired cognition and AD-related dementia [35]. Severely decreased phosphorylation of insulin receptors has been found in patient brains from both AD and diabetes [36]. The disturbance in insulin signaling could contribute to making the CNS environment more vulnerable to metabolic stress and, therefore, accelerate the neuronal dysfunction [37]. Diabetes is associated with islet amyloid polypeptide (IAPP) accumulation in the pancreatic islets. The IAPP is concurrently secreted with insulin from the pancreas. In diabetic and AD patients, the IAPP is found to be misfolded and elevated [38], accompanied by elevated Aβ accumulation, hyper-phosphorylated tau, and impaired fasting glucose as comorbidities [39].

Substantial evidence indicates that patients with obesity and diabetes are more susceptible to develop AD-related cognitive degeneration. Several longitudinal [40,41] and epidemiological studies [42–45] have established a significant association between midlife large waist-hip ratios to AD-related dementia and decreased hippocampal volume in later life. Moreover, the common pathways of neurodegeneration in the AD brain resemble similar pathologies observed in the brains of individuals with diabetes. Obesity, AD, and diabetes concomitantly share common features like brain atrophy, reduced cerebral glucose, and CNS insulin resistance [46].

4. Obesity, Diabetes, and Subsequent Systemic and Neuro-Inflammation

Obesity, diabetes, and AD attributes to a common shared chronic inflammatory process. Both epidemiological and observational studies suggested that neuro-inflammation is an early-stage marker of AD pathogenesis [47]. A higher plasma and CNS levels of inflammatory markers known as Interleukin-6 (IL-6), Interleukin 1β (IL-1β), transforming growth factor-β (TGF-β), and tumor necrosis factor-α (TNF-α) has been reported in AD patients, which indicates the potential role of inflammatory markers in AD pathogenesis [48]. Insulin resistance and inflammation have a bidirectional relation with AD. In the chronic peripheral inflammatory process in obesity and diabetes, the production of inflammatory cytokines can lead to serine phosphorylation of insulin receptor substrate-1 (IRS-1), which can inhibit the downstream signaling pathways like kappa B kinase (IKK), c-Jun N-terminal kinase (JNK), and extracellular signal regulated kinase 2 (ERK2). These can block the intracellular insulin signaling by downregulating the insulin receptor-mediated signaling [49]. Additionally, the systemic inflammation can damage and cross the blood-brain barrier (BBB) and enter into the brain, which might trigger the brain-specific inflammatory response [50]. These circulating cytokines can increase the apoptosis (cell death) rate, reduce synaptic function, and inhibit the neurogenesis and, thus, causing neuronal death [51]. Moreover, systemic inflammatory processes, e.g., IL-6, TNF-α, and C-reactive proteins (CRP), inhibit the transfer of Aβ from the CNS to the periphery [52]. Thus, Aβ oligomers accumulation can activate brain microglia that secrete the pro-inflammatory cytokines (IL-1β, IL-6, TNF-α), which can phosphorylate insulin receptor substrate (IRS) in multiple sites by activating the IRS-1 serine kinase upon binding with the respective receptors and alter brain insulin signaling [53]. Although the precise mechanisms are yet to be understood, the putative mechanisms for systemic and neuro-inflammation caused by obesity and diabetes are as follows.

4.1. *Systemic Inflammation and AD*

The circulating pro-inflammatory molecules either increase the permeability of the BBB or gain access via the area that lacks effective BBB to initiate neuro-inflammation in the hypothalamus [54,55]. The mechanism of BBB disruption is multifaceted and includes changes in the structural components like pericyte dysfunction, tight junction, and elevated endothelial oxidative stress [56]. HFD can elevate the expression and activation of pro-inflammatory cytokines and corresponding transcription factors, such as NF-*k*B, in the hypothalamus [57]. This pro-inflammatory action (a) will increase the microglial (brain's residing macrophage) infiltration and activation in the hypothalamus resulting in the local inflammatory mediators such as cytokines [57,58]. In addition, the elevated free fatty acids (FFA) enters the arcuate nucleus and increases TLR-4, a molecular pattern recognition receptor, on microglia and astrocytes and initiates the inflammatory response centrally [59]. (b) The circulating cytokines have limited spread and activate the hypothalamic cytokine receptors. This action can augment the brain inflammation [28]. (c) The direct entry of cytokines, chemokines, and FFA in systemic circulation can also propagate neuro-inflammation by initiating pro-inflammatory cytokines and prostaglandin production [60]. Collectively, this pro-inflammatory milieu can disrupt the hypothalamic function by inducing synaptic remodeling, neuronal cell apoptosis, and disturbed neurogenesis [61]. The hypothalamus has a potential role in cognitive function related to feeding, metabolism, stress regulation, and cardiovascular function along with cognition, attention, and memory function [62]. The remodeling of the hypothalamic circuit leads to dysregulation in the hypothalamic-pituitary-adrenal (HPA) axis resulting in increased production of glucocorticoids, which are related to impaired cognition and memory including depression, Cushing's syndrome, and AD [63]. Moreover, the chronic HPA axis activation and elevated glucocorticoid level is also associated with dendritic atrophy, hippocampal volume reduction, and reduced synaptic plasticity [64]. One of the characteristic features of AD is the hippocampus and cerebral cortex atrophy [65]. All these possible events collectively can lead to neurodegeneration and eventually AD.

4.2. Neuro-Inflammation in AD

The brain was thought to be unaffected by systemic inflammation and, thus, regarded as an "immune-privileged" organ not susceptible to inflammation for many years. However, this notion changed after extensive neuro-immune research that explored the central nervous system interaction with the peripheral system through hormonal and paracrine action [66]. In the case of the AD brain, Aβ deposition triggered by systemic inflammation initiates a series of immune-responses intended to reduce the Aβ plaques and the aggregates by activating the innate immunity to elicit the inflammatory response from microglia and astrocytes [67,68]. These pathological adaptations incite the release of pro-inflammatory cytokines including IL-6, IL-1β, or TNF-α along with other pro-inflammatory molecules including macrophage inflammatory proteins, monocyte chemoattractant proteins, coagulating factors, reactive oxygen species (ROS), nitric oxide, proteases, protease inhibitors, prostaglandins, thromboxanes, leukotrienes, and CRP from glial cells [52,69–71]. The aggravated environment induces additional phosphorylation of tau, accumulation of Aβ, and pro-inflammatory molecules [52], which, consequently, release reactive substances like nitric oxide, proteolytic enzymes, excitatory amino acids, and complementary factors, and damage the adjacent healthy neurons [72]. Therefore, the well-intended initial response to assist Aβ clearance, in turn, also secretes mediators that cause damage and leads to neurodegeneration [73]. An elevated level of IL-1β was found in serum, cerebrospinal fluids, and in the brain region [74,75], particularly astrocytes of the cortex and hippocampus [76] of patients with AD. The IL-1β secreted from astrocytes increases the neurotoxic Aβ and APP production [76,77]. The IL-1β also activates microglia to induce pro-inflammatory cytokine release that can lead to neurotoxicity [78]. Additionally, oxidative damage and alteration in tau phosphorylation in neurons, along with chronic low-grade inflammatory states, collectively lead to compromised brain integrity [79].

4.3. RAGE-Mediated Inflammation in AD

Dyslipidemia and chronic hyperglycemia caused by disturbance of insulin signaling in obesity can lead to glucolipotoxicity, which can play a pivotal role in AD. Hyperglycemia also generates advanced glycation end products (AGE), which is a senescent macro-protein derivative that can be identified in both senile plaques and NFTs as a possible link between AD and diabetes. AGEs are the derivatives of proteins, lipids, or nucleic acids modified by non-enzymatic glycosylation and tend to increase the production and accumulation during aging, diabetes, or obesity [80,81]. Advanced glycation end products (AGE) and its pattern recognition receptors (RAGE) induce a chronic, persistent inflammatory response that propagates vascular injuries [81–83]. RAGE is also a putative receptor for Aβ [84] and is found to be expressed in neurons, microglia, and astrocytes [85,86]. Aβ is a ligand for RAGE that interacts with the N-terminal domain. Neurons and microglia of the hippocampus and inferior frontal cortex area of the AD brain have reported expressing an elevated level of RAGE [85,87].

The Aβ-RAGE interaction in the neuronal cells leads to an ROS mediated cellular response and activation of NF-kB that induce elevated inflammatory milieu [87]. RAGE dependent Aβ-induced migration has been shown in both in-vitro Aβ plaque models and postmortem human microglia cell culture experiments [85]. It was reported that Aβ-RAGE dependent microglial activation elevates the RAGE and microglial colony-stimulating factors (M-CSF), while inhibition of RAGE using anti-RAGE F(ab′)$_2$ inhibits the microglial chemotactic response against Aβ_{42} [85]. Moreover, increased production of IL-1β or TNF-α, enhanced microglial infiltration in Aβ plaques, reduced acetylcholine esterase activity, and impaired spatial and learning memory observed in double transgenic mouse models when compared to APP or RAGE mouse models [88]. Elevated levels of AGE in the brain and plasma are associated with the cognitive dysfunction in AD patients [89,90]. AGE, along with increasing Aβ cytotoxicity, supports fibrillary tangles and Aβ plaque formation, which contributes to the pathogenesis of AD [91].

5. Inflammation Mediated Impaired Mitochondrial Health in AD

Mitochondria, which is the powerhouse of cells that provides energy by utilizing ATP, is also responsible for cellular processes including energy metabolism, ROS generation, calcium ion (Ca^{2+}) homeostasis, cell survival, and apoptosis [92]. Mitochondria maintain the normal functioning through regulated quality control even in the presence of persistent insults. However, any failure of quality control results in mechanical defects and damages that cause mitochondrial dysfunction [93]. It can lead to metabolic disorders. The major metabolic organs like liver, muscle, and adipose tissue are the active contributors in this process. During obesity and diabetes, excess lipid accumulation and hyperglycemia induced insulin resistance can lead to abnormal mitochondrial function via altering the ATP synthesis activity of mitochondria, beta-oxidation, and elevated oxidative stress [94]. Adipocyte differentiation drastically increases the activity and biogenesis of mitochondria, pointing towards a link between mitochondria and obesity. Mitochondrial dysfunction is correlated with a reduced size and number of mitochondria [95], oxidative capacity [96], reduced oxygen consumption, and oxidative phosphorylation related gene expression [97], which have been observed in individuals with obesity [90]. In mature adipocytes, mitochondrial dysfunction has been linked to fatty acid oxidation [98], adipokine secretion [99], and impaired glucose homeostasis [100]. Additionally, in obese mice, the expression of mitochondrial DNA (mtDNA), mtDNA transcription factor A (Tfam), and respiratory proteins are also significantly reduced [92]. HFD increases the production of ROS and oxidative stress in mouse adipocytes [101]. HFD consumption or excess calorie intake results in an excess mitochondrial load that hinders the effective dissipation of the proton gradient, which increases ROS generation, mtDNA mutation, and apoptosis [102].

There are several ways obesity and diabetes-induced inflammation affects mitochondrial functioning.

5.1. *Inflammation and Energy Metabolism*

Neuronal glucose metabolism consists of mechanisms that regulate uptake of glucose, insulin, and insulin signaling pathways, glucose transporters (GLUTs), and entry of glycolytic end-products into mitochondria that eventually metabolize and generate ATP via oxidative phosphorylation [103]. Mitochondria participates and modulates several metabolic signaling pathways including cytosolic signaling, redox-sensitive signaling, JNK, and 5′ AMP-activated protein kinase (AMPK) signaling [104]. These signaling pathways along with the associated metabolites, transporters, receptors, and enzymes ensure proper neuronal energy metabolism. Mitochondria-centered altered glucose metabolism manifested by impaired insulin signaling, altered receptors activity, and reduced glucose uptake is one of the key features of AD [104]. Mitochondria regulate the tricarboxylic acid (TCA) cycle, which is the principal regulator of cellular respiration. The TCA cycle generates adenosine triphosphate (ATP) via a series of enzyme-catalyzed chemical reactions and any malfunction in the enzymes involved in this cycle leads to impaired cellular respiration and ATP production [104].

Inflammatory processes mediated by infiltrated immune cells from the periphery and activated microglia initiate an intracellular signaling cascade that modifies the mitochondrial energy metabolism [105]. The activated microglia and astrocytes release pro-inflammatory cytokines, particularly TNF-α, and induce oxidative phosphorylation impairment, ATP production, and ROS production [105]. In one study, loss of mitochondrial transmembrane potential and reduction in intracellular ATP upon treatment with IL-1β in the retinal neuronal cells has also been reported [106]. Moreover, IL-1β and TNF-α are reported in decreasing the pyruvate dehydrogenase (PDH) enzyme activity in vivo [107], particularly in cardiomyocytes [108]. Reduced glucose oxidation in cultured human dermal fibroblast [109] reduced skeletal muscle [110,111], hepatic PDH activity [107], and complex I and II activity reported in the presence of inflammatory cytokines [105]. Impaired PDH activity has been found in the postmortem AD brain along with increased IL-6, IL-1β, or TNF-α, which suggests a compromised TCA cycle activity in the inflamed CNS of mild cognitive impairment and AD patients [105]. A significant reduction of neuronal complex I and III along with several other nuclear-encoded subunits of the Electron Transport Chain (ETC) has also been reported [112]. A reduction of ATP production and basal respiration upon TNF-α exposure has been shown in a dose-dependent manner in the mouse hippocampal cell line and primary neuronal cell culture [113]. TNF-α administration also reduces the peroxisome proliferator-activated receptor (PPAR)-γ co-activator 1α (PGC-1α) in myoblasts [114] and human cardiomyocytes [115] even though the effect of TNF-α on neuronal cells of various neurodegenerative diseases has not yet been reported. PGC-1α plays an important role in many cellular and metabolic processes including energy metabolism, cardiovascular diseases, and neurodegenerative diseases [116].

It has been reported that, in the AD brain, the levels of mitochondrial enzymes including PDH, cytochrome oxidase (COX), and α-ketoglutarate dehydrogenase complex are all decreased [117]. Proteomics studies on AD brains reveal that enzymes involved in metabolic pathways of the Kreb's cycle and glycolysis including malate dehydrogenase, glyceraldehyde 3-phosphate dehydrogenase (GAPDH), fructose-bis-phosphate-enolase, alpha-enolase (ENO1), and ATP synthase are oxidized [46]. The oxidation of these enzymes is related to dysfunctional cerebral glucose metabolism and reduction in ATP synthesis, which leads to loss of synaptic function [118]. These oxidative changes can lead to inflammation and eventually compromise metabolic function. The exact mechanism of how neuro-inflammation affects the metabolic function of mitochondria is yet to be understood. However, cellular and biochemical studies revealed that APP, Aβ, tau, and presenilin are associated with impaired mitochondrial energy metabolism [119,120]. It has been proposed that Aβ interacts with mitochondrial proteins disrupting ETC, increases ROS production, and free superoxide radicals that preclude the cellular ATP generation [121]. It has also been proposed that the hyper-phosphorylated tau and Aβ aggregates can block mitochondria and other cell organelles from nerve terminals, synapsis, and other brain regions with high ATP demands [122], which might lead to starvation of dendritic spines and synapsis due to severe mitochondrial ATP depletion [123].

5.2. *Inflammation and Altered Mitochondrial Dynamics*

Mitochondria are organelles that exist in dynamic networks, migrate throughout the cell, continuously fuse, divide, and undergo regulated turnover as the metabolic environment demands [124]. Mitochondrial dynamics can change the size and shape and adapt to the challenges [125]. Mitochondrial fission and fusion are two distinct processes that mediate the mitochondrial dynamic morphology and integrity [126]. In healthy neurons, mitochondria need to maintain the fusion and fission mechanism in a balanced way for the normal functioning of the synapses [125]. The enzymes involved in the fusion process are mitofusion 1 (Mfn1), mitofusion 2 (Mfn2), and optic atrophy protein 1 (OPA1). The proteins involved in the fission process are dynamin-related protein-1 (Drp1) and fission 1 (Fis1).

Mitochondrial biogenesis is the cellular process of producing new mitochondria and increasing the mitochondrial mass [127]. The regulation of biogenesis is modulated by nuclear factors including a set of nuclear transcription factors 1 and 2 (NRF 1 and NRF2), which control the cytochrome c and COX gene expression [128]. Any dysregulation in the mitochondrial dynamics and biogenesis might lead to excessive mitochondrial fragmentation and altered mitochondrial function resulting in mitochondrial dysfunction and eventually contribute to AD progression [129,130].

In astrocytes, impaired respiration rate and increased mitochondrial fragmentation (Drp1) have been reported upon IL-1β exposure [131]. In 3T3L1 adipocytes, TNF-α treatment alters mitochondrial morphology [132], along with smaller condensed mitochondria attributed by an increased level of Fis1 and decreased level of mitochondrial OPA1 [133,134]. In another in-vivo study, IL-6 downregulated Mfn1/Mfn2 and Fis1, which suggests neurotoxic effects of IL-6 [135]. In HFD mice, a decreased level of mitochondrial fusion genes (OPA1, Mfn1) and elevated expression of fission genes (Fis1, Drp1) along with increased pro-inflammatory cytokines has been reported [136]. Perturbation in mitochondrial function and release of mitochondrial contents in extracellular milieu activates the innate immune system, which can exacerbate the inflammatory response and alter the mitochondrial function. The production of ROS can provoke inflammation, and further mitochondrial dysfunction can lead to the production of pro-inflammatory IL-1β [137]. These studies suggested that inflammation and mitochondrial dysfunction operate in a synergic autotoxic feedback loop.

5.3. *Inflammation and Mitochondrial Oxidative Stress*

As a major source of ROS, mitochondria regulate the oxidative stress process [138]. Oxidative stress results from the imbalance between ROS production and detoxification in biological systems. ROS production is an important physiological by-product of the ETC. In the respiratory chain, while transferring the electron to molecular oxygen, about 0.4% to 5% of electrons lose their way and generate superoxide radicals ($O_2\bullet^-$), which, in turn, activates the mitochondrial permeability transition pore and results in apoptosis [139]. The brain is a highly susceptible organ to oxidative stress when compared to other organs due to the high demand for energy and oxygen, high levels of peroxidizable polyunsaturated fatty acids, the relative paucity of antioxidants, and anti-oxidant defense mechanisms and relative abundance of potent ROS catalyst iron [140]. During obesity and HFD consumption, adipose tissue propagates the inflammation and secretes pro-inflammatory cytokines including TNF-α, IL-6, and IL-1β, which also induce ROS production [141]. The activation of these cytokines promotes nitric oxide and ROS generation by macrophages and monocytes. HFD consumption propagates the lipid peroxidation in the brain by elevated levels of ROS via a similar mechanism that has been found in the non-neuronal tissue [142]. In mice, upon HFD consumption, elevated expression of ERK, and inducible nitric oxide synthase (i-NOS) are associated with oxidative stress [143,144]. The occurrence of oxidative stress has been shown as one of the early events in AD development and plays a major role in the pathogenesis of AD [118,145,146], whereas oxidative damage has been estimated to occur before other prognoses including the onset of Aβ aggregates, tau pathologies, or inflammation in the AD brain [147,148]. The activation of these cytokines promotes nitrogen and ROS generation by macrophages and monocytes. It has also been shown that oxidative stress is related to the hippocampal dysfunction in obese mice [146,149]. In the AD brain, excessive levels of ROS production indicated by the presence of an increased level of oxidative stress markers including oxidized lipid, protein, and DNA has been noticed [118,146].

Aβ generates hydrogen peroxide (H_2O_2) by reducing metal ions and increasing the free radical production by zinc, iron, and copper, which is highly concentrated in the core and periphery of Aβ deposits [150]. Aβ plaques can lead to a cytosolic calcium ions overload by depleting Ca^{2+} storage in the endoplasmic reticulum (ER). Increased Ca^{2+} leads to decreased endogenous glutathione (GSH) levels and increased accumulation of ROS inside the cell [151]. ROS potentially can mediate the JNK/stress-activated protein kinase pathways that can be associated with tau hyper-phosphorylation [152]. Aβ can also initiate free radical formation upon Nicotinamide adenine dinucleotide phosphate hydrogen (NADPH) oxidase activation, which leads to over-accumulation of ROS. The Aβ-induced ROS can initiate tau hyper-phosphorylation and modify cellular signaling via p38 mitogen-activated protein kinase (MAPK) activation [153]. Aβ can generate free radicals when interacting with metal ions. Cu^{2+}/Zn^{2+}-bound Aβ has been found to possess a similar structure to the antioxidant superoxide dismutase (SOD) [154].

Figure 1 provides an overview of how obesity and diabetes associated with elevated free fatty acids and impaired endocrine function leads to insulin resistance and systemic inflammation. This systemic inflammation triggers neuro-inflammation, which eventually hinders the metabolic and regulatory function of the brain mitochondria and leads to neuronal damage.

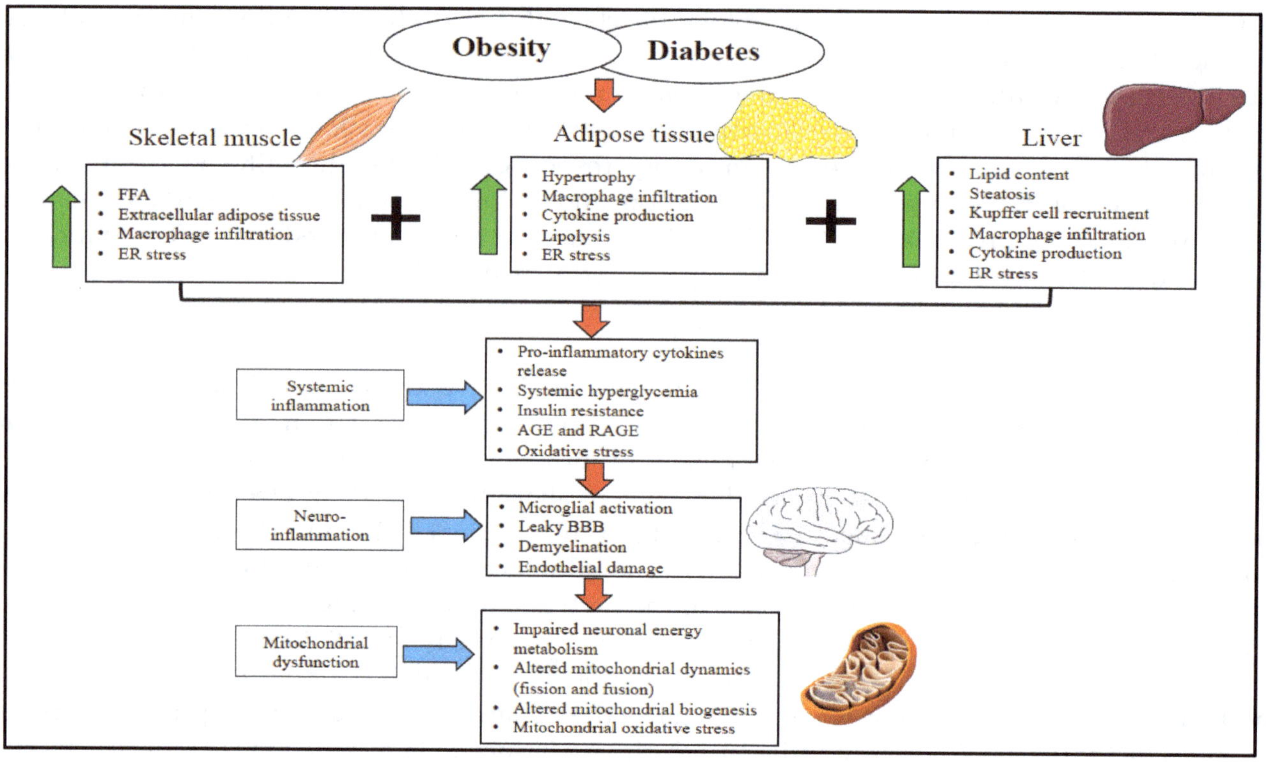

Figure 1. Overview of the diverse mechanism involved in obesity and diabetes-induced systemic and neuro-inflammation in mitochondrial and brain health. Skeletal muscle, adipose tissue, and liver are involved in glucose and lipid metabolism and play a vital role in developing adipose tissue dysfunction and insulin resistance during the obese condition. In obesity and diabetes, elevated free fatty acid, increased secretion of pro-inflammatory cytokines and macrophage infiltration, AGE and RAGE generation, and ER stress induce systemic inflammation. Systemic inflammation progressively initiates microglial activation, endothelial damage, and BBB disruption, which eventually leads to neuro-inflammation. These unfavorable inflammatory events alter the mitochondrial energy metabolism, mitochondrial dynamics, and biogenesis to escalate the mitochondrial oxidative stress collectively and trigger the mitochondrial assault. This gradually results in synapsis loss and neuronal death. FFA—Free Fatty Acid. ER—Endoplasmic Reticulum. AGE—Advanced Glycation End Products. RAGE—pattern recognition receptors of AGE. BBB—Blood-Brain Barrier.

Collectively, it has been proposed that the development of AD in the brain is the consequence of increased oxidative stress derived from several mechanisms: (a) elevated lipid peroxidation, (b) increased protein and DNA oxidation, (c) reduced energy metabolism and activity of COX, (d) ability of Aβ to generate free radicals in the form of increased accumulation of some metal ions like mercury, iron, and aluminum, which can stimulate free radical formation by the Fenton and Haber-Weiss pathway, and increased advanced glycation end products, SOD-1, and malonaldehyde in NFT and senile plaques [155].

5.4. *Inflammation and Cognitive Impairment*

The association between inflammation and cognitive decline has been reported in several cross-sectional studies [156–158]. However, the data were limited by the number of subjects [156–158], lack of adequate follow-up duration [156], or enough inflammatory markers [156] or subjects who were more than 80 years old. Elevated IL-6 in midlife is associated with cognitive decline whereas increased CRP levels did not predict the concurrent cognitive decline [159]. One neuroimaging study found that IL-6 is consistently associated with cognitive decline. In a follow-up study, increased circulating IL-6 level was found to be associated with accelerated cognitive decline after a 10-year follow up [160]. In another study, IL-6 was found strongly associated with the higher volume of white matter hyper-intensities, decreased gray matter, and reduced hippocampal volume whereas, in the case of CRP, the association was weaker than IL-6. This suggests that an inflammatory process could be associated with alteration of the brain [161]. Animal studies indicate declined cognition associated with elevated inflammation and Aβ deposition [162]. However, some studies found a minor association between cognition and inflammation [156–158,163]. In the Rotterdam Study, elevated levels of pro-inflammatory cytokines including IL-6 and CRP were found to be associated with cognitive decline and executive function. In the Leiden 85-plus study, a systematic level of IL-6 was found to be associated with declined cognition and memory function after adjustment for Apolipoprotein E ε4 (APOE ε4) carriers [164]. On the other hand, the Amsterdam Longitudinal Aging Study did not find any association between inflammation and cognitive decline after adjusting for APOE ε4 [157]. Furthermore, cerebral small vessel disease (SVD) refers to intracranial vascular disease associated with clinical manifestation and neuroimaging features caused by any changes in the morphology of cerebral vessels, which are crucial for adequate cerebral blood flow and brain parenchyma [165]. SVD causes decreased cerebral blood flow, increased BBB permeability, impaired cerebral autoregulation, brain functionality loss, and cognitive decline in the elderly [165]. SVD has often detected the parenchymal alteration based on four different features in magnetic resonance imaging (MRI), which include white matter hyperintensities, lacunes, cerebral microbleeds, and enlarged perivascular spaces [166–168]. A detailed systematic review suggested a robust association of inflammation with SVD represented by the presence of increased vascular inflammatory markers, especially among patients with stroke, which indicates an alteration in the endothelium and BBB [169]. Mounting evidence also indicates the potential role of inflammation and cerebral SVD in neurodegeneration and related disorders in recent years [168,170].

6. Conclusions and Future Direction

In this review, we discussed how obesity and diabetes can lead to systemic and neuro-inflammation, and whether inflammation affects the overall mitochondrial functioning, dynamics, oxidative stress, and cognitive decline in patients with AD. After cautiously considering the facts, we can suggest (but not conclude) that obesity or diabetes-induced inflammation is associated with impaired mitochondrial health. However, the question remains regarding to what extent the systemic or neuro-inflammation directly affect the brain mitochondrial health and subsequent AD pathogenesis. The association between inflammation and cognitive decline could be the consequence of underlying disease conditions triggered by diabetes, obesity, or cardiovascular disease and their consequent comorbidities. If the answer to this question can be addressed, it would be easier to decide whether targeting anti-inflammatory agents alone will be an effective and valid approach to combat AD. It seems even an anti-inflammatory approach is not the central focus for fighting AD but will support the mainstream treatment options including inhibiting Aβ production and tau hyper-phosphorylation. If the anti-inflammatory approach effectively improves the systemic neuro-inflammation, which is one of the events in AD that happens before memory loss, it is possible to improve the progressive Aβ deposition and tau hyper-phosphorylation. However, it is impossible to differentiate the effects of inflammation from other pathologies that occur concomitantly. One of the known modulators for the immune system is diet [171]. Diet high in sugar and saturated fat (SFA) is associated with cognitive impairment especially in learning and memory function both in humans and animal models, independent of obesity or associated metabolic changes [172–175]. High consumption of sugar and SFA results in substantial memory deficits in animals and humans, however, the impact of relative consumption remains unclear due to variability between human consumption and the controlled diet feeding in animal studies [176–178]. The ketogenic diet could be one way to counteract the inflammation and improve mitochondrial biogenesis [179]. The ketogenic diet was tested on subjects with a mild cognitive impairment syndrome and found to be associated with reduced inflammation, enhanced energy metabolism, and potentially improved neurocognitive function [180]. Dietary administration of a medium-chain triglyceride supplement was found to improve cognitive performance [181,182]. The ketogenic diet has been reported to be helpful in reducing the frequency of epilepsy in children [183]. Similar findings have been reported in animal studies where mice fed a ketogenic diet improved neuro-inflammation represented by reduced brain mRNA levels of TNFα, IL-6, and IL-1β and increased the PGC1β mRNA levels indicating ketone bodies related changes [184,185]. Moreover, the Mediterranean diet (MD) has been used as a potential dietary intervention to combat AD-related dementia due to its anti-inflammatory potential [186,187]. Numerous neuroimaging studies reported that the MD has protective effects on the neuronal structure and AD-related morphological changes [188–192].

Notably, several epidemiological studies effectively demonstrate the protective effects of NSAIDs in combating AD via its anti-inflammatory actions along with Aβ lowering properties whereas clinical studies did not support such an improvement [193–197]. More research is needed to conclude if obesity and diabetes associated with chronic inflammation and induced mitochondrial dysfunction can be identified as a biomarker that affects AD pathogenesis and whether the anti-inflammatory approach is a suitable therapeutic option to combat AD.

Author Contributions: Conceptualization, M.S.H.K. and V.H. Writing—original draft preparation, M.S.H.K. Writing—review and editing, V.H. Supervision, V.H. All authors have read and agreed to the published version of the manuscript.

References

1. Schapira, A.H. Mitochondria in the etiology of Parkinson's disease. *Handb. Clin. Neurol.* **2007**, *83*, 479–491.
2. Alzheimer's Association. 2018 Alzheimer's disease facts and figures. *Alzheimers Dement.* **2018**, *14*, 367–429.
3. Gaugler, J.; James, B.; Johnson, T.; Marin, A.; Weuve, J. 2019 Alzheimer's disease facts and figures. *Alzheimers Dement.* **2019**, *15*, 321–387.
4. Hebert, L.E.; Beckett, L.A.; Scherr, P.A.; Evans, D.A. Annual incidence of Alzheimer disease in the United States projected to the years 2000 through 2050. *Alzheimer Dis. Assoc. Disord.* **2001**, *15*, 169–173. [CrossRef]
5. Mokdad, A.H.; Ballestros, K.; Echko, M.; Glenn, S.; Olsen, H.E.; Mullany, E.; Lee, A.; Khan, A.R.; Ahmadi, A.; Ferrari, A.J. The state of US health, 1990-2016: Burden of diseases, injuries, and risk factors among US states. *JAMA* **2018**, *319*, 1444–1472.
6. Lei, X.; Seldin, M.M.; Little, H.C.; Choy, N.; Klonisch, T.; Wong, G.W. C1q/TNF-related protein 6 (CTRP6) links obesity to adipose tissue inflammation and insulin resistance. *J. Biol. Chem.* **2017**, *292*, 14836–14850. [CrossRef]
7. Naznin, F.; Toshinai, K.; Waise, T.Z.; NamKoong, C.; Moin, A.S.M.; Sakoda, H.; Nakazato, M. Diet-induced obesity causes peripheral and central ghrelin resistance by promoting inflammation. *J. Endocrinol.* **2015**, *226*, 81. [CrossRef]
8. Rigotto, G.; Basso, E. Mitochondrial Dysfunctions: A Thread Sewing Together Alzheimer's Disease, Diabetes, and Obesity. *Oxidative Med. Cell. Longev.* **2019**, *2019*. [CrossRef]
9. Yoo, M.-H.; Gu, X.; Xu, X.-M.; Kim, J.-Y.; Carlson, B.A.; Patterson, A.D.; Cai, H.; Gladyshev, V.N.; Hatfield, D.L. Delineating the role of glutathione peroxidase 4 in protecting cells against lipid hydroperoxide damage and in Alzheimer's disease. *Antioxid. Redox Signal.* **2010**, *12*, 819–827. [CrossRef]

10. Riemer, J.; Kins, S. Axonal transport and mitochondrial dysfunction in Alzheimer's disease. *Neurodegener. Dis.* **2013**, *12*, 111–124. [CrossRef]
11. Reddy, P.H.; Yin, X.; Manczak, M.; Kumar, S.; Pradeepkiran, J.A.; Vijayan, M.; Reddy, A.P. Mutant APP and amyloid beta-induced defective autophagy, mitophagy, mitochondrial structural and functional changes and synaptic damage in hippocampal neurons from Alzheimer's disease. *Hum. Mol. Genet.* **2018**, *27*, 2502–2516. [CrossRef]
12. Jiang, Y.; Mullaney, K.A.; Peterhoff, C.M.; Che, S.; Schmidt, S.D.; Boyer-Boiteau, A.; Ginsberg, S.D.; Cataldo, A.M.; Mathews, P.M.; Nixon, R.A. Alzheimer's-related endosome dysfunction in Down syndrome is Aβ-independent but requires APP and is reversed by BACE-1 inhibition. *Proc. Natl. Acad. Sci. USA* **2010**, *107*, 1630–1635. [CrossRef]
13. Zetterberg, H.; Blennow, K.; Hanse, E. Amyloid β and APP as biomarkers for Alzheimer's disease. *Exp. Gerontol.* **2010**, *45*, 23–29. [CrossRef]
14. Younkin, S.G. The role of Aβ42 in Alzheimer's disease. *J. Physiol.-Paris* **1998**, *92*, 289–292. [CrossRef]
15. Kneynsberg, A.; Combs, B.; Christensen, K.; Morfini, G.; Kanaan, N.M. Axonal degeneration in tauopathies: Disease relevance and underlying mechanisms. *Front. Neurosci.* **2017**, *11*, 572. [CrossRef]
16. Mandelkow, E.-M.; Biernat, J.; Drewes, G.; Gustke, N.; Trinczek, B.; Mandelkow, E. Tau domains, phosphorylation, and interactions with microtubules. *Neurobiol. Aging* **1995**, *16*, 355–362. [CrossRef]
17. Kocahan, S.; Doğan, Z. Mechanisms of Alzheimer's disease pathogenesis and prevention: The brain, neural pathology, N-methyl-D-aspartate receptors, tau protein and other risk factors. *Clin. Psychopharmacol. Neurosci.* **2017**, *15*, 1. [CrossRef]
18. Greenberg, A.S.; Obin, M.S. Obesity and the role of adipose tissue in inflammation and metabolism. *Am. J. Clin. Nutr.* **2006**, *83*, 461S–465S. [CrossRef]
19. D O'Brien, P.; Hinder, L.M.; Callaghan, B.C.; Feldman, E.L. Neurological consequences of obesity. *Lancet Neurol.* **2017**, *16*, 465–477. [CrossRef]
20. Mraz, M.; Haluzik, M. The role of adipose tissue immune cells in obesity and low-grade inflammation. *J. Endocrinol.* **2014**, *222*, R113–R127. [CrossRef]
21. Noeman, S.A.; Hamooda, H.E.; Baalash, A.A. Biochemical study of oxidative stress markers in the liver, kidney and heart of high fat diet induced obesity in rats. *Diabetol. Metab. Syndr.* **2011**, *3*, 17. [CrossRef]
22. Matsuda, M.; Shimomura, I. Increased oxidative stress in obesity: Implications for metabolic syndrome, diabetes, hypertension, dyslipidemia, atherosclerosis, and cancer. *Obes. Res. Clin. Pract.* **2013**, *7*, e330–e341. [CrossRef]
23. Heinonen, S.; Buzkova, J.; Muniandy, M.; Kaksonen, R.; Ollikainen, M.; Ismail, K.; Hakkarainen, A.; Lundbom, J.; Lundbom, N.; Vuolteenaho, K. Impaired mitochondrial biogenesis in adipose tissue in acquired obesity. *Diabetes* **2015**, *64*, 3135–3145. [CrossRef]
24. De Pauw, A.; Tejerina, S.; Raes, M.; Keijer, J.; Arnould, T. Mitochondrial (dys) function in adipocyte (de) differentiation and systemic metabolic alterations. *Am. J. Pathol.* **2009**, *175*, 927–939. [CrossRef]
25. Altshuler-Keylin, S.; Kajimura, S. Mitochondrial homeostasis in adipose tissue remodeling. *Sci. Signal.* **2017**, *10*, eaai9248. [CrossRef]
26. Montgomery, M.K.; Turner, N. Mitochondrial dysfunction and insulin resistance: An update. *Endocr. Connect.* **2015**, *4*, R1–R15. [CrossRef]
27. Vernochet, C.; Damilano, F.; Mourier, A.; Bezy, O.; Mori, M.A.; Smyth, G.; Rosenzweig, A.; Larsson, N.-G.; Kahn, C.R. Adipose tissue mitochondrial dysfunction triggers a lipodystrophic syndrome with insulin resistance, hepatosteatosis, and cardiovascular complications. *FASEB J.* **2014**, *28*, 4408–4419. [CrossRef]
28. Cai, D.; Liu, T. Inflammatory cause of metabolic syndrome via brain stress and NF-κB. *Aging* **2012**, *4*, 98. [CrossRef]
29. Ho, L.; Qin, W.; Pompl, P.N.; Xiang, Z.; Wang, J.; Zhao, Z.; Peng, Y.; Cambareri, G.; Rocher, A.; Mobbs, C.V. Diet-induced insulin resistance promotes amyloidosis in a transgenic mouse model of Alzheimer's disease. *FASEB J.* **2004**, *18*, 902–904. [CrossRef]
30. Schubert, M.; Gautam, D.; Surjo, D.; Ueki, K.; Baudler, S.; Schubert, D.; Kondo, T.; Alber, J.; Galldiks, N.; Küstermann, E. Role for neuronal insulin resistance in neurodegenerative diseases. *Proc. Natl. Acad. Sci. USA* **2004**, *101*, 3100–3105. [CrossRef]
31. Stanley, M.; Macauley, S.L.; Holtzman, D.M. Changes in insulin and insulin signaling in Alzheimer's disease: Cause or consequence? *J. Exp. Med.* **2016**, *213*, 1375–1385. [CrossRef] [PubMed]

32. Arnold, S.E.; Arvanitakis, Z.; Macauley-Rambach, S.L.; Koenig, A.M.; Wang, H.-Y.; Ahima, R.S.; Craft, S.; Gandy, S.; Buettner, C.; Stoeckel, L.E. Brain insulin resistance in type 2 diabetes and Alzheimer disease: Concepts and conundrums. *Nat. Rev. Neurol.* **2018**, *14*, 168. [CrossRef] [PubMed]
33. Ferreira, S.T.; Lourenco, M.V.; Oliveira, M.M.; De Felice, F.G. Soluble amyloid-b oligomers as synaptotoxins leading to cognitive impairment in Alzheimer's disease. *Front. Cell. Neurosci.* **2015**, *9*, 191. [CrossRef]
34. D'Ercole, A.J.; Ye, P.; Calikoglu, A.S.; Gutierrez-Ospina, G. The role of the insulin-like growth factors in the central nervous system. *Mol. Neurobiol.* **1996**, *13*, 227–255. [CrossRef]
35. Neumann, K.F.; Rojo, L.; Navarrete, L.P.; Farías, G.; Reyes, P.; Maccioni, R.B. Insulin resistance and Alzheimer's disease: Molecular links & clinical implications. *Curr. Alzheimer Res.* **2008**, *5*, 438–447.
36. Liu, Y.; Liu, F.; Grundke-Iqbal, I.; Iqbal, K.; Gong, C.X. Deficient brain insulin signalling pathway in Alzheimer's disease and diabetes. *J. Pathol.* **2011**, *225*, 54–62. [CrossRef]
37. Kim, B.; Feldman, E.L. Insulin resistance in the nervous system. *Trends Endocrinol. Metab.* **2012**, *23*, 133–141. [CrossRef]
38. Jackson, K.; Barisone, G.A.; Diaz, E.; Jin, L.w.; DeCarli, C.; Despa, F. Amylin deposition in the brain: A second amyloid in Alzheimer disease? *Ann. Neurol.* **2013**, *74*, 517–526. [CrossRef]
39. Miklossy, J.; Qing, H.; Radenovic, A.; Kis, A.; Vileno, B.; Làszló, F.; Miller, L.; Martins, R.N.; Waeber, G.; Mooser, V. Beta amyloid and hyperphosphorylated tau deposits in the pancreas in type 2 diabetes. *Neurobiol. Aging* **2010**, *31*, 1503–1515. [CrossRef]
40. Whitmer, R.; Gustafson, D.; Barrett-Connor, E.; Haan, M.; Gunderson, E.; Yaffe, K. Central obesity and increased risk of dementia more than three decades later. *Neurology* **2008**, *71*, 1057–1064. [CrossRef]
41. Jagust, W.; Harvey, D.; Mungas, D.; Haan, M. Central obesity and the aging brain. *Arch. Neurol.* **2005**, *62*, 1545–1548. [CrossRef] [PubMed]
42. Fitzpatrick, A.L.; Kuller, L.H.; Lopez, O.L.; Diehr, P.; O'Meara, E.S.; Longstreth, W.; Luchsinger, J.A. Midlife and late-life obesity and the risk of dementia: Cardiovascular health study. *Arch. Neurol.* **2009**, *66*, 336–342. [CrossRef] [PubMed]
43. Hassing, L.B.; Dahl, A.K.; Thorvaldsson, V.; Berg, S.; Gatz, M.; Pedersen, N.L.; Johansson, B. Overweight in midlife and risk of dementia: A 40-year follow-up study. *Int. J. Obes.* **2009**, *33*, 893–898. [CrossRef]
44. Whitmer, R.A.; Gunderson, E.P.; Barrett-Connor, E.; Quesenberry, C.P.; Yaffe, K. Obesity in middle age and future risk of dementia: A 27 year longitudinal population based study. *BMJ* **2005**, *330*, 1360. [CrossRef]
45. Qizilbash, N.; Gregson, J.; Johnson, M.E.; Pearce, N.; Douglas, I.; Wing, K.; Evans, S.J.; Pocock, S.J. BMI and risk of dementia in two million people over two decades: A retrospective cohort study. *Lancet Diabetes Endocrinol.* **2015**, *3*, 431–436. [CrossRef]
46. Verdile, G.; Fuller, S.J.; Martins, R.N. The role of type 2 diabetes in neurodegeneration. *Neurobiol. Dis.* **2015**, *84*, 22–38. [CrossRef]
47. Bhamra, M.S.; Ashton, N.J. Finding a pathological diagnosis for A lzheimer's disease: Are inflammatory molecules the answer? *Electrophoresis* **2012**, *33*, 3598–3607. [CrossRef]
48. Swardfager, W.; Lanctôt, K.; Rothenburg, L.; Wong, A.; Cappell, J.; Herrmann, N. A meta-analysis of cytokines in Alzheimer's disease. *Biol. Psychiatry* **2010**, *68*, 930–941. [CrossRef]
49. Nakamura, M.; Watanabe, N. Ubiquitin-like protein MNSFβ/endophilin II complex regulates Dectin-1-mediated phagocytosis and inflammatory responses in macrophages. *Biochem. Biophys. Res. Commun.* **2010**, *401*, 257–261. [CrossRef]
50. Banks, W.A.; Kastin, A.J.; Broadwell, R.D. Passage of cytokines across the blood-brain barrier. *Neuroimmunomodulation* **1995**, *2*, 241–248. [CrossRef]
51. Rosenberg, P.B. Clinical aspects of inflammation in Alzheimer's disease. *Int. Rev. Psychiatry* **2005**, *17*, 503–514. [CrossRef]
52. Chiroma, S.M.; Baharuldin, M.T.H.; Taib, C.; Amom, Z.; Jagadeesan, S.; Moklas, M. Inflammation in Alzheimer's disease: A friend or foe? *Biomed. Res. Ther.* **2018**, *5*, 2552–2564. [CrossRef]
53. Ma, Q.-L.; Yang, F.; Rosario, E.R.; Ubeda, O.J.; Beech, W.; Gant, D.J.; Chen, P.P.; Hudspeth, B.; Chen, C.; Zhao, Y. β-amyloid oligomers induce phosphorylation of tau and inactivation of insulin receptor substrate via c-Jun N-terminal kinase signaling: Suppression by omega-3 fatty acids and curcumin. *J. Neurosci.* **2009**, *29*, 9078–9089. [CrossRef]
54. Pickup, J.; Crook, M. Is type II diabetes mellitus a disease of the innate immune system? *Diabetologia* **1998**, *41*, 1241–1248. [CrossRef]

55. Weisberg, S.P.; McCann, D.; Desai, M.; Rosenbaum, M.; Leibel, R.L.; Ferrante, A.W. Obesity is associated with macrophage accumulation in adipose tissue. *J. Clin. Investig.* **2003**, *112*, 1796–1808. [CrossRef]
56. Tucsek, Z.; Toth, P.; Sosnowska, D.; Gautam, T.; Mitschelen, M.; Koller, A.; Szalai, G.; Sonntag, W.E.; Ungvari, Z.; Csiszar, A. Obesity in aging exacerbates blood–brain barrier disruption, neuroinflammation, and oxidative stress in the mouse hippocampus: Effects on expression of genes involved in beta-amyloid generation and Alzheimer's disease. *J. Gerontol. Ser. A Biomed. Sci. Med Sci.* **2014**, *69*, 1212–1226. [CrossRef]
57. De Souza, C.T.; Araujo, E.P.; Bordin, S.; Ashimine, R.; Zollner, R.L.; Boschero, A.C.; Saad, M.J.; Velloso, L.C.A. Consumption of a fat-rich diet activates a proinflammatory response and induces insulin resistance in the hypothalamus. *Endocrinology* **2005**, *146*, 4192–4199. [CrossRef]
58. Thaler, J.P.; Yi, C.-X.; Schur, E.A.; Guyenet, S.J.; Hwang, B.H.; Dietrich, M.O.; Zhao, X.; Sarruf, D.A.; Izgur, V.; Maravilla, K.R. Obesity is associated with hypothalamic injury in rodents and humans. *J. Clin. Investig.* **2012**, *122*, 153–162. [CrossRef]
59. Milanski, M.; Degasperi, G.; Coope, A.; Morari, J.; Denis, R.; Cintra, D.E.; Tsukumo, D.M.; Anhe, G.; Amaral, M.E.; Takahashi, H.K. Saturated fatty acids produce an inflammatory response predominantly through the activation of TLR4 signaling in hypothalamus: Implications for the pathogenesis of obesity. *J. Neurosci.* **2009**, *29*, 359–370. [CrossRef]
60. Blatteis, C.M. The onset of fever: New insights into its mechanism. *Prog. Brain Res.* **2007**, *162*, 3–14.
61. Miller, A.A.; Spencer, S.J. Obesity and neuroinflammation: A pathway to cognitive impairment. *Brain Behav. Immun.* **2014**, *42*, 10–21. [CrossRef]
62. Koessler, S.; Engler, H.; Riether, C.; Kissler, J. No retrieval-induced forgetting under stress. *Psychol. Sci.* **2009**, *20*, 1356–1363. [CrossRef]
63. Raber, J. Detrimental effects of chronic hypothalamic—Pituitary—Adrenal axis activation. *Mol. Neurobiol.* **1998**, *18*, 1–22. [CrossRef]
64. MacQueen, G.; Frodl, T. The hippocampus in major depression: Evidence for the convergence of the bench and bedside in psychiatric research? *Mol. Psychiatry* **2011**, *16*, 252–264. [CrossRef]
65. Alves, L.; Correia, A.S.A.; Miguel, R.; Alegria, P.; Bugalho, P. Alzheimer's disease: A clinical practice-oriented review. *Front. Neurol.* **2012**, *3*, 63. [CrossRef]
66. Wärnberg, J.; Gomez-Martinez, S.; Romeo, J.; Díaz, L.E.; Marcos, A. Nutrition, inflammation, and cognitive function. *Ann. N. Y. Acad. Sci.* **2009**, *1153*, 164–175.
67. Eikelenboom, P.; Veerhuis, R.; Van Exel, E.; Hoozemans, J.J.M.; Rozemuller, A.J.M.; van Gool, W.A. The early involvement of the innate immunity in the pathogenesis of lateonset Alzheimer's disease: Neuropathological, epidemiological and genetic evidence. *Curr. Alzheimer Res.* **2011**, *8*, 142–150. [CrossRef]
68. Morales, I.; Guzmán-Martínez, L.; Cerda-Troncoso, C.; Farías, G.A.; Maccioni, R.B. Neuroinflammation in the pathogenesis of Alzheimer's disease. A rational framework for the search of novel therapeutic approaches. *Front. Cell. Neurosci.* **2014**, *8*, 112. [CrossRef]
69. Tuppo, E.E.; Arias, H.R. The role of inflammation in Alzheimer's disease. *Int. J. Biochem. Cell Biol.* **2005**, *37*, 289–305. [CrossRef]
70. Akiyama, H.; Barger, S.; Barnum, S.; Bradt, B.; Bauer, J.; Cole, G.M.; Cooper, N.R.; Eikelenboom, P.; Emmerling, M.; Fiebich, B.L. Inflammation and Alzheimer's disease. *Neurobiol. Aging* **2000**, *21*, 383–421. [CrossRef]
71. Mrak, R.E.; Sheng, J.G.; Griffin, W.S.T. Glial cytokines in Alzheimer's disease: Review and pathogenic implications. *Hum. Pathol.* **1995**, *26*, 816–823. [CrossRef]
72. Halliday, G.; Robinson, S.R.; Shepherd, C.; Kril, J. Alzheimer's disease and inflammation: A review of cellular and therapeutic mechanisms. *Clin. Exp. Pharmacol. Physiol.* **2000**, *27*, 1–8. [CrossRef] [PubMed]
73. Minter, M.R.; Taylor, J.M.; Crack, P.J. The contribution of neuroinflammation to amyloid toxicity in Alzheimer's disease. *J. Neurochem.* **2016**, *136*, 457–474. [CrossRef] [PubMed]
74. Déniz-Naranjo, M.; Muñoz-Fernandez, C.; Alemany-Rodríguez, M.; Pérez-Vieitez, M.; Aladro-Benito, Y.; Irurita-Latasa, J.; Sánchez-García, F. Cytokine IL-1 beta but not IL-1 alpha promoter polymorphism is associated with Alzheimer disease in a population from the Canary Islands, Spain. *Eur. J. Neurol.* **2008**, *15*, 1080–1084. [CrossRef]
75. Li, C.; Zhao, R.; Gao, K.; Wei, Z.; Yaoyao Yin, M.; Ting Lau, L.; Chui, D.; Cheung Hoi Yu, A. Astrocytes: Implications for neuroinflammatory pathogenesis of Alzheimer's disease. *Curr. Alzheimer Res.* **2011**, *8*, 67–80. [CrossRef]

76. Wyss-Coray, T. Inflammation in Alzheimer disease: Driving force, bystander or beneficial response? *Nat. Med.* **2006**, *12*, 1005–1015.
77. Griffin, W.S.T.; Liu, L.; Li, Y.; Mrak, R.E.; Barger, S.W. Interleukin-1 mediates Alzheimer and Lewy body pathologies. *J. Neuroinflammation* **2006**, *3*, 5. [CrossRef]
78. Liu, L.; Chan, C. The role of inflammasome in Alzheimer's disease. *Ageing Res. Rev.* **2014**, *15*, 6–15. [CrossRef]
79. Milionis, H.J.; Florentin, M.; Giannopoulos, S. Metabolic syndrome and Alzheimer's disease: A link to a vascular hypothesis? *CNS Spectr.* **2008**, *13*, 606–613. [CrossRef]
80. Chellan, P.; Nagaraj, R.H. Protein crosslinking by the Maillard reaction: Dicarbonyl-derived imidazolium crosslinks in aging and diabetes. *Arch. Biochem. Biophys.* **1999**, *368*, 98–104. [CrossRef]
81. Thorpe, S.R.; Baynes, J.W. Role of the Maillard reaction in diabetes mellitus and diseases of aging. *Drugs Aging* **1996**, *9*, 69–77. [CrossRef]
82. Hori, O.; Yan, S.D.; Ogawa, S.; Kuwabara, K.; Matsumoto, M.; Stern, D.; Schmidt, A.M. The receptor for advanced glycation end-products has a central role in mediating the effects of advanced glycation end-products on the development of vascular disease in diabetes mellitus. *Nephrol. Dial. Transplant.* **1996**, *11*, 13–16. [CrossRef]
83. Ulrich, P.; Cerami, A. Protein glycation, diabetes, and aging. *Recent Prog. Horm. Res.* **2001**, *56*, 1–22. [CrossRef]
84. Srikanth, V.; Maczurek, A.; Phan, T.; Steele, M.; Westcott, B.; Juskiw, D.; Münch, G. Advanced glycation endproducts and their receptor RAGE in Alzheimer's disease. *Neurobiol. Aging* **2011**, *32*, 763–777. [CrossRef]
85. Lue, L.-F.; Walker, D.G.; Brachova, L.; Beach, T.G.; Rogers, J.; Schmidt, A.M.; Stern, D.M.; Du Yan, S. Involvement of microglial receptor for advanced glycation endproducts (RAGE) in Alzheimer's disease: Identification of a cellular activation mechanism. *Exp. Neurol.* **2001**, *171*, 29–45. [CrossRef]
86. Sasaki, N.; Toki, S.; Chowei, H.; Saito, T.; Nakano, N.; Hayashi, Y.; Takeuchi, M.; Makita, Z. Immunohistochemical distribution of the receptor for advanced glycation end products in neurons and astrocytes in Alzheimer's disease. *Brain Res.* **2001**, *888*, 256–262. [CrossRef]
87. Lue, L.-F.; Andrade, C.; Sabbagh, M.; Walker, D. Is there inflammatory synergy in type II diabetes mellitus and Alzheimer's disease? *Int. J. Alzheimer's Dis.* **2012**, *2012*. [CrossRef]
88. Fang, F.; Lue, L.-F.; Yan, S.; Xu, H.; Luddy, J.S.; Chen, D.; Walker, D.G.; Stern, D.M.; Yan, S.; Schmidt, A.M. RAGE-dependent signaling in microglia contributes to neuroinflammation, Aβ accumulation, and impaired learning/memory in a mouse model of Alzheimer's disease. *FASEB J.* **2010**, *24*, 1043–1055. [CrossRef]
89. Beeri, M.S.; Moshier, E.; Schmeidler, J.; Godbold, J.; Uribarri, J.; Reddy, S.; Sano, M.; Grossman, H.T.; Cai, W.; Vlassara, H. Serum concentration of an inflammatory glycotoxin, methylglyoxal, is associated with increased cognitive decline in elderly individuals. *Mech. Ageing Dev.* **2011**, *132*, 583–587. [CrossRef]
90. Pugazhenthi, S.; Qin, L.; Reddy, P.H. Common neurodegenerative pathways in obesity, diabetes, and Alzheimer's disease. *Biochim. Et Biophys. Acta BBA-Mol. Basis Dis.* **2017**, *1863*, 1037–1045. [CrossRef]
91. Kasten, T.; Zhang, L.; Goate, A.; Morris, J.C.; Holtzman, D.; Bateman, R.J. Age and Amyloid Effects on Human CNS Amyloid-Beta Kinetics. *Ann. Neurol.* **2015**, *78*, 439–453. [CrossRef]
92. Bhatti, J.; Kumar, S.; Vijayan, M.; Bhatti, G.; Reddy, P.H. Therapeutic strategies for mitochondrial dysfunction and oxidative stress in age-related metabolic disorders. In *Progress in Molecular Biology and Translational Science*; Elsevier: Amsterdam, The Netherlands, 2017; Volume 146, pp. 13–46.
93. Yoo, S.-M.; Park, J.; Kim, S.-H.; Jung, Y.-K. Emerging perspectives on mitochondrial dysfunction and inflammation in Alzheimer's disease. *BMB Rep.* **2020**, *53*, 35. [CrossRef]
94. Bournat, J.C.; Brown, C.W. Mitochondrial dysfunction in obesity. *Curr. Opin. Endocrinol. Diabetes Obes.* **2010**, *17*, 446. [CrossRef]
95. Ritov, V.B.; Menshikova, E.V.; He, J.; Ferrell, R.E.; Goodpaster, B.H.; Kelley, D.E. Deficiency of subsarcolemmal mitochondria in obesity and type 2 diabetes. *Diabetes* **2005**, *54*, 8–14. [CrossRef]
96. Mogensen, M.; Sahlin, K.; Fernström, M.; Glintborg, D.; Vind, B.F.; Beck-Nielsen, H.; Højlund, K. Mitochondrial respiration is decreased in skeletal muscle of patients with type 2 diabetes. *Diabetes* **2007**, *56*, 1592–1599. [CrossRef]
97. Richardson, D.K.; Kashyap, S.; Bajaj, M.; Cusi, K.; Mandarino, S.J.; Finlayson, J.; DeFronzo, R.A.; Jenkinson, C.P.; Mandarino, L.J. Lipid infusion decreases the expression of nuclear encoded mitochondrial genes and increases the expression of extracellular matrix genes in human skeletal muscle. *J. Biol. Chem.* **2005**, *280*, 10290–10297. [CrossRef]

98. Bogacka, I.; Xie, H.; Bray, G.A.; Smith, S.R. Pioglitazone induces mitochondrial biogenesis in human subcutaneous adipose tissue in vivo. *Diabetes* **2005**, *54*, 1392–1399. [CrossRef]
99. Gao, C.-L.; Zhu, C.; Zhao, Y.-P.; Chen, X.-H.; Ji, C.-B.; Zhang, C.-M.; Zhu, J.-G.; Xia, Z.-K.; Tong, M.-L.; Guo, X.-R. Mitochondrial dysfunction is induced by high levels of glucose and free fatty acids in 3T3-L1 adipocytes. *Mol. Cell. Endocrinol.* **2010**, *320*, 25–33. [CrossRef]
100. Koh, E.H.; Park, J.-Y.; Park, H.-S.; Jeon, M.J.; Ryu, J.W.; Kim, M.; Kim, S.Y.; Kim, M.-S.; Kim, S.-W.; Park, I.S. Essential role of mitochondrial function in adiponectin synthesis in adipocytes. *Diabetes* **2007**, *56*, 2973–2981. [CrossRef]
101. Sparks, L.M.; Xie, H.; Koza, R.A.; Mynatt, R.; Hulver, M.W.; Bray, G.A.; Smith, S.R. A high-fat diet coordinately downregulates genes required for mitochondrial oxidative phosphorylation in skeletal muscle. *Diabetes* **2005**, *54*, 1926–1933. [CrossRef]
102. Lin, Y.; Berg, A.H.; Iyengar, P.; Lam, T.K.; Giacca, A.; Combs, T.P.; Rajala, M.W.; Du, X.; Rollman, B.; Li, W. The hyperglycemia-induced inflammatory response in adipocytes the role of reactive oxygen species. *J. Biol. Chem.* **2005**, *280*, 4617–4626. [CrossRef]
103. Yin, F.; Sancheti, H.; Patil, I.; Cadenas, E. Energy metabolism and inflammation in brain aging and Alzheimer's disease. *Free Radic. Biol. Med.* **2016**, *100*, 108–122. [CrossRef]
104. Yin, F.; Boveris, A.; Cadenas, E. Mitochondrial energy metabolism and redox signaling in brain aging and neurodegeneration. *Antioxid. Redox Signal.* **2014**, *20*, 353–371. [CrossRef]
105. van Horssen, J.; van Schaik, P.; Witte, M. Inflammation and mitochondrial dysfunction: A vicious circle in neurodegenerative disorders? *Neurosci. Lett.* **2019**, *710*, 132931. [CrossRef]
106. Abcouwer, S.F.; Shanmugam, S.; Gomez, P.F.; Shushanov, S.; Barber, A.J.; Lanoue, K.F.; Quinn, P.G.; Kester, M.; Gardner, T.W. Effect of IL-1β on survival and energy metabolism of R28 and RGC-5 retinal neurons. *Investig. Ophthalmol. Vis. Sci.* **2008**, *49*, 5581–5592. [CrossRef]
107. Tredget, E.E.; Yu, Y.M.; Zhong, S.; Burini, R.; Okusawa, S.; Gelfand, J.A.; Dinarello, C.A.; Young, V.; Burke, J. Role of interleukin 1 and tumor necrosis factor on energy metabolism in rabbits. *Am. J. Physiol.-Endocrinol. Metab.* **1988**, *255*, E760–E768. [CrossRef]
108. Zell, R.; Geck, P.; Werdan, K.; Boekstegers, P. TNF-α and IL-1α inhibit both pyruvate dehydrogenase activity and mitochondrial function in cardiomyocytes: Evidence for primary impairment of mitochondrial function. *Mol. Cell. Biochem.* **1997**, *177*, 61–67. [CrossRef]
109. Taylor, D.; Faragher, E.; Evanson, J. Inflammatory cytokines stimulate glucose uptake and glycolysis but reduce glucose oxidation in human dermal fibroblasts in vitro. *Circ. Shock* **1992**, *37*, 105–110.
110. Vary, T.C.; Siegel, J.H.; Nakatani, T.; Sato, T.; Aoyama, H. Effect of sepsis on activity of pyruvate dehydrogenase complex in skeletal muscle and liver. *Am. J. Physiol.-Endocrinol. Metab.* **1986**, *250*, E634–E640. [CrossRef]
111. Vary, T.; Martin, L. Potentiation of decreased pyruvate dehydrogenase activity by inflammatory stimuli in sepsis. *Circ. Shock* **1993**, *39*, 299–305.
112. Dutta, R.; McDonough, J.; Yin, X.; Peterson, J.; Chang, A.; Torres, T.; Gudz, T.; Macklin, W.B.; Lewis, D.A.; Fox, R.J. Mitochondrial dysfunction as a cause of axonal degeneration in multiple sclerosis patients. *Ann. Neurol.* **2006**, *59*, 478–489. [CrossRef]
113. Doll, D.N.; Rellick, S.L.; Barr, T.L.; Ren, X.; Simpkins, J.W. Rapid mitochondrial dysfunction mediates TNF-alpha-induced neurotoxicity. *J. Neurochem.* **2015**, *132*, 443–451. [CrossRef]
114. Tang, K.; Wagner, P.D.; Breen, E.C. TNF-α-mediated reduction in PGC-1α may impair skeletal muscle function after cigarette smoke exposure. *J. Cell. Physiol.* **2010**, *222*, 320–327. [CrossRef]
115. Palomer, X.; Álvarez-Guardia, D.; Rodríguez-Calvo, R.; Coll, T.; Laguna, J.C.; Davidson, M.M.; Chan, T.O.; Feldman, A.M.; Vázquez-Carrera, M. TNF-α reduces PGC-1 α expression through NF-κB and p38 MAPK leading to increased glucose oxidation in a human cardiac cell model. *Cardiovasc. Res.* **2009**, *81*, 703–712. [CrossRef]
116. Zhang, Y.; Chen, C.; Jiang, Y.; Wang, S.; Wu, X.; Wang, K. PPARγ coactivator-1α (PGC-1α) protects neuroblastoma cells against amyloid-beta (Aβ) induced cell death and neuroinflammation via NF-κB pathway. *BMC Neurosci.* **2017**, *18*, 1–8. [CrossRef]
117. Gibson, G.; Sheu, K.-F.; Blass, J. Abnormalities of mitochondrial enzymes in Alzheimer disease. *J. Neural Transm.* **1998**, *105*, 855–870. [CrossRef]

118. Butterfield, D.A.; Poon, H.F.; Clair, D.S.; Keller, J.N.; Pierce, W.M.; Klein, J.B.; Markesbery, W.R. Redox proteomics identification of oxidatively modified hippocampal proteins in mild cognitive impairment: Insights into the development of Alzheimer's disease. *Neurobiol. Dis.* **2006**, *22*, 223–232. [CrossRef]
119. Caspersen, C.; Wang, N.; Yao, J.; Sosunov, A.; Chen, X.; Lustbader, J.W.; Xu, H.W.; Stern, D.; McKhann, G.; Yan, S.D. Mitochondrial Aβ: A potential focal point for neuronal metabolic dysfunction in Alzheimer's disease. *FASEB J.* **2005**, *19*, 2040–2041. [CrossRef]
120. Lustbader, J.W.; Cirilli, M.; Lin, C.; Xu, H.W.; Takuma, K.; Wang, N.; Caspersen, C.; Chen, X.; Pollak, S.; Chaney, M. ABAD directly links Aß to mitochondrial toxicity in Alzheimer's disease. *Science* **2004**, *304*, 448–452. [CrossRef]
121. Reddy, P.H.; Beal, M.F. Amyloid beta, mitochondrial dysfunction and synaptic damage: Implications for cognitive decline in aging and Alzheimer's disease. *Trends Mol. Med.* **2008**, *14*, 45–53. [CrossRef]
122. Reddy, P.H.; Beal, M.F. Are mitochondria critical in the pathogenesis of Alzheimer's disease? *Brain Res. Rev.* **2005**, *49*, 618–632. [CrossRef] [PubMed]
123. Thies, E.; Mandelkow, E.-M. Missorting of tau in neurons causes degeneration of synapses that can be rescued by the kinase MARK2/Par-1. *J. Neurosci.* **2007**, *27*, 2896–2907. [CrossRef] [PubMed]
124. Chan, D.C. Mitochondria: Dynamic organelles in disease, aging, and development. *Cell* **2006**, *125*, 1241–1252. [CrossRef] [PubMed]
125. Suen, D.-F.; Norris, K.L.; Youle, R.J. Mitochondrial dynamics and apoptosis. *Genes Dev.* **2008**, *22*, 1577–1590. [CrossRef] [PubMed]
126. J Bonda, D.; A Smith, M.; Perry, G.; Lee, H.-G.; Wang, X.; Zhu, X. The mitochondrial dynamics of Alzheimer's disease and Parkinson's disease offer important opportunities for therapeutic intervention. *Curr. Pharm. Des.* **2011**, *17*, 3374–3380. [CrossRef]
127. Valero, T. Editorial (thematic issue: Mitochondrial biogenesis: Pharmacological approaches). *Curr. Pharm. Des.* **2014**, *20*, 5507–5509. [CrossRef]
128. Wenz, T. Regulation of mitochondrial biogenesis and PGC-1α under cellular stress. *Mitochondrion* **2013**, *13*, 134–142. [CrossRef]
129. Wang, X.; Su, B.; Siedlak, S.L.; Moreira, P.I.; Fujioka, H.; Wang, Y.; Casadesus, G.; Zhu, X. Amyloid-β overproduction causes abnormal mitochondrial dynamics via differential modulation of mitochondrial fission/fusion proteins. *Proc. Natl. Acad. Sci. USA* **2008**, *105*, 19318–19323. [CrossRef]
130. Wang, X.; Su, B.; Lee, H.-G.; Li, X.; Perry, G.; Smith, M.A.; Zhu, X. Impaired balance of mitochondrial fission and fusion in Alzheimer's disease. *J. Neurosci.* **2009**, *29*, 9090–9103. [CrossRef]
131. Motori, E.; Puyal, J.; Toni, N.; Ghanem, A.; Angeloni, C.; Malaguti, M.; Cantelli-Forti, G.; Berninger, B.; Conzelmann, K.-K.; Götz, M. Inflammation-induced alteration of astrocyte mitochondrial dynamics requires autophagy for mitochondrial network maintenance. *Cell Metab.* **2013**, *18*, 844–859. [CrossRef]
132. Chen, X.-H.; Zhao, Y.-P.; Xue, M.; Ji, C.-B.; Gao, C.-L.; Zhu, J.-G.; Qin, D.-N.; Kou, C.-Z.; Qin, X.-H.; Tong, M.-L. TNF-α induces mitochondrial dysfunction in 3T3-L1 adipocytes. *Mol. Cell. Endocrinol.* **2010**, *328*, 63–69. [CrossRef]
133. Anusree, S.; Nisha, V.; Priyanka, A.; Raghu, K. Insulin resistance by TNF-α is associated with mitochondrial dysfunction in 3T3-L1 adipocytes and is ameliorated by punicic acid, a PPARγ agonist. *Mol. Cell. Endocrinol.* **2015**, *413*, 120–128. [CrossRef] [PubMed]
134. Hahn, W.S.; Kuzmicic, J.; Burrill, J.S.; Donoghue, M.A.; Foncea, R.; Jensen, M.D.; Lavandero, S.; Arriaga, E.A.; Bernlohr, D.A. Proinflammatory cytokines differentially regulate adipocyte mitochondrial metabolism, oxidative stress, and dynamics. *Am. J. Physiol.-Endocrinol. Metab.* **2014**, *306*, E1033–E1045. [CrossRef] [PubMed]
135. White, J.P.; Puppa, M.J.; Sato, S.; Gao, S.; Price, R.L.; Baynes, J.W.; Kostek, M.C.; Matesic, L.E.; Carson, J.A. IL-6 regulation on skeletal muscle mitochondrial remodeling during cancer cachexia in the Apc Min/+ mouse. *Skelet. Muscle* **2012**, *2*, 14. [CrossRef] [PubMed]
136. Miotto, P.M.; LeBlanc, P.J.; Holloway, G.P. High-fat diet causes mitochondrial dysfunction as a result of impaired ADP sensitivity. *Diabetes* **2018**, *67*, 2199–2205. [CrossRef] [PubMed]
137. Zhou, R.; Yazdi, A.S.; Menu, P.; Tschopp, J. A role for mitochondria in NLRP3 inflammasome activation. *Nature* **2011**, *469*, 221–225. [CrossRef]
138. Brookes, P.S.; Yoon, Y.; Robotham, J.L.; Anders, M.; Sheu, S.-S. Calcium, ATP, and ROS: A mitochondrial love-hate triangle. *Am. J. Physiol.-Cell Physiol.* **2004**, *287*, C817–C833. [CrossRef]

139. Reddy, P.H. Amyloid precursor protein-mediated free radicals and oxidative damage: Implications for the development and progression of Alzheimer's disease. *J. Neurochem.* **2006**, *96*, 1–13. [CrossRef]
140. Wang, X.; Wang, W.; Li, L.; Perry, G.; Lee, H.-G.; Zhu, X. Oxidative stress and mitochondrial dysfunction in Alzheimer's disease. *Biochim. Et Biophys. Acta BBA-Mol. Basis Dis.* **2014**, *1842*, 1240–1247. [CrossRef]
141. Fernández-Sánchez, A.; Madrigal-Santillán, E.; Bautista, M.; Esquivel-Soto, J.; Morales-González, Á.; Esquivel-Chirino, C.; Durante-Montiel, I.; Sánchez-Rivera, G.; Valadez-Vega, C.; Morales-González, J.A. Inflammation, oxidative stress, and obesity. *Int. J. Mol. Sci.* **2011**, *12*, 3117–3132. [CrossRef]
142. Amin, K.A.; Nagy, M.A. Effect of Carnitine and herbal mixture extract on obesity induced by high fat diet in rats. *Diabetol. Metab. Syndr.* **2009**, *1*, 17. [CrossRef]
143. Brown, G.C. Nitric oxide and neuronal death. *Nitric Oxide* **2010**, *23*, 153–165. [CrossRef] [PubMed]
144. Zhang, L.; Bruce-Keller, A.J.; Dasuri, K.; Nguyen, A.; Liu, Y.; Keller, J.N. Diet-induced metabolic disturbances as modulators of brain homeostasis. *Biochim. Et Biophys. Acta (BBA)-Mol. Basis Dis.* **2009**, *1792*, 417–422. [CrossRef] [PubMed]
145. Nunomura, A.; Perry, G.; Aliev, G.; Hirai, K.; Takeda, A.; Balraj, E.K.; Jones, P.K.; Ghanbari, H.; Wataya, T.; Shimohama, S. Oxidative damage is the earliest event in Alzheimer disease. *J. Neuropathol. Exp. Neurol.* **2001**, *60*, 759–767. [CrossRef] [PubMed]
146. Morrison, C.D.; Pistell, P.J.; Ingram, D.K.; Johnson, W.D.; Liu, Y.; Fernandez-Kim, S.O.; White, C.L.; Purpera, M.N.; Uranga, R.M.; Bruce-Keller, A.J. High fat diet increases hippocampal oxidative stress and cognitive impairment in aged mice: Implications for decreased Nrf2 signaling. *J. Neurochem.* **2010**, *114*, 1581–1589. [CrossRef]
147. Reddy, P.H.; McWeeney, S.; Park, B.S.; Manczak, M.; Gutala, R.V.; Partovi, D.; Jung, Y.; Yau, V.; Searles, R.; Mori, M. Gene expression profiles of transcripts in amyloid precursor protein transgenic mice: Up-regulation of mitochondrial metabolism and apoptotic genes is an early cellular change in Alzheimer's disease. *Hum. Mol. Genet.* **2004**, *13*, 1225–1240. [CrossRef]
148. Manczak, M.; Park, B.S.; Jung, Y.; Reddy, P.H. Differential expression of oxidative phosphorylation genes in patients with Alzheimer's disease. *Neuromolecular Med.* **2004**, *5*, 147–162. [CrossRef]
149. Pistell, P.J.; Morrison, C.D.; Gupta, S.; Knight, A.G.; Keller, J.N.; Ingram, D.K.; Bruce-Keller, A.J. Cognitive impairment following high fat diet consumption is associated with brain inflammation. *J. Neuroimmunol.* **2010**, *219*, 25–32. [CrossRef]
150. Butterfield, D.A.; Drake, J.; Pocernich, C.; Castegna, A. Evidence of oxidative damage in Alzheimer's disease brain: Central role for amyloid β-peptide. *Trends Mol. Med.* **2001**, *7*, 548–554. [CrossRef]
151. Ferreiro, E.; Oliveira, C.R.; Pereira, C.M. The release of calcium from the endoplasmic reticulum induced by amyloid-beta and prion peptides activates the mitochondrial apoptotic pathway. *Neurobiol. Dis.* **2008**, *30*, 331–342. [CrossRef]
152. Shelat, P.B.; Chalimoniuk, M.; Wang, J.H.; Strosznajder, J.B.; Lee, J.C.; Sun, A.Y.; Simonyi, A.; Sun, G.Y. Amyloid beta peptide and NMDA induce ROS from NADPH oxidase and AA release from cytosolic phospholipase A2 in cortical neurons. *J. Neurochem.* **2008**, *106*, 45–55. [CrossRef] [PubMed]
153. Liu, Z.; Zhou, T.; Ziegler, A.C.; Dimitrion, P.; Zuo, L. Oxidative stress in neurodegenerative diseases: From molecular mechanisms to clinical applications. *Oxidative Med. Cell. Longev.* **2017**, *2017*. [CrossRef] [PubMed]
154. Curtain, C.C.; Ali, F.; Volitakis, I.; Cherny, R.A.; Norton, R.S.; Beyreuther, K.; Barrow, C.J.; Masters, C.L.; Bush, A.I.; Barnham, K.J. Alzheimer's disease amyloid-β binds copper and zinc to generate an allosterically ordered membrane-penetrating structure containing superoxide dismutase-like subunits. *J. Biol. Chem.* **2001**, *276*, 20466–20473. [CrossRef] [PubMed]
155. Rojas-Gutierrez, E.; Muñoz-Arenas, G.; Treviño, S.; Espinosa, B.; Chavez, R.; Rojas, K.; Flores, G.; Díaz, A.; Guevara, J. Alzheimer's disease and metabolic syndrome: A link from oxidative stress and inflammation to neurodegeneration. *Synapse* **2017**, *71*, e21990. [CrossRef] [PubMed]
156. Weaver, J.; Huang, M.-H.; Albert, M.; Harris, T.; Rowe, J.; Seeman, T.E. Interleukin-6 and risk of cognitive decline: MacArthur studies of successful aging. *Neurology* **2002**, *59*, 371–378. [CrossRef] [PubMed]
157. Dik, M.; Jonker, C.; Hack, C.; Smit, J.; Comijs, H.; Eikelenboom, P. Serum inflammatory proteins and cognitive decline in older persons. *Neurology* **2005**, *64*, 1371–1377. [CrossRef]
158. Teunissen, C.; Van Boxtel, M.; Bosma, H.; Bosmans, E.; Delanghe, J.; De Bruijn, C.; Wauters, A.; Maes, M.; Jolles, J.; Steinbusch, H. Inflammation markers in relation to cognition in a healthy aging population. *J. Neuroimmunol.* **2003**, *134*, 142–150. [CrossRef]

159. Singh-Manoux, A.; Dugravot, A.; Brunner, E.; Kumari, M.; Shipley, M.; Elbaz, A.; Kivimaki, M. Interleukin-6 and C-reactive protein as predictors of cognitive decline in late midlife. *Neurology* **2014**, *83*, 486–493. [CrossRef]
160. Ozawa, M.; Shipley, M.; Kivimaki, M.; Singh-Manoux, A.; Brunner, E.J. Dietary pattern, inflammation and cognitive decline: The Whitehall II prospective cohort study. *Clin. Nutr.* **2017**, *36*, 506–512. [CrossRef]
161. Satizabal, C.; Zhu, Y.; Mazoyer, B.; Dufouil, C.; Tzourio, C. Circulating IL-6 and CRP are associated with MRI findings in the elderly: The 3C-Dijon Study. *Neurology* **2012**, *78*, 720–727. [CrossRef]
162. Kyrkanides, S.; Tallents, R.H.; Jen-nie, H.M.; Olschowka, M.E.; Johnson, R.; Yang, M.; Olschowka, J.A.; Brouxhon, S.M.; O'Banion, M.K. Osteoarthritis accelerates and exacerbates Alzheimer's disease pathology in mice. *J. Neuroinflammation* **2011**, *8*, 112. [CrossRef] [PubMed]
163. Ravaglia, G.; Forti, P.; Maioli, F.; Brunetti, N.; Martelli, M.; Servadei, L.; Bastagli, L.; Bianchin, M.; Mariani, E. Serum C-reactive protein and cognitive function in healthy elderly Italian community dwellers. *J. Gerontol. Ser. A Biol. Sci. Med Sci.* **2005**, *60*, 1017–1021. [CrossRef] [PubMed]
164. Schram, M.T.; Euser, S.M.; De Craen, A.J.; Witteman, J.C.; Frölich, M.; Hofman, A.; Jolles, J.; Breteler, M.M.; Westendorp, R.G. Systemic markers of inflammation and cognitive decline in old age. *J. Am. Geriatr. Soc.* **2007**, *55*, 708–716. [CrossRef] [PubMed]
165. Li, Q.; Yang, Y.; Reis, C.; Tao, T.; Li, W.; Li, X.; Zhang, J.H. Cerebral small vessel disease. *Cell Transplant.* **2018**, *27*, 1711–1722. [CrossRef] [PubMed]
166. Staals, J.; Booth, T.; Morris, Z.; Bastin, M.E.; Gow, A.J.; Corley, J.; Redmond, P.; Starr, J.M.; Deary, I.J.; Wardlaw, J.M. Total MRI load of cerebral small vessel disease and cognitive ability in older people. *Neurobiol. Aging* **2015**, *36*, 2806–2811. [CrossRef] [PubMed]
167. Staals, J.; Makin, S.D.; Doubal, F.N.; Dennis, M.S.; Wardlaw, J.M. Stroke subtype, vascular risk factors, and total MRI brain small-vessel disease burden. *Neurology* **2014**, *83*, 1228–1234. [CrossRef]
168. Wardlaw, J.M.; Smith, C.; Dichgans, M. Mechanisms of sporadic cerebral small vessel disease: Insights from neuroimaging. *Lancet Neurol.* **2013**, *12*, 483–497. [CrossRef]
169. Low, A.; Mak, E.; Rowe, J.B.; Markus, H.S.; O'Brien, J.T. Inflammation and cerebral small vessel disease: A systematic review. *Ageing Res. Rev.* **2019**, 100916. [CrossRef]
170. Vemuri, P.; Lesnick, T.G.; Przybelski, S.A.; Knopman, D.S.; Preboske, G.M.; Kantarci, K.; Raman, M.R.; Machulda, M.M.; Mielke, M.M.; Lowe, V.J. Vascular and amyloid pathologies are independent predictors of cognitive decline in normal elderly. *Brain* **2015**, *138*, 761–771. [CrossRef]
171. Calder, P.C.; Bosco, N.; Bourdet-Sicard, R.; Capuron, L.; Delzenne, N.; Doré, J.; Franceschi, C.; Lehtinen, M.J.; Recker, T.; Salvioli, S. Health relevance of the modification of low grade inflammation in ageing (inflammageing) and the role of nutrition. *Ageing Res. Rev.* **2017**, *40*, 95–119. [CrossRef]
172. Benito-León, J.; Mitchell, A.; Hernández-Gallego, J.; Bermejo-Pareja, F. Obesity and impaired cognitive functioning in the elderly: A population-based cross-sectional study (NEDICES). *Eur. J. Neurol.* **2013**, *20*, 899-e877. [CrossRef] [PubMed]
173. Darling, J.; Ross, A.; Bartness, T.; Parent, M. Predicting the effects of a high-energy diet on fatty liver and hippocampal-dependent memory in male rats. *Obesity* **2013**, *21*, 910–917. [CrossRef]
174. Kanoski, S.E.; Zhang, Y.; Zheng, W.; Davidson, T.L. The effects of a high-energy diet on hippocampal function and blood-brain barrier integrity in the rat. *J. Alzheimer's Dis.* **2010**, *21*, 207–219. [CrossRef] [PubMed]
175. Kanoski, S.E.; Davidson, T.L. Different patterns of memory impairments accompany short-and longer-term maintenance on a high-energy diet. *J. Exp. Psychol. Anim. Behav. Process.* **2010**, *36*, 313. [CrossRef] [PubMed]
176. Francis, H.; Stevenson, R. The longer-term impacts of Western diet on human cognition and the brain. *Appetite* **2013**, *63*, 119–128. [CrossRef]
177. Freeman, L.R.; Haley-Zitlin, V.; Rosenberger, D.S.; Granholm, A.-C. Damaging effects of a high-fat diet to the brain and cognition: A review of proposed mechanisms. *Nutr. Neurosci.* **2014**, *17*, 241–251. [CrossRef]
178. Martin, A.A.; Davidson, T.L. Human cognitive function and the obesogenic environment. *Physiol. Behav.* **2014**, *136*, 185–193. [CrossRef]
179. M Wilkins, H.; H Swerdlow, R. Relationships between mitochondria and neuroinflammation: Implications for Alzheimer's disease. *Curr. Top. Med. Chem.* **2016**, *16*, 849–857. [CrossRef]
180. Krikorian, R.; Shidler, M.D.; Dangelo, K.; Couch, S.C.; Benoit, S.C.; Clegg, D.J. Dietary ketosis enhances memory in mild cognitive impairment. *Neurobiol. Aging* **2012**, *33*, 425.e19–425.e27. [CrossRef]
181. Reger, M.A.; Henderson, S.T.; Hale, C.; Cholerton, B.; Baker, L.D.; Watson, G.; Hyde, K.; Chapman, D.; Craft, S. Effects of β-hydroxybutyrate on cognition in memory-impaired adults. *Neurobiol. Aging* **2004**, *25*,

311–314. [CrossRef]

182. Henderson, S.T.; Vogel, J.L.; Barr, L.J.; Garvin, F.; Jones, J.J.; Costantini, L.C. Study of the ketogenic agent AC-1202 in mild to moderate Alzheimer's disease: A randomized, double-blind, placebo-controlled, multicenter trial. *Nutr. Metab.* **2009**, *6*, 31. [CrossRef]
183. Neal, E.G.; Chaffe, H.; Schwartz, R.H.; Lawson, M.S.; Edwards, N.; Fitzsimmons, G.; Whitney, A.; Cross, J.H. The ketogenic diet for the treatment of childhood epilepsy: A randomised controlled trial. *Lancet Neurol.* **2008**, *7*, 500–506. [CrossRef]
184. Selfridge, J.E.; Wilkins, H.M.; Lezi, E.; Carl, S.M.; Koppel, S.; Funk, E.; Fields, T.; Lu, J.; Tang, E.P.; Slawson, C. Effect of one month duration ketogenic and non-ketogenic high fat diets on mouse brain bioenergetic infrastructure. *J. Bioenerg. Biomembr.* **2015**, *47*, 1–11. [CrossRef]
185. Rutledge, A.C.; Adeli, K. Fructose and the metabolic syndrome: Pathophysiology and molecular mechanisms. *Nutr. Rev.* **2007**, *65*, S13–S23. [CrossRef]
186. Casas, R.; Sacanella, E.; Urpí-Sardà, M.; Corella, D.; Castaner, O.; Lamuela-Raventos, R.-M.; Salas-Salvadó, J.; Martínez-González, M.-A.; Ros, E.; Estruch, R. Long-term immunomodulatory effects of a mediterranean diet in adults at high risk of cardiovascular disease in the PREvención con DIeta MEDiterránea (PREDIMED) randomized controlled trial. *J. Nutr.* **2016**, *146*, 1684–1693. [CrossRef]
187. Casas, R.; Urpi-Sardà, M.; Sacanella, E.; Arranz, S.; Corella, D.; Castañer, O.; Lamuela-Raventós, R.-M.; Salas-Salvadó, J.; Lapetra, J.; Portillo, M.P. Anti-inflammatory effects of the Mediterranean diet in the early and late stages of atheroma plaque development. *Mediat. Inflamm.* **2017**, *2017*. [CrossRef]
188. Berti, V.; Walters, M.; Sterling, J.; Quinn, C.G.; Logue, M.; Andrews, R.; Matthews, D.C.; Osorio, R.S.; Pupi, A.; Vallabhajosula, S. Mediterranean diet and 3-year Alzheimer brain biomarker changes in middle-aged adults. *Neurology* **2018**, *90*, e1789–e1798. [CrossRef]
189. Luciano, M.; Corley, J.; Cox, S.R.; Hernández, M.C.V.; Craig, L.C.; Dickie, D.A.; Karama, S.; McNeill, G.M.; Bastin, M.E.; Wardlaw, J.M. Mediterranean-type diet and brain structural change from 73 to 76 years in a Scottish cohort. *Neurology* **2017**, *88*, 449–455. [CrossRef]
190. Staubo, S.C.; Aakre, J.A.; Vemuri, P.; Syrjanen, J.A.; Mielke, M.M.; Geda, Y.E.; Kremers, W.K.; Machulda, M.M.; Knopman, D.S.; Petersen, R.C. Mediterranean diet, micronutrients and macronutrients, and MRI measures of cortical thickness. *Alzheimer's Dement.* **2017**, *13*, 168–177. [CrossRef]
191. Rainey-Smith, S.R.; Gu, Y.; Gardener, S.L.; Doecke, J.D.; Villemagne, V.L.; Brown, B.M.; Taddei, K.; Laws, S.M.; Sohrabi, H.R.; Weinborn, M. Mediterranean diet adherence and rate of cerebral Aβ-amyloid accumulation: Data from the Australian Imaging, Biomarkers and Lifestyle Study of Ageing. *Transl. Psychiatry* **2018**, *8*, 1–7. [CrossRef]
192. Gu, Y.; Scarmeas, N.; Stern, Y.; Manly, J.J.; Schupf, N.; Mayeux, R.; Brickman, A.M. Mediterranean diet is associated with slower rate of hippocampal atrophy: A longitudinal study in cognitively normal older adults. *Alzheimer's Dement. J. Alzheimer's Assoc.* **2016**, *12*, P193–P194. [CrossRef]
193. Beher, D.; Clarke, E.E.; Wrigley, J.D.; Martin, A.C.; Nadin, A.; Churcher, I.; Shearman, M.S. Selected Non-steroidal Anti-inflammatory Drugs and Their Derivatives Target γ-Secretase at a Novel Site EVIDENCE FOR AN ALLOSTERIC MECHANISM. *J. Biol. Chem.* **2004**, *279*, 43419–43426. [CrossRef]
194. Eriksen, J.L.; Sagi, S.A.; Smith, T.E.; Weggen, S.; Das, P.; McLendon, D.; Ozols, V.V.; Jessing, K.W.; Zavitz, K.H.; Koo, E.H. NSAIDs and enantiomers of flurbiprofen target γ-secretase and lower Aβ42 in vivo. *J. Clin. Investig.* **2003**, *112*, 440–449. [CrossRef]
195. Jantzen, P.T.; Connor, K.E.; DiCarlo, G.; Wenk, G.L.; Wallace, J.L.; Rojiani, A.M.; Coppola, D.; Morgan, D.; Gordon, M.N. Microglial activation and β-amyloid deposit reduction caused by a nitric oxide-releasing nonsteroidal anti-inflammatory drug in amyloid precursor protein plus presenilin-1 transgenic mice. *J. Neurosci.* **2002**, *22*, 2246–2254. [CrossRef]
196. Weggen, S.; Eriksen, J.L.; Sagi, S.A.; Pietrzik, C.U.; Ozols, V.; Fauq, A.; Golde, T.E.; Koo, E.H. Evidence that nonsteroidal anti-inflammatory drugs decrease amyloid β42 production by direct modulation of γ-secretase activity. *J. Biol. Chem.* **2003**, *278*, 31831–31837. [CrossRef]
197. Weggen, S.; Eriksen, J.L.; Sagi, S.A.; Pietrzik, C.U.; Golde, T.E.; Koo, E.H. Aβ42-lowering nonsteroidal anti-inflammatory drugs preserve intramembrane cleavage of the amyloid precursor protein (APP) and ErbB-4 receptor and signaling through the APP intracellular domain. *J. Biol. Chem.* **2003**, *278*, 30748–30754. [CrossRef]

6

miRNA-34c Overexpression Causes Dendritic Loss and Memory Decline

Yu-Chia Kao [1,2], I-Fang Wang [1,3] and Kuen-Jer Tsai [1,4,*]

1 Institute of Clinical Medicine, College of Medicine, National Cheng Kung University, Tainan 704, Taiwan; yukanomail2006@yahoo.com.tw (Y.-C.K.); e_fung0207@hotmail.com (I.-F.W.)
2 Department of Pediatrics, E-Da Hospital, Kaohsiung 824, Taiwan
3 Institute of Molecular Biology, Academia Sinica, Taipei 115, Taiwan
4 Research Center of Clinical Medicine, National Cheng Kung University Hospital, College of Medicine, National Cheng Kung University, Tainan 704, Taiwan
* Correspondence: kjtsai@mail.ncku.edu.tw

Abstract: Microribonucleic acids (miRNAs) play a pivotal role in numerous aspects of the nervous system and are increasingly recognized as key regulators in neurodegenerative diseases. This study hypothesized that miR-34c, a miRNA expressed in mammalian hippocampi whose expression level can alter the hippocampal dendritic spine density, could induce memory impairment akin to that of patients with Alzheimer's disease (AD) in mice. In this study, we showed that miR-34c overexpression in hippocampal neurons negatively regulated dendritic length and spine density. Hippocampal neurons transfected with miR-34c had shorter dendrites on average and fewer filopodia and spines than those not transfected with miR-34c (control mice). Because dendrites and synapses are key sites for signal transduction and fundamental structures for memory formation and storage, disrupted dendrites can contribute to AD. Therefore, we supposed that miR-34c, through its effects on dendritic spine density, influences synaptic plasticity and plays a key role in AD pathogenesis.

Keywords: miR-34c; dendritic spine; Alzheimer's disease

---

1. Introduction

Alzheimer's disease (AD) is a neurodegenerative disorder characterized by memory loss and cognitive decline due to extracellular accumulation of beta-amyloid peptide and intracellular accumulation of tau; it is also a consequence of dysfunction and loss of synapses [1]. From a pathological perspective, although neurofibrillary tangles and extracellular amyloid accumulations—defined as neuritic plaques—are the main hallmarks of AD, synaptic loss is the best predictor of clinical symptoms of AD [1].

Microribonucleic acids (miRNAs) are small noncoding RNAs composed of 19–25 nucleotides, which mediate the post-transcriptional regulation of gene expression. These non-coding RNAs function by binding to the 3′ untranslated regions of target messenger RNAs (mRNAs) (within the RNA-induced silencing complex), silencing their target mRNAs, and downregulating protein translation [2]. Each miRNA contains seed sequences crucial for recognizing and binding to target mRNAs. Some miRNAs participate in key neuronal functions, such as cell signaling, transcription, and axonal guidance [3]. More than three miRNAs, including miR-124, miR-34, and miR-132, are key to hippocampal function [4,5]. miR-124 expression in the medial prefrontal cortex could partially rescue the behavioral deficits associated with frontotemporal dementia [6]. Zovoilis et al. found that miR-34c was upregulated in AD patients [7] Bhatnagar et al. showed that there was a strong correlation between the expression level of miR-34c and scores of mini-mental state examination [8]. Other studies have observed that miR-132 is downregulated in patients with mild cognitive impairment [9], and the miR-132 level is reduced in AD-affected brains [10]. Therefore, miR-124, miR-34, and miR-132 are regarded as memory miRNAs, which play a key role in neurodegenerative diseases such as AD, Parkinson's disease, and Huntington's disease [5].

miR-34 is a markedly conserved miRNA of the let-7 family, with an identical seed sequence of orthologues in flies, *Caenorhabditis elegans*, mice, and humans [11]. The miR-34 family consists of three members: miR-34a, miR-34b, and miR-34c. Of these, miR-34a and miR-34c have identical seed sequences, whereas the seed sequence of miR-34b is similar, but not identical. This suggests that miR-34a and miR-34c share similar mRNA targets, whereas those of miR-34b might be slightly different [12]. Although miR-34b and miR-34c are co-transcribed from the same chromosome, they differ in amount and may regulate different targets in a particular brain region [13]. In mice, miR-34a is ubiquitously expressed, with its highest levels appearing in the brain, whereas miR-34b and miR-34c are expressed mainly in the brain, lungs, testes, and ovaries [14].

The miR-34 family is essential for normal brain development [14]; miR-34 has been linked to neurogenesis, spine morphology, neurite outgrowth, neurodegeneration, and hippocampal memory formation [15]. In zebrafish, the repression of miR-34 led to developmental defects in the neuronal system with an enlargement of the hindbrain during early embryonic development [16]. Moreover, miR-34/449 controls mitotic spindle orientation during mammalian cortex development [17]. Furthermore, miR-34 has been implicated in brain disorders and aging; in *Drosophila*, loss of miR-34 decreased survival and accelerated brain aging and degeneration, whereas miR-34 upregulation extended survival and diminished neurodegeneration due to human pathogenic polyglutamine disease protein [11]. In addition to being present in neurons, miR-34 is expressed in glial cells [4].

Zovoilis et al. showed that miR-34c was elevated in the hippocampi of AD patients, aging mice, and APPPS1-21, a model of amyloid pathology linked to AD. The researchers demonstrated that miR-34c constrained memory consolidation, and miR-34c-mediated memory impairment was regulated, at least in part, by decreased hippocampal sirtuin-1 (SIRT1) levels [7]. Similarly, the expression of another miR-34 family member—miR-34a—was elevated in APPswe/PSΔE9 (AD mouse model) mice compared with control mice [18]. However, a contradictory correlation between miR-34 and cognitive function was also observed. A study that used Adeno-associated virus-delivered sponges in mice revealed that miR-34 inhibition impaired reference memory during the Morris water maze [4]. In *Drosophila*, loss of miR-34 accelerated brain aging and late-onset brain degeneration. miR-34 mutant flies were born with typical brains but showed dramatic vacuolization with age, whereas miR-34 upregulation extended their median lifespan and mitigated neurodegeneration [11]. Because AD is a neurodegenerative disorder associated with aging, we were unsure why loss of miR-34 accelerated brain aging in *Drosophila* while its overexpression caused memory impairment in mammals. Dickson et al. observed that miR-34a inhibited expression of endogenous tau, a crucial intraneuronal aggregate of AD [19]. In addition, Wu et al. found that overexpression of miR-34c downregulated tau expression in gastric cancer cells [20], although the researchers did not perform experiments to test cognitive function or analyze tau proteins in neural cells, the results were confusing in that the decreased tau expression associated with miR-34a and miR-34c overexpression contradicted AD pathogenesis. Therefore, miR-34 seems to play a mutual role in neurodegeneration; it can be protective or causative. For this reason, we wanted to study the role of miR-34c in memory function in mammals.

Dendritic spines are tiny protrusions along dendrites that constitute major postsynaptic sites for synaptic transmission [21]. These spines are highly dynamic structures that can undergo remodeling even in adults. Spine remodeling and new synapse formation, termed "plasticity", underlie the basis for learning and memory [22]. Loss or alteration of these structures was described in patients with neurodegenerative disorders such as AD [23], and synaptic reduction is the feature most closely related with decline in memory and cognition [24]. In one study, the density of neocortical synapses revealed highly powerful correlations with cognitive alterations in AD—the lower the mental status scores, the greater was the loss of synapses [25]. In another study, only weak correlations were observed between psychometric indices and plaques and tangles [26]. Thus, AD is primarily considered to be a synaptopathy [27].

Based on previous reports regarding the importance of particular hippocampal miRNAs in memory function, we studied the influence of miR-34c on memory function and compared dendritic spines between hippocampal neurons overexpressing miR-34c and controls, given that dendritic spines are the fundamental elements of synapses that form the basis of learning and memory.

2. Results

2.1. *Overexpression of miR-34c Caused Memory Impairment*

Using the Morris water maze task, we found that mice overexpressing miR-34c exhibited markedly increased latency compared with vector-transfected (control) mice (Figure 1A), indicating that the mice overexpressing miR-34c exhibited memory impairment. We used quantitative polymerase chain reaction (PCR) to measure the expression level of miR-34c in the hippocampi of miR-34c and control mice. The miR-34c expression level of the miR-34c-transfected mice was five times higher than that of the control mice (Figure 1B).

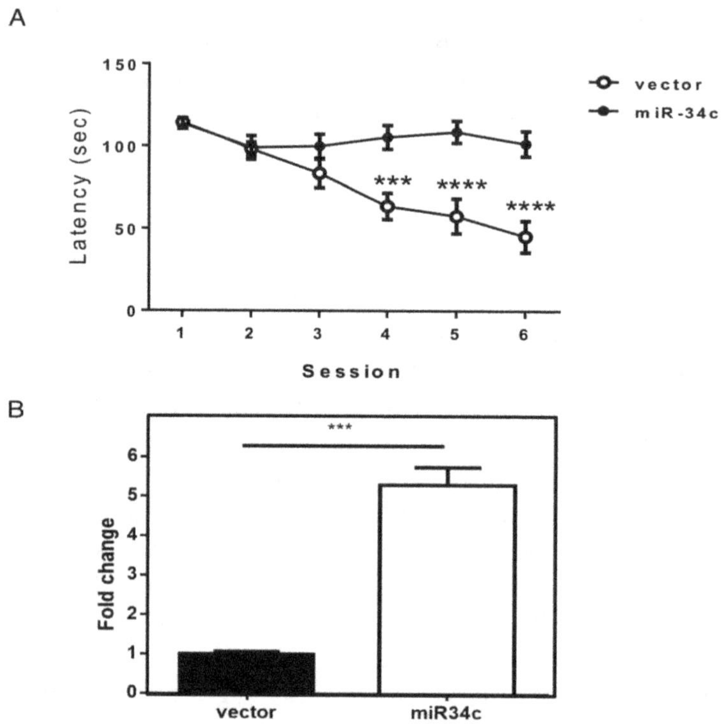

Figure 1. Overexpression of miR-34c caused memory impairment. (**A**) Escape latencies of mice overexpressing miR-34c and control vector (vec) mice ($n = 16$ in each group) in the Morris water maze. The asterisks represent the level of statistical significance calculated by a two-way analysis of variance (*** $p < 0.001$, **** $p < 0.0001$); (**B**) Hippocampal miR-34c expression levels were determined by quantitative PCR in mice transfected with miR-34c construct or mice transfected with the control vector and calculated using a two-tailed Student's t-test (*** $p < 0.001$).

2.2. *Expression Level of miR-34c in the Hippocampus*

The miR-34c construct was transfected into primary hippocampal cells to investigate the role of miR-34c in neuronal morphology. The transfection efficiency of miR-34c was identified on the seventh day of culture (DIV7) through immunofluorescence staining. Cells that co-expressed green fluorescence (from green fluorescent protein $GFP^{+/-}$ mice) and red fluorescence (from miR-34c-transfected cells) were selected, and neural dendrites were confirmed using the microtubule-associated protein 2 (Map2) antibody, which stained the soma and dendrites, but not the axons (Figure 2A). The expression levels of miR-34c in the transfected and control cells were detected using reverse transcription PCR (RT-PCR). Of the hippocampal primary cells, the expression of miR-34c was nearly four times higher in the miR-34c-transfected cells than in the control cells (Figure 2B).

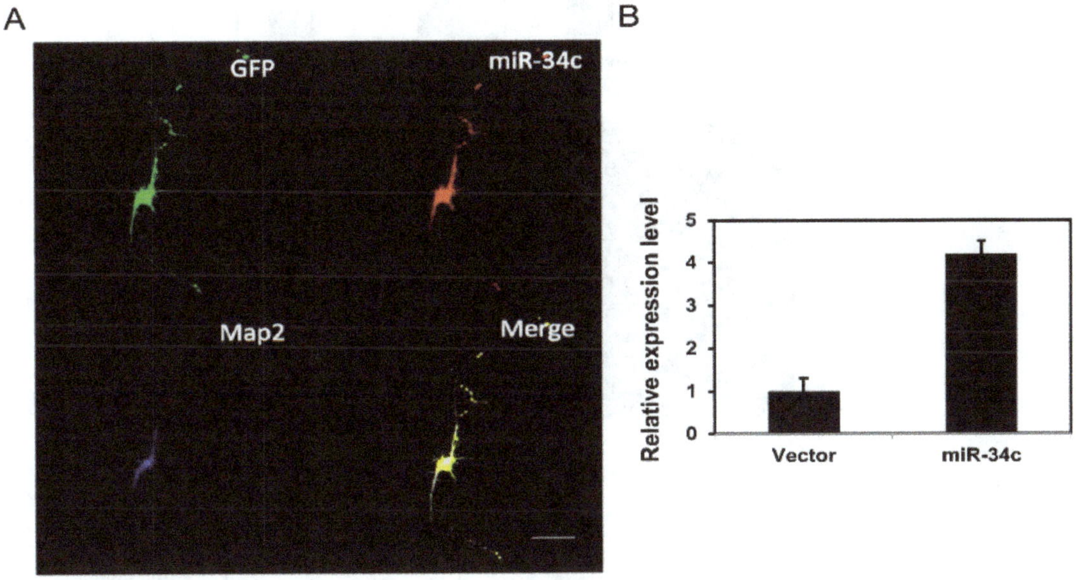

Figure 2. We observed that miR-34c was expressed in cultured hippocampal neurons. (**A**) Transfection of miR-34c was identified on DIV7 through immunofluorescence staining. Cells co-expressing green fluorescence (from GFP$^{+/-}$ mice) and red fluorescence (from miR-34c-transfected cells) were selected, and neural dendrites were confirmed using the Map2 antibody. Scale bar = 50 μm; (**B**) The expression level of miR-34c in the cultured hippocampal cells transfected with the miR-34c construct or control vector were detected using RT-PCR and calculated using a two-tailed Student's *t*-test.

2.3. *Overexpression of miR-34c Reduced Dendritic Length and Branch Numbers*

To investigate the effect of miR-34c on neuronal morphology, we measured the total dendritic length, dendritic main shaft, and dendritic branch numbers of the hippocampi two days after transfection. In the earlier stage—DIV 7—it appeared that miR-34c suppressed the outgrowth and branching of dendrites; however, this result was nonsignificant (Figure 3A). In the later stage—at DIV 14—the total dendritic length of neurons with miR-34c overexpression had a shorter dendritic length than did the neurons transfected with the control vector (Figure 3B). The numbers of dendritic shafts and branches were slightly decreased in the miR-34c-overexpression group; however, this result was nonsignificant. Therefore, miR-34c partially inhibited dendritic outgrowth but did not affect dendritic branching.

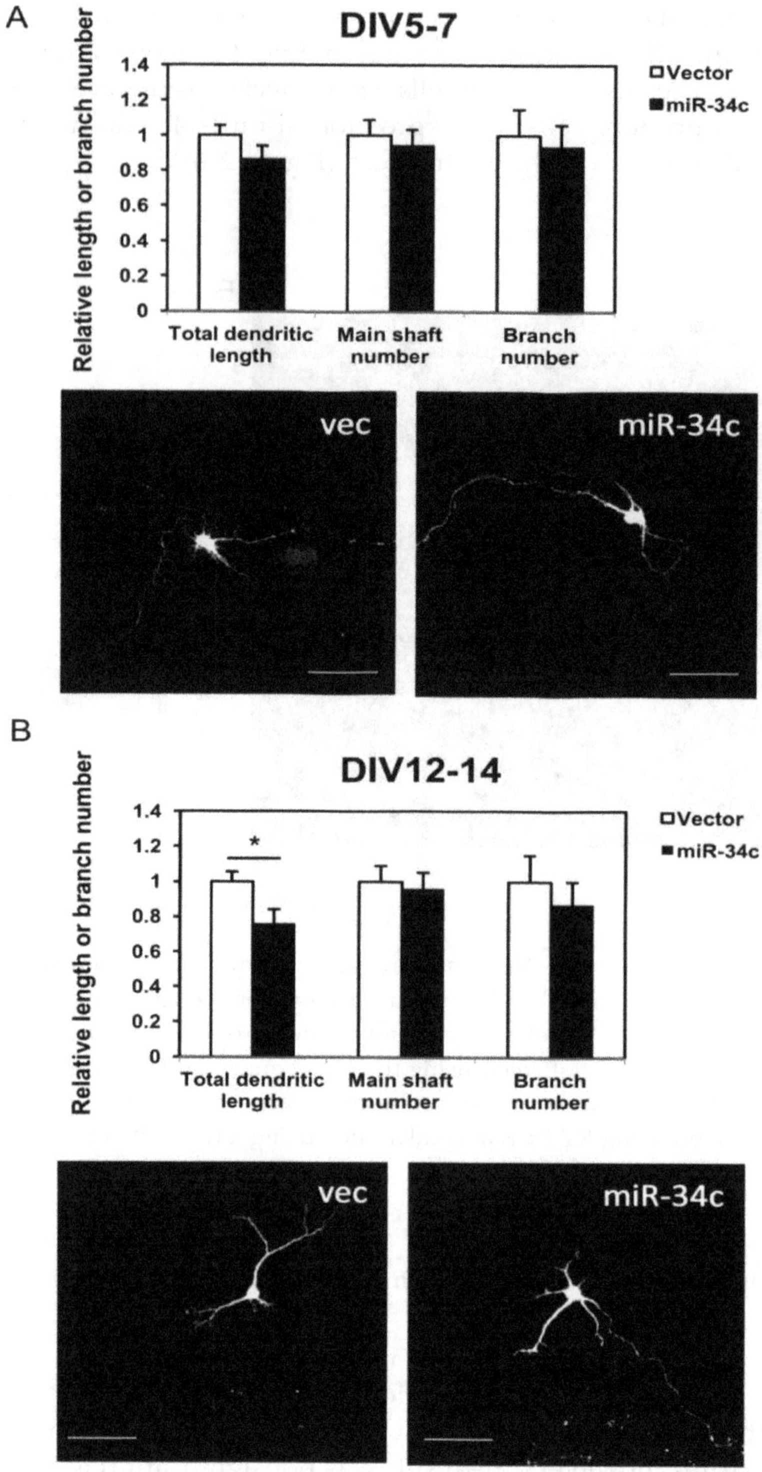

Figure 3. We observed that miR-34c affected the dendritic length of hippocampal neurons. Immunostaining with GFP, red fluorescent protein, and the Map2 antibody was performed on (**A**) DIV 7 (Scale bar = 100 μm) and (**B**) DIV 14. The total dendritic length, shaft number, and branch number of miR-34c hippocampal neurons and vector-transfected (vec) hippocampal neurons (n = 18 in each group) were counted under a fluorescence and confocal microscope (20× magnification) and calculated using a two-tailed Student's t-test (* $p < 0.05$). Scale bar = 100 μm.

2.4. *Effects of miR-34c Overexpression on Neurite Protrusion Density*

Protrusions of neurites develop at an early stage of neuronal development and later differentiate into mature spines. This process requires electrical signals from other neurons. The density of protrusions reflects not only the morphological state of the neurons, but also the physiological function. Therefore, we investigated the status of these protrusions by categorizing them into spines and filopodia, and measured the total protrusions, defined as the summation of spines and filopodia. Spines were defined as short extensions from the membranes of dendrite, with mushroom-like heads or extensions with an obscure neck. Filopodia were slender protrusions mostly twice longer as spines, and were identified as protrusions without an apparent shallow head; they were considered the immature form of protrusions. On DIV7, when the protrusions had not developed completely, neurons transfected with miR-34c had a significantly lower spine density and total number of protrusions (Figure 4A). On DIV14, the neurons transfected with miR-34c exhibited declines in spines and filopodia, as well as in total protrusions compared with the controls (Figure 4B).

2.5. *Effects of miR-34c Overexpression on Protrusion Density in Various Dendritic Areas*

To gain a better understanding of the effects of miR-34c on dendritic protrusion, each dendrite was divided into three equal segments of 40 μm for further analysis, starting from the soma as the proximal segment and followed by the middle and distal segments. The results revealed various density patterns in the spines and filopodia (Figure 5A). Spine density and total protrusions in all three segments of the miR-34c-transfected cells remained lower than those in the controls (Figure 5B,D). In addition, the reductions in spine density and total protrusions were proportional to their distance from the soma, meaning that in the miR-34c-overexpressing neurons, the farther the dendrites were from the soma, the lower was the number of spines. By contrast, no such change was observed in the filopodia along the dendrites (Figure 5C). Based on these findings, we assumed that miR-34c participated in the formation (turnover) of dendritic protrusions and may have acted as a negative regulator in the maturation of dendritic protrusions from filopodia into spines. While the spine density increased with the distance of dendrites from the soma in the control group, the miR-34c-transfected cells exhibited reduced spine density away from the soma.

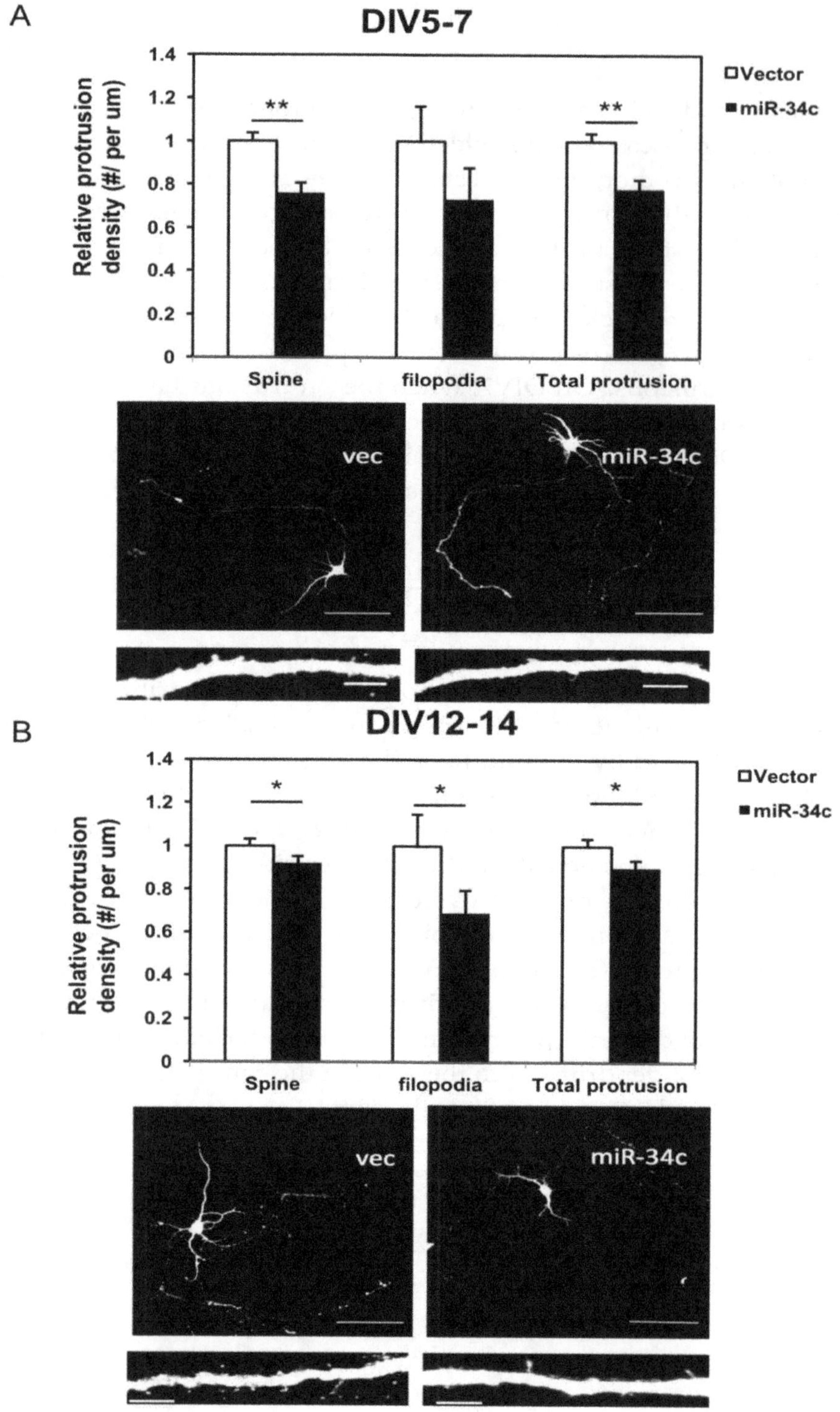

Figure 4. We observed that miR-34c lowered dendritic spine density and total protrusion density. Quantification of the protrusion density of neurites including mature spines, immature filopodia, and the summation of both using immunostaining on the (**A**) DIV 7 (Scale bar of upper panel = 100 μm; lower panel = 5 μm) and (**B**) DIV 14 in miR-34c and vector-transfected (vec) cells (n = 28 in each group) was conducted under 100× magnification and calculated using a two-tailed Student's t-test (* $p < 0.05$, ** $p < 0.01$). Scale bar of upper panel = 100 μm; lower panel = 5 μm.

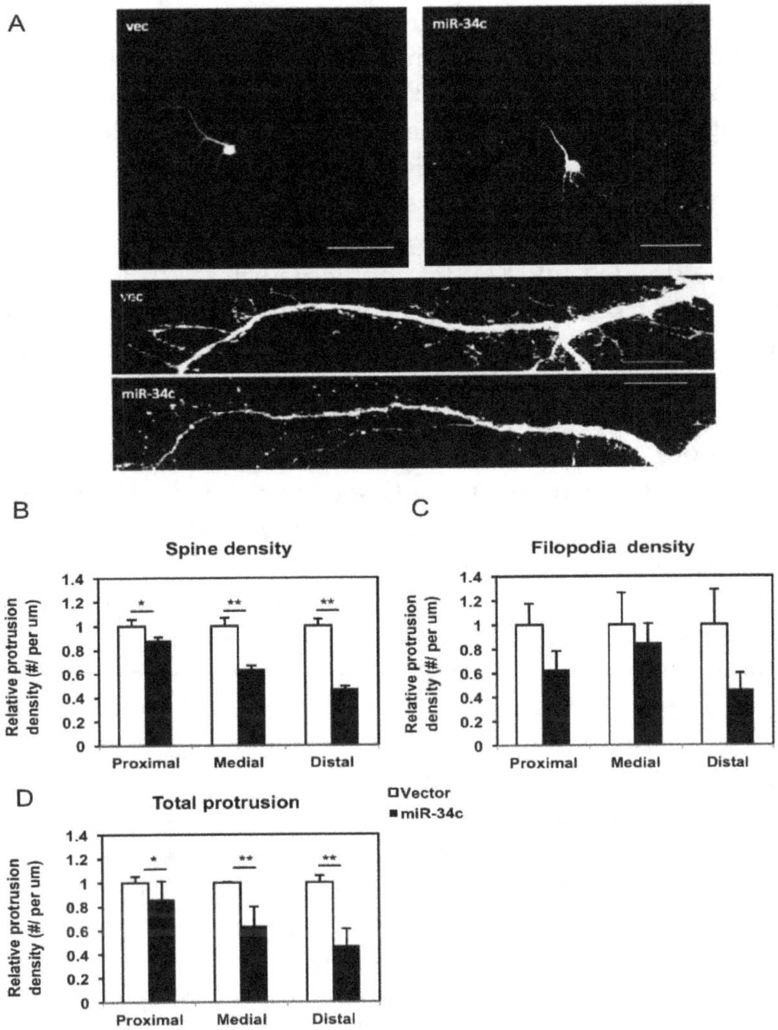

Figure 5. We observed that miR-34c exerted a negative effect on spine density along the dendrites. (**A**) Low- and high-power fields (20× in upper panels and 100× in lower panels) were used for counting. Scale bar of upper panel = 100 μm, lower panel = 20 μm. Quantification of the densities of (**B**) spines, (**C**) filopodia, and (**D**) total protrusions was conducted by dividing each dendrite into three equal segments of 40-μm in length, starting from the soma as the proximal segment (0–40 μm) and followed by the middle (40–80 μm) and distal (80–120 μm) segments, and calculated using a two-tailed Student's *t*-test (* $p < 0.05$, ** $p < 0.01$).

3. Discussion

The present study showed that mice overexpressing miR-34c exhibited significant memory impairment and hippocampal dendritic spine loss. In our study, miR-34c partially inhibited dendritic outgrowth as the total dendritic length was shorter. In addition, miR-34c resulted in reduced numbers of dendritic spines and total protrusions at an early stage (DIV 7). Subsequently, the miR-34c-transfected cells exhibited loss of filopodia and spines; in these cells, the farther the dendrites were from the soma, the lower was the number of spines; however, no such change was observed among filopodia. A study on the acoustic and visual cortices of autopsied AD patients revealed a marked decrease in the number of dendritic spines and loss of distal spines. However, the branches of the apical part of the dendritic tree and basal arborizations appeared to be equally affected by spine depletion [28]. The hippocampus contains two types of dendrites on pyramidal cells: apical and basal dendrites. Apical dendrites can be further divided into distal and proximal parts. Pyramidal cells segregate their inputs by using proximal apical dendrites, which project radially to local pyramidal cells and interneurons, while distal apical dendrites form non-local synapses by receiving inputs from distant cortical and thalamic locations [29]. CA1 neurons receive inputs at the distal tuft from the entorhinal cortex through the perforant path and from the thalamic nucleus reuniens, whereas the basal and apical dendrites receive inputs from the CA3 through the Schaffer collaterals. Based on the finding of more prominent distal dendritic spinal loss in the miR-34c cells in our study, we assumed that miR-34c might disrupt the perforant path from the entorhinal cortex of the memory circuit in mammalian brains.

Dendritic abnormalities in AD are widespread and occur in early stages of the disease; such abnormalities can be divided into (1) dystrophic neurites, (2) dendritic complexity reduction, and (3) dendritic spine loss. Marked dendritic spine loss is the final major dendritic abnormality found in AD patients, and the cortex and hippocampus are the two areas most affected by spine loss [30,31]. In APPxPS1-KI (an AD mouse model), an alteration of spine morphology occurred before reduction of synapses and neuronal density. The researchers observed a reduction in spine length and enlargement its neck, giving the spines a more "stubby" appearance [32].

Filopodia are the smallest structures protruding from dendrites [33]. Filopodia-like protrusions are highly unstable and can form and be removed within hours, whereas larger mushroom-type spines are more likely to remain stable for months to years. In both cell culture and in vivo, filopodia can form, stabilize, and grow into larger spines; this suggests that they represent an early stage of spine formation [34]. Transitions in spine size and stability—from immature and unstable filopodia to mature and stable spines—accompany the maturation and strengthening of synaptic contacts on spines [33]. An in vivo imaging study on the rodent neocortex demonstrated that small spines were NMDAR-dominated and highly motile, whereas large spines were AMPAR-dominated and highly stable. These findings led to the hypothesis that small thin spines are learning spines, whereas larger mushroom spines are memory spines [35]. Changes in the shapes of spine heads (morphogenesis) were actin-dependent and likely regulated by synaptic stimulation in response to a variety of stimuli [36]. In the present study, in the miR-34c-transfected mice, the number of spines were decreased compared with the control mice at an early stage and the filopodia remained unaffected, whereas immature filopodia and mature spines were lost at a later stage; thus, we speculated that miR-34c might disrupt the maturation of spines at an earlier stage and eventually destroy all dendritic spines, thereby affecting learning and memory consolidation.

Studies by Zovoilis and Bhatnagar et al. showed that miR-34c was increased in AD patients' brains and they pointed out one specific target—SIRT1—that contributed to memory decline [7,8]. Codocedo et al. later proved that SIRT1 overexpression was sufficient to change dendritic morphogenesis in the hippocampi and offer certain resistance against the cytotoxic damage induced by Aβ and avoid neuritic dystrophy [37]. Hence, the causal relationship between miR-34c and changes in dendritic spines in our study can be verified. Future research is required to investigate the pathogenic mechanism underlying the association between miR-34c and dendritic spine loss and to search for other possible miR-34c targets.

Structural changes in spines were driven by remodeling of the actin cytoskeleton [38]. Small Rho GTPases were deemed as central regulators of cell cytoarchitecture and played key roles in modulating cell migration, neurite outgrowth, survival, and synapse formation in neurons [39]. Cell division cycle 42 (Cdc42), ras-related C3 botulinum toxin substrate 1 (Rac1), and ras homolog family member A (RhoA) are the most frequently studied members of the small Rho GTPase family [40]. Rac and Rho are crucial to the maintenance of dendritic spines and branches in hippocampal pyramidal neurons [41] and appear to be critical in the formation and maintenance of memory [42]. Activation of Rac1 facilitated the formation of dendritic spines and increased spine head volume. By contrast, RhoA activation prevented spine formation and induced spine shortening [43]. As mentioned, miR-124, miR-34, and miR-132 are regarded as memory miRNAs. Both miR-124 and miR-132 have been reported to be associated with changes in dendritic spines through Rho GTPases, which underlie the stabilization of memory. In one study, miR-124 reduced the expression of Rho GTPs, thereby inhibiting axonal and dendritic branching via Rac1 and Cdc42 signaling, respectively [44]. Moreover, miR-132 activated Rac1 and promoted spine formation [45]. Thus far, no relationship between miR-34 and Rho GTPases in neurons has been reported. Since SIRT1 activators (RES) could modulates the dendritic arborization through the inhibition of Rho-associated protein kinase (ROCK) [37]—downstream effector of Rho GTPases—this served as indirect evidence for the association between miR-34c and Rho GTPases. Besides, one study investigated the roles of miR-34 and Rho GTPases in cancer cells; Huang et al. demonstrated that two key mechanisms involved in cancer metastasis—epithelial-to-mesenchymal transition and mesenchymal-to-amoeboid transition—were coupled through two miRNAs, namely miR-200 and miR-34, both of which inhibited RhoA and Rac1 [46]. This implies that Rho GTPase-dependent cytoskeletal changes might occur in the dendritic spines of miR-34-expressing hippocampal neurons, and thus underlie memory impairment.

Because postsynaptic density protein 95 (PSD-95) is the hallmark of a mature and stable glutamatergic synapse associated with memory consolidation [33], miR-34c might be associated with PSD-95. Bustos et al. designed an epigenetic editing strategy by using a zinc finger construct to control Dlg4/PSD-95 expression in the hippocampus and validate PSD-95 as a key player in plasticity and memory. PSD-95-6ZF-VP64 transduction could increase PSD-95 levels and recover learning and memory deficits in aged and AbPPswe/PS-1 (AD model) mice [47]. Whether synaptic changes in memory miRNAs are also related to PSD-95 requires further investigation.

4. Materials and Methods

4.1. Animals

C57BL/6JNarl (B6) mice were kept in a ventilated room under controlled conditions with a 12-h/12-h light/dark cycle and a maintained temperature of 22 $\pm$ 2 °C. The animals were given access to food and water ad libitum. This study was approved by the University Institutional Animal Care and Use Committee of National Cheng Kung University (NCKU) (Project code-106073, date of approval-23/12/2016). The experimental procedures for handling the mice were in accordance with the guidelines of the Institutional Animal Care and Use Committee of NCKU. Transgenic mice with $GFP^{+/-}$ expression and B6 mice were provided by the national laboratory animal center.

4.2. Deoxyribonucleic Acid Constructions

To produce the miRNA constructs, the genomic deoxyribonucleic acid (DNA) from a B6-wild type mouse was used as the complementary template to amplify the precursor of miR-34c by PCR, with the forward primer: 5′-GCA GTG TAA TTA GCT GAT TGT AGT G-3′, and reverse primer: 5′-ATA TTA GGA AAC CAG CTG GT TTT AA-3′. After PCR amplification, the precursor miR-34c product was separated by electrophoresis and eluted from the agarose gel, ligated into a lentiviral construct-pFUGW, driven by a ubiquitin promoter, with a red fluorescent protein gene (dsRed) for co-expression.

4.3. Lentivirus Production

The lentivirus was produced by the RNAi core laboratory of Academia Sinica, Taipei, Taiwan with a 100$\times$ concentration.

4.4. Stereotaxic Hippocampal Injections

Male B6 mice were placed in the induction chambers. The oxygen flowmeter was adjusted to approximately 0.1–0.3 L/min. Isoflurane vaporizer was adjusted to 5% for anesthesia induction and 1.5–3.5% for maintenance. The anesthetized mice were then mounted in a stereotactic apparatus for intra-hippocampal injections. Concentrated lentivirus (1 $\times$ 10^7 in 2 μL) was injected into the dentate gyrus of bilateral hippocampus (−2.0 mm anterior–posterior, 1.8 mm medial–lateral, and −2.3 mm dorsal–ventral relative to the bregma) using a Hamilton micro-syringe (Hamilton Company, Reno, Nevada). After each injection, the needle was left in situ for 8 min to prevent regurgitation of the virus during removal. Control groups were injected with the same volume of control lentivirus. A Morris Water Maze test was performed 30 days after the injection.

4.5. Morris Water Maze Test

miR-34c-expressing and control vector-infected male B6 mice, $n = 16$ in each group, were tested 30 days after hippocampal injections of viral particles. The swimming pool is divided into four quadrants and contains an escape platform placed beneath the water. The mice were trained with four consecutive trials per day for six days. When released, the mice swam around the pool in search of an exit and on subsequent trials the mice were able to locate the platform more rapidly. Each trial lasted until the mice found the platform or for a maximum of 2 min. The time to locate the platform was recorded and the average latency calculated from the values of four trials each day. The swimming speed and probe test were recorded on video for further analysis.

4.6. Primary Hippocampal Culture

The embryos from B6 wild-type pregnant female mice were used for hippocampal primary culture. Pregnant B6 wild-type mice were dissected at embryonic day 16.5, and the hippocampi were separated from embryonic brains. The hippocampal tissues were washed with 1× Hank's balanced salt solution (HBSS) twice and digested with papain for about 10 min at 37 °C. Then, the aggregated tissues were washed with 1× HBSS twice, followed by resuspension in 1 ml Neurobasal medium with 1× B27 (Invitrogen, Thermo Fisher Scientific, Waltham, MA, USA), 1× Penicillin Streptomycin (P/S) antibiotics (Invitrogen), and 1× GlutaMax (Invitrogen). Cell viability was counted by an Invitrogen countess automatic cell counter. Cells were plated at 2×10^5 cells/well on poly-D-lysine-coated coverslips in six-well plates and incubated at 37 °C/5% CO_2. After 2 h, the medium was changed to a new Neurobasal medium to prevent contamination. Cells were cultured until DIV5 and DIV12 to perform miRNA transfection.

4.7. Transfection

Cells plated in six-well plates were transfected at DIV5 or DIV12. Thirty minutes before transfection, the medium was replaced with P/S antibiotics-free Neurobasal medium. The ubiquitin promoter-driven miR-34c plasmid, or vector only, were transfected into hippocampal primary culture with Lipofectamine 2000 (Invitrogen) for 2 h. The transfected cells were cultured for two days and analyzed by confocal microscopy for neuronal morphology or collected to extract RNA samples.

4.8. Immunofluorescence Staining

The transfected cells were washed twice with phosphate-buffered saline (PBS) and fixed with 4% paraformaldehyde (Electron Microscopy Sciences, Hatfield, UK). The cells were blocked for 1 h (blocking solution: 10% goat serum/PBS) at room temperature. The primary antibody was Map2 (Invitrogen) with 1% goat serum. All images were visualized using a Zeiss laser confocal microscope (LSM510, Zeiss, Oberkochen, Germany) and a fluorescence microscope (DeltaVision, GE Healthcare Life Sciences, London, UK), with a single optical section.

4.9. Image Analysis

Neural cells emitted green fluorescence because of the inherited GFP protein. All images were at the same resolution of 1024 pixels × 1024 pixels. Confocal z sectioning was used, and images were overlapped to have full signals. Each neuron was captured under the low-power field (20× objective, NA 1.4, respectively) for both soma and neurites. These low power images were used to measure the neuritic length and branch numbers, owing to the whole cell coverage with this larger visual field. Dendritic spines were focused on under high magnification (40× and 100× objective) in order to count spine numbers and observe spine morphology, specifically for measuring (1) total dendritic length, defined as the summation of all dendritic length in a neuron; (2) main dendritic shaft number, defined as the numbers of dendritic outgrowth from one soma; (3) dendritic branch number, defined as the total branch numbers from the primary dendrites; and (4) dendritic spine density, expressed as the average number of spines per μm of dendritic length. The total dendritic length and branch numbers were measured using the software NeuronJ (provided by Dr. Erik Meijering, Biomedical Imaging Group Rotterdam of Erasmus University Medical Center, Rotterdam, The Netherlands), whereas the numbers of different protrusions (spines, filopodia, and total protrusions) were counted using ImageJ (provided by Dr. Erik Meijering, Biomedical Imaging Group Rotterdam of Erasmus University Medical Center, Rotterdam, The Netherlands) in various areas divided by their distance from the soma (proximal: 0–40 μm, middle: 40–80 μm, distal: 80–120 μm).

4.10. Reverse Transcription PCR (RT-PCR)

The total RNA products extracted from the hippocampal primary culture or hippocampi in the brain were then reverse-transcribed to complementary DNA (cDNA) by SuperScript II RT (Invitrogen) following the Universal ProbeLibrary (UPL; Roche, Basel, Switzerland) protocol, and the expression levels of miR-34c were then detected by UPL probe #21, according to the manufacturer's protocol. Primer sequences used were as followed, miR-34c UPL RT primer: GTT GGC TCT GGT GCA GGG TCC GAG GTA TTC GC ACCAGAGCCAACGCAATC, miR-34c forward primer: 5′-CGG CGA GGC AGT GTA GTT AGC T-3′, universal reverse primer: 5′-GTG CAG GGT CCG AGG T-3′.

4.11. Statistics

Data were analyzed using SPSS and the Morris water maze was analyzed using a two-way analysis of variance. Mean values were analyzed using a two-tailed Student's *t*- test. All results are represented as mean ± standard error of the mean and were first examined using an *f*-test to identify the homogeneity of variance. A probability level of <0.05 was accepted as statistically significant and degrees of significance are presented as * $p < 0.05$, ** $p < 0.01$, *** $p < 0.001$, **** $p < 0.0001$.

5. Conclusions

We established miR-34c expression constructs and transfected miR-34c into primary hippocampal cells. The present study revealed that miR-34c overexpression resulted in memory decline, accompanied by a decrease in dendritic spine density. Our data suggested that miR-34c plays a pivotal role in cognitive decline and therapies targeting miR-34c may restore synaptic defects and shed further light on AD.

Author Contributions: Conceptualization, K.-J.T.; Data curation, Y.-C.K. and I.-F.W.; Funding acquisition, K.-J.T.; Investigation, K.-J.T.; Methodology, Y.-C.K. and I.-F.W.; Project administration, K.-J.T.; Resources, K.-J.T.; Supervision, K.-J.T.; Validation, Y.-C.K. and I.-F.W.; Writing—original draft, Y.-C.K.; Writing—review & editing, K.-J.T.

References

1. Forner, S.; Baglietto-Vargas, D.; Martini, A.C.; Trujillo-Estrada, L.; LaFerla, F.M. Synaptic impairment in Alzheimer's disease: A dysregulated symphony. *Trends Neurosci.* **2017**, *40*, 347–357. [CrossRef] [PubMed]
2. Pillai, R.S.; Bhattacharyya, S.N.; Filipowicz, W. Repression of protein synthesis by mirnas: How many mechanisms? *Trends Cell Biol.* **2007**, *17*, 118–126. [CrossRef] [PubMed]
3. Malmevik, J.; Petri, R.; Klussendorf, T.; Knauff, P.; Akerblom, M.; Johansson, J.; Soneji, S.; Jakobsson, J. Identification of the mirna targetome in hippocampal neurons using rip-seq. *Sci. Rep.* **2015**, *5*, 12609. [CrossRef] [PubMed]
4. Malmevik, J.; Petri, R.; Knauff, P.; Brattas, P.L.; Akerblom, M.; Jakobsson, J. Distinct cognitive effects and underlying transcriptome changes upon inhibition of individual mirnas in hippocampal neurons. *Sci. Rep.* **2016**, *6*, 19879. [CrossRef] [PubMed]
5. Hernandez-Rapp, J.; Rainone, S.; Hebert, S.S. MicroRNAs underlying memory deficits in neurodegenerative disorders. *Prog. Neuro-Psychopharmacol. Biol. Psychiatry* **2017**, *73*, 79–86. [CrossRef] [PubMed]

6. Gascon, E.; Lynch, K.; Ruan, H.; Almeida, S.; Verheyden, J.M.; Seeley, W.W.; Dickson, D.W.; Petrucelli, L.; Sun, D.; Jiao, J.; et al. Alterations in microRNA-124 and ampa receptors contribute to social behavioral deficits in frontotemporal dementia. *Nat. Med.* **2014**, *20*, 1444–1451. [CrossRef] [PubMed]
7. Zovoilis, A.; Agbemenyah, H.Y.; Agis-Balboa, R.C.; Stilling, R.M.; Edbauer, D.; Rao, P.; Farinelli, L.; Delalle, I.; Schmitt, A.; Falkai, P.; et al. MicroRNA-34c is a novel target to treat dementias. *EMBO J.* **2011**, *30*, 4299–4308. [CrossRef] [PubMed]
8. Bhatnagar, S.; Chertkow, H.; Schipper, H.M.; Yuan, Z.; Shetty, V.; Jenkins, S.; Jones, T.; Wang, E. Increased microRNA-34c abundance in Alzheimer's disease circulating blood plasma. *Front. Mol. Neurosci.* **2014**, *7*, 2. [CrossRef] [PubMed]
9. Xie, B.; Zhou, H.; Zhang, R.; Song, M.; Yu, L.; Wang, L.; Liu, Z.; Zhang, Q.; Cui, D.; Wang, X.; et al. Serum mir-206 and mir-132 as potential circulating biomarkers for mild cognitive impairment. *J. Alzheimers Dis.* **2015**, *45*, 721–731. [CrossRef] [PubMed]
10. Lau, P.; Frigerio, C.S.; de Strooper, B. Variance in the identification of microRNAs deregulated in Alzheimer's disease and possible role of lincrnas in the pathology: The need of larger datasets. *Ageing Res. Rev.* **2014**, *17*, 43–53. [CrossRef] [PubMed]
11. Liu, N.; Landreh, M.; Cao, K.; Abe, M.; Hendriks, G.J.; Kennerdell, J.R.; Zhu, Y.; Wang, L.S.; Bonini, N.M. The microRNA mir-34 modulates ageing and neurodegeneration in drosophila. *Nature* **2012**, *482*, 519–523. [CrossRef] [PubMed]
12. Rokavec, M.; Li, H.; Jiang, L.; Hermeking, H. The p53/mir-34 axis in development and disease. *J. Mol. Cell Biol.* **2014**, *6*, 214–230. [CrossRef] [PubMed]
13. Jauhari, A.; Singh, T.; Singh, P.; Parmar, D.; Yadav, S. Regulation of mir-34 family in neuronal development. *Mol. Neurobiol.* **2018**, *55*, 936–945. [CrossRef] [PubMed]
14. Wu, J.; Bao, J.; Kim, M.; Yuan, S.; Tang, C.; Zheng, H.; Mastick, G.S.; Xu, C.; Yan, W. Two mirna clusters, mir-34b/c and mir-449, are essential for normal brain development, motile ciliogenesis, and spermatogenesis. *Proc. Nat.Acad. Sci. USA* **2014**, *111*, E2851–E2857. [CrossRef] [PubMed]
15. Agostini, M.; Tucci, P.; Steinert, J.R.; Shalom-Feuerstein, R.; Rouleau, M.; Aberdam, D.; Forsythe, I.D.; Young, K.W.; Ventura, A.; Concepcion, C.P.; et al. MicroRNA-34a regulates neurite outgrowth, spinal morphology, and function. *Proc. Nat.Acad. Sci. USA* **2011**, *108*, 21099–21104. [CrossRef] [PubMed]
16. Soni, K.; Choudhary, A.; Patowary, A.; Singh, A.R.; Bhatia, S.; Sivasubbu, S.; Chandrasekaran, S.; Pillai, B. Mir-34 is maternally inherited in drosophila melanogaster and danio rerio. *Nucleic Acids Res.* **2013**, *41*, 4470–4480. [CrossRef] [PubMed]
17. Fededa, J.P.; Esk, C.; Mierzwa, B.; Stanyte, R.; Yuan, S.; Zheng, H.; Ebnet, K.; Yan, W.; Knoblich, J.A.; Gerlich, D.W. MicroRNA-34/449 controls mitotic spindle orientation during mammalian cortex development. *EMBO J.* **2016**, *35*, 2386–2398. [CrossRef] [PubMed]
18. Wang, X.; Liu, P.; Zhu, H.; Xu, Y.; Ma, C.; Dai, X.; Huang, L.; Liu, Y.; Zhang, L.; Qin, C. miR-34a, a microRNA up-regulated in a double transgenic mouse model of Alzheimer's disease, inhibits bcl2 translation. *Brain Res. Bull.* **2009**, *80*, 268–273. [CrossRef] [PubMed]
19. Dickson, J.R.; Kruse, C.; Montagna, D.R.; Finsen, B.; Wolfe, M.S. Alternative polyadenylation and mir-34 family members regulate tau expression. *J. Neurochem.* **2013**, *127*, 739–749. [CrossRef] [PubMed]
20. Wu, H.; Huang, M.; Lu, M.; Zhu, W.; Shu, Y.; Cao, P.; Liu, P. Regulation of microtubule-associated protein tau (mapt) by mir-34c-5p determines the chemosensitivity of gastric cancer to paclitaxel. *Cancer Chemother. Pharmacol.* **2013**, *71*, 1159–1171. [CrossRef] [PubMed]
21. Uchizono, K. Characteristics of excitatory and inhibitory synapses in the central nervous system of the cat. *Nature* **1965**, *207*, 642–643. [CrossRef] [PubMed]
22. Attardo, A.; Fitzgerald, J.E.; Schnitzer, M.J. Impermanence of dendritic spines in live adult ca1 hippocampus. *Nature* **2015**, *523*, 592–596. [CrossRef] [PubMed]
23. Takashima, S.; Ieshima, A.; Nakamura, H.; Becker, L.E. Dendrites, dementia and the down syndrome. *Brain Dev.* **1989**, *11*, 131–133. [CrossRef]
24. Spires-Jones, T.; Knafo, S. Spines, plasticity, and cognition in Alzheimer's model mice. *Neural Plast.* **2012**, *2012*, 319836. [CrossRef] [PubMed]
25. DeKosky, S.T.; Scheff, S.W. Synapse loss in frontal cortex biopsies in Alzheimer's disease: Correlation with cognitive severity. *Ann. Neurol.* **1990**, *27*, 457–464. [CrossRef] [PubMed]

26. Terry, R.D.; Masliah, E.; Salmon, D.P.; Butters, N.; DeTeresa, R.; Hill, R.; Hansen, L.A.; Katzman, R. Physical basis of cognitive alterations in Alzheimer's disease: Synapse loss is the major correlate of cognitive impairment. *Ann. Neurol.* **1991**, *30*, 572–580. [CrossRef] [PubMed]
27. Selkoe, D.J. Alzheimer's disease is a synaptic failure. *Science* **2002**, *298*, 789–791. [CrossRef] [PubMed]
28. Baloyannis, S.J. Dendritic pathology in Alzheimer's disease. *J. Neurol. Sci.* **2009**, *283*, 153–157. [CrossRef] [PubMed]
29. Spruston, N. Pyramidal neurons: Dendritic structure and synaptic integration. *Nat. Rev. Neurosci.* **2008**, *9*, 206–221. [CrossRef] [PubMed]
30. Catala, I.; Ferrer, I.; Galofre, E.; Fabregues, I. Decreased numbers of dendritic spines on cortical pyramidal neurons in dementia. A quantitative golgi study on biopsy samples. *Hum. Neurobiol.* **1988**, *6*, 255–259. [PubMed]
31. Einstein, G.; Buranosky, R.; Crain, B.J. Dendritic pathology of granule cells in Alzheimer's disease is unrelated to neuritic plaques. *J. Neurosci.* **1994**, *14*, 5077–5088. [CrossRef] [PubMed]
32. Androuin, A.; Potier, B.; Nagerl, U.V.; Cattaert, D.; Danglot, L.; Thierry, M.; Youssef, I.; Triller, A.; Duyckaerts, C.; El Hachimi, K.H.; et al. Evidence for altered dendritic spine compartmentalization in Alzheimer's disease and functional effects in a mouse model. *Acta Neuropathol.* **2018**, *135*, 839–854. [CrossRef] [PubMed]
33. Berry, K.P.; Nedivi, E. Spine dynamics: Are they all the same? *Neuron* **2017**, *96*, 43–55. [CrossRef] [PubMed]
34. Zuo, Y.; Lin, A.; Chang, P.; Gan, W.B. Development of long-term dendritic spine stability in diverse regions of cerebral cortex. *Neuron* **2005**, *46*, 181–189. [CrossRef] [PubMed]
35. Kasai, H.; Matsuzaki, M.; Noguchi, J.; Yasumatsu, N.; Nakahara, H. Structure-stability-function relationships of dendritic spines. *Trends Neurosci.* **2003**, *26*, 360–368. [CrossRef]
36. Tada, T.; Sheng, M. Molecular mechanisms of dendritic spine morphogenesis. *Curr. Opin. Neurobiol.* **2006**, *16*, 95–101. [CrossRef] [PubMed]
37. Codocedo, J.F.; Allard, C.; Godoy, J.A.; Varela-Nallar, L.; Inestrosa, N.C. Sirt1 regulates dendritic development in hippocampal neurons. *PLoS ONE* **2012**, *7*, e47073. [CrossRef] [PubMed]
38. Lamprecht, R.; LeDoux, J. Structural plasticity and memory. *Nat. Rev. Neurosci.* **2004**, *5*, 45–54. [CrossRef] [PubMed]
39. Haditsch, U.; Leone, D.P.; Farinelli, M.; Chrostek-Grashoff, A.; Brakebusch, C.; Mansuy, I.M.; McConnell, S.K.; Palmer, T.D. A central role for the small gtpase rac1 in hippocampal plasticity and spatial learning and memory. *Mol. Cell. Neurosci.* **2009**, *41*, 409–419. [CrossRef] [PubMed]
40. Vadodaria, K.C.; Jessberger, S. Maturation and integration of adult born hippocampal neurons: Signal convergence onto small rho gtpases. *Front. Synaptic Neurosci.* **2013**, *5*, 4. [CrossRef] [PubMed]
41. Nakayama, A.Y.; Harms, M.B.; Luo, L. Small gtpases rac and rho in the maintenance of dendritic spines and branches in hippocampal pyramidal neurons. *J. Neurosci.* **2000**, *20*, 5329–5338. [CrossRef] [PubMed]
42. Hedrick, N.G.; Yasuda, R. Regulation of rho gtpase proteins during spine structural plasticity for the control of local dendritic plasticity. *Curr. Opin. Neurobiol.* **2017**, *45*, 193–201. [CrossRef] [PubMed]
43. Nakayama, A.Y.; Luo, L. Intracellular signaling pathways that regulate dendritic spine morphogenesis. *Hippocampus* **2000**, *10*, 582–586. [CrossRef]
44. Schumacher, S.; Franke, K. miR-124-regulated RhoG: A conductor of neuronal process complexity. *Small GTPases* **2013**, *4*, 42–46. [CrossRef] [PubMed]
45. Castaneda, P.; Munoz, M.; Garcia-Rojo, G.; Ulloa, J.L.; Bravo, J.A.; Marquez, R.; Garcia-Perez, M.A.; Arancibia, D.; Araneda, K.; Rojas, P.S.; et al. Association of n-cadherin levels and downstream effectors of rho gtpases with dendritic spine loss induced by chronic stress in rat hippocampal neurons. *J. Neurosci. Res.* **2015**, *93*, 1476–1491. [CrossRef] [PubMed]
46. Huang, B.; Jolly, M.K.; Lu, M.; Tsarfaty, I.; Ben-Jacob, E.; Onuchic, J.N. Modeling the transitions between collective and solitary migration phenotypes in cancer metastasis. *Sci. Rep.* **2015**, *5*, 17379. [CrossRef] [PubMed]
47. Bustos, F.J.; Ampuero, E.; Jury, N.; Aguilar, R.; Falahi, F.; Toledo, J.; Ahumada, J.; Lata, J.; Cubillos, P.; Henriquez, B.; et al. Epigenetic editing of the *Dlg4*/PSD95 gene improves cognition in aged and Alzheimer's disease mice. *Brain* **2017**, *140*, 3252–3268. [CrossRef] [PubMed]

7

Semantic Priming in Mild Cognitive Impairment and Healthy Subjects: Effect of Different Time of Presentation of Word-Pairs

Valeria Guglielmi [1], Davide Quaranta [1,*], Ilaria Mega [2], Emanuele Maria Costantini [2], Claudia Carrarini [2], Alice Innocenti [2] and Camillo Marra [2,3]

1 Neurology Unit, Fondazione Policlinico Agostino Gemelli-IRCCS, 00168 Rome, Italy; valeria.guglielmi@policlinicogemelli.it
2 Department of Neuroscience, Catholic University of Sacred Heart, 00168 Rome, Italy; ilaria.mega@gmail.com (I.M.); emanule.m.costantini@gmail.com (E.M.C.); claudia.carrarini@live.it (C.C.); linceinnocenti@gmail.com (A.I.); camillo.marra@policlinicogemelli.it (C.M.)
3 Memory Clinic, Fondazione Policlinico Universitario Agostino Gemelli-IRCCS, 00168 Rome, Italy
* Correspondence: davide.quaranta@policlinicogemelli.it

Abstract: Introduction: Semantic memory is impaired in mild cognitive impairment (MCI). Two main hypotheses about this finding are debated and refer to the degradation of stored knowledge versus the impairment of semantic access mechanisms. The aim of our study is to evaluate semantic impairment in MCI versus healthy subjects (HS) by an experiment evaluating semantic priming. **Methods**: We enrolled 27 MCI and 20 HS. MCI group were divided, according to follow up, into converters-MCI and non converters-MCI. The semantic task consisted of 108 pairs of words, 54 of which were semantically associated. Stimuli were presented 250 or 900 ms later the appearance of the target in a randomized manner. Data were analyzed using factorial ANOVA. **Results**: Both HS and MCI answered more quickly for word than for non-word at both stimulus onset asynchrony (SOA) intervals. At 250 ms, both MCI and HS experienced a shorter time of response for related-word than for unrelated words (priming effect), while only the converters-MCI subgroup lost the priming effect. Further, we observed a rather larger Cohen's d effect size in non converters-MCI than in converters-MCI. **Conclusion**: Our data, and in particular the absence of a semantic priming effect in converters-MCI, could reflect the impairment of semantic knowledge rather than the accessibility of semantic stores in MCI individuals that progress to dementia.

Keywords: Alzheimer disease; semantic priming; mild cognitive impairment

---

1. Introduction

Alzheimer's disease (AD) is a degenerative process that, in its typical evolution, proceeds in the early stages from the medial perirhinal cortex to the entorhinal, and finally, the hippocampus cortex [1]. Memory disorders are consequently the first symptoms of the disease and episodic memory has been always considered a neuropsychological diagnostic marker of AD. Since the medial perirhinal cortex is deeply involved in the organization of item recollection and general knowledge, it is conceivable that impairment of semantic memory could precede that of episodic memory in the early stages of AD [2]. As a matter of fact, subjects with mild AD experienced lower scores on tests of object naming [3–5], and categorical verbal fluency [2,6–8]. Moreover, low performances in different semantic memory tasks have been also reported in mild AD [9–12], with categorical verbal fluency tasks being found impaired in mild cognitive impairment (MCI) [13,14]. Some authors focused on specific deficits of semantic memory emphasizing the presence of an early and specific deficit in naming and knowing of famous people in MCI patients [15]. Other authors explored specific linguistic markers of degradation of the semantic system, such as frequency, age of acquisition (AoA), familiarity and typicality of the words produced in both category fluency tasks [16–18] or procedural speaking in famous writers [19]. Most studies have shown that AD and MCI patients tend to produce, as the disease progresses, more frequent, more typical and early acquired words [20–24].

Nevertheless, the nature of semantic impairment in the early stage of AD is still controversial. Two main hypotheses have been suggested. The first refers the semantic memory deficits to progressive degradation of the stored knowledge; the second suggests an inability of patients to timely recollect the semantic knowledge cause of a deficit of the mechanism that guarantees the access to the information. In this latter case, executive and phonological verbal mechanisms are hypothesized, and worse category fluency was interpreted as a deficit in access to semantic system [25].

The two explanation are not mutually exclusive and probably describe a simple progression of the degradation of the semantic system. Duong et al. studied both automatic and intentional access to the semantic system in a cohort of MCI and AD subjects. They found that the MCI group was only impaired on tasks of intentional access while the AD group was impaired on both types of tasks. This study would suggest that impaired access to the semantic system in MCI precede semantic store degradation observed in AD.

On the other hand, some authors sustain the hypothesis of early semantic degradation from the beginning [9,26–29]. The disproportionate impairment in category fluency relative to letter-based fluency—that is particularly sensitive to executive damage [5,30]—come out on the side of this.

We have previously investigated some aspects of the semantic system, regarding semantic fluency, specifically the typicality of words produced in a semantic verbal fluency task [23]. Our results showed that the MCI group produced more typical words in comparison with the healthy group, while no differences in typicality were observed within the MCI and AD group. These results were interpreted in term of a progressive disruption of semantic system organization, leading the patients to retrieve more typical items of specific categories in respect to less prototypical elements. Our groups also reported that MCI individuals who will eventually progress to dementia produce words that are less related than the ones produced by healthy controls and stable MCI in a category fluency test [31]. This evidence can be interpreted as an effect of reduced strength of conceptual links between items belonging to a given category.

In previous works, semantic priming (SP) has been used to explore the semantic system automatically; SP is an experimental condition of a lexical decision based on the fact that subjects are faster and more accurate in recognizing a target word when it follows a related word as a prime than when it follows an unrelated word [32]. When it happens in a brief interstimulus interval (250 ms or less), the priming effect is automatic and is not influenced by preparatory or intentional strategies [33]. The prime word automatically and diffusely activates the semantic network, allowing a faster recognition of the target word. Several explanations of the priming effect have been proposed. According to the classical spread-activation hypothesis, the retrieval of an item from memory requires the activation of its conceptual representation. The activation can spread to related concepts, that in turn will be more easily retrieved [34]. The compound-cue models claim that a cue to memory contains the target item and other items of the surrounding context. In this model, a relevant effect of familiarity on priming effect is predicted, since cues formed by related words will be more familiar than cues formed by unrelated words, explaining the shorter reaction times in the case of related words [34]. Finally, distributed network models have been developed. According to the so-called proximity models, priming is observed because related primes and targets are close to each other in a high-dimensional semantic space [35]. The semantic proximity models claim that concepts are represented by patterns of activity over interconnected conceptual units, and that related concepts share similar patterns of activity. The other category of distributed models, referred to as learning models [34], attributes SP to incremental learning. In fact, each presentation of a word causes an alteration of the network connections, increasing the probability of producing the same response to the same input, including semantically related targets. According to this class of models, the decay of learning can be very slow, and may cause SP also over long SOAs. The models of SP are embedded in general conceptualizations of semantic memory based on observations obtained from other typologies of investigations. In Alzheimer's disease and MCI, previous studies suggest that spread-activation models or more complex proximity models could be satisfactory to explain the disruption of lexical-semantic system [31,36].

The previous studies on SP in AD have reported contrasting results. Some authors found less-than-normal priming (hypo-priming) in Alzheimer's disease patients compared with controls [37–39], while others reported no differences on priming in AD vs. Healthy subjects [40,41] or even paradoxical increased priming effects (hyper-priming) in Alzheimer's disease patients [42–47]. These opposed results may reflect some differences in the methods used, and also clinical heterogeneity in the samples of individuals studied. The severity of dementia, and therefore of semantic deficits, differed from one study to another, leading to different results in semantic tasks, SP included. Furthermore, the type of paradigm between the prime and the target, that maybe, superordinate, coordinate, or attribute, seems able to influence the priming effects observed. When the semantic relationship is based on the superordinate category, a normal priming effect was observed [41,48,49], while hypo-priming is more frequently reported in experiments in which the target is an attribute of the prime [48,50,51]. Finally, when the prime and the target belong to the same category (coordinate condition) [46,48,49] hypo- or hyper priming is observed.

Few studies have investigated SP in mild cognitive impairment. Duong et al. [25] reported that MCI and healthy individuals both reported SP effect. The same authors, instead, reported that the MCI group was impaired on tasks that required intentional access to the semantic system, suggesting that in early stages of AD, the involvement of the semantic system concerns access to its first.

The aim of the present study is to clarify the subtle semantic impairment in the MCI condition by studying the behavior to an SP paradigm in comparison to a population of healthy subjects (HS). First, we want to verify if a different behavior can be observed in MCI compared with HS and to understand the meaning of the observed behavior. From a theoretical point of view, if in MCI condition patients experienced an early degradation of the semantic system, consequently they do not benefit from SP. On the contrary, if there is difficult access to the semantic system, the semantic facilitation of priming allows a faster time of answer, especially at the brief, pre-attentional interstimulus interval.

2. Materials and Methods

We enrolled 27 individuals with amnestic MCI and 20 age- and education-matched HS. In the patient groups, all subjects underwent a clinical evaluation including medical history, physical and neurological examination, and an extensive neuropsychological evaluation and MRI scans. All the subjects of our sample were native Italian speakers and none of them had a history of traumatic head injury, alcoholism, epilepsy, stroke, nor other relevant neurologic, psychiatric, and general medical diseases. MCI was diagnosed following clinical criteria [52]; the diagnosis of Alzheimer's Disease was based on current clinical criteria [53]. MCI subjects were evaluated after 12 and 24 months. At follow up, patients were assessed according to the clinical dementia rating scale and activity daily living scales. Dementia was diagnosed when CDR >1 and functional impairment were found. Eleven MCI progressed to overt dementia at the 24 months follow-up.

2.1. Neuropsychological Examination

Patients were diagnosed as amnesic MCI after administration of the Mini Mental State examination and a comprehensive battery including learning and long term memory (Rey's Auditory Verbal Learning test- RAVLT) [54]; executive functions (Stroop's test; [55]); visual search and attention (Multiple Features Target Cancellation, MFTC; [56]); working memory (digit span forwards and backwards; [57]); abstract reasoning (Raven's progressive matrices, PM'47; [54]); constructional praxis (copy of figures without and with Landmarks; [54]). Verbal fluency was examined by phonological [54] and categorical verbal fluency tasks [58].

2.2. *Lexical and Semantic Priming Procedure*

The task consisted of 216 pairs of stimuli (prime-target). Each target stimulus was a word or a non-word preceded by a prime word. Patients were required to decide if the target was a word or not as fast as possible. In total, 108 pairs were a word–non word couple and 108 pairs were a word–word couple. In total, 54 out of the 108 word–word couples were semantically related. The primer–target couples were controlled for word frequency [59]. Stimuli were presented at different intervals of response to the prime and the appearance of the target (SOA) of 250 and 900 ms (Figure 1). The order of appearance of the pairs of word–non word and word–word at different SOA was randomized for each subject. Words were presented in Italian (English translation of the words is reported in the Appendix A). Our task was built with OpenSesame software and was administered by means of a 15″ laptop posed at 0.5 mt from the individual, who had to respond by pressing one out of two buttons marked with a "yes" or "no" label. Time of response for each item was recorded.

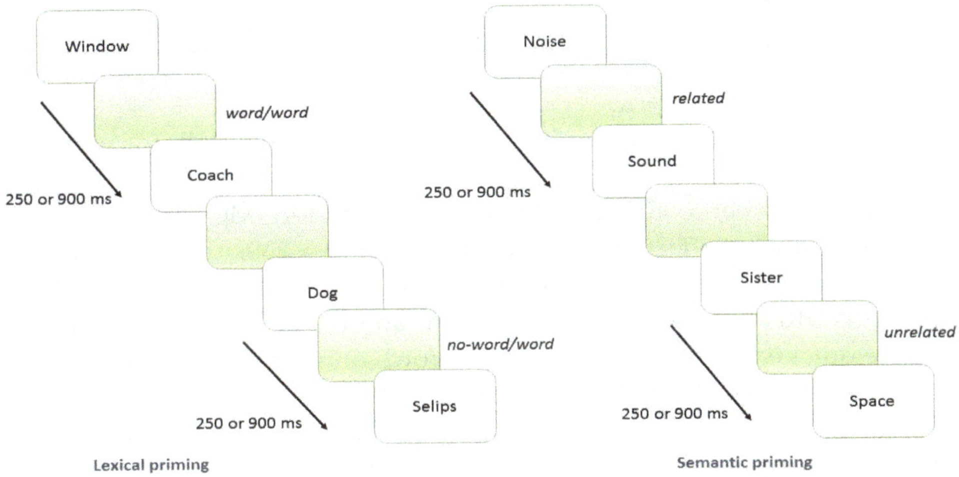

Figure 1. Assessment of the lexical and semantic priming tasks.

We evaluated the 'lexicality effect'; that is, the faster recognition of words compared to non-words. The lexicality effect has been computed as the difference between the mean reaction time between response after that the priming was a word. The 'SP effect' was calculated as the difference in the mean reaction time to word that was preceded by semantically related or semantically unrelated word.

3. Results

MCI and HS were similar in age (MCI: mean age = 72.79; DS = 5.090; HS: mean age = 69.44; DS = 5.515; p = 0.115) and educational level (MCI: mean = 11.61; DS = 2.909; HS: mean = 13.12; DS = 2.711; p = 0.193). At 24 months follow up, 11 subjects (45.8%) were diagnosed as affected by Alzheimer Disease. Then, according to the progression or not to dementia, we divided MCI group in non converters-MCI (*n.* 13) and converters-MCI (*n.* 11).

3.1. *Lexicality Effect*

Both at 250 ms and 900 ms, the factorial ANOVAs comparing MCI vs. HS showed a significant effect of the GROUP factors (F = 458; p <0.001 and F = 441; p<0.001 respectively), WORD factors (word vs. non-word) (F = 1072; $p < 0.001$ and F = 1166; $p < 0.001$ respectively) and of interaction GROUP × WORD (F = 23; $p < 0.001$ and F = 42; $p < 0.001$, respectively).

Table 1 shows response times of the two groups at 250 and 900 ms. Both HS and MCI answered more quickly for word than for non-word, regardless of the presence of a semantic connection between prime and target.

Table 1. Lexicality effect.

	HS		MCI			Non Converters-MCI		Converters-MCI		
SOA 250 ms										
	Mean	**SD**	**Mean**	**SD**	*P*	**Mean**	**SD**	**Mean**	**SD**	*p*
Words	813.37	248.266	1046.15	375.320	<0.001	1052.94	366.878	1036.24	387.545	n.s.
No words	1205.38	483.902	1573.38	471.991	<0.001	1547.61	480.800	1610.85	456.888	n.s.
p	<0.001		<0.001			<0.001		<0.001		
SOA 900 ms										
	Mean	**SD**	**Mean**	**SD**	*P*	**Mean**	**SD**	**Mean**	**SD**	*p*
Words	808.15	247.161	1002.23	331.279	<0.001	996.86	323.493	1010.02	342.552	n.s.
No words	1177.64	460.944	1543.75	462.437	<0.001	1519.25	468.131	1579.34	452.266	n.s.
p	<0.001		<0.001			<0.001		<0.001		

Similarly, patients with MCI were significantly slower than HS both for words ($p < 0.001$) and non-words ($p < 0.001$).

In the comparison between converters-MCI, non converters-MCI and HS at 250 and 900 ms, ANOVA confirmed a significant effect of the GROUP factors ($F = 230$; $p < 0.001$ at 250 ms and $F = 223$; $p < 0.001$ at 900 ms), WORD ($F = 1144$; $p < 0.001$ at 250 ms, and $F = 1267$; $p < 0.001$ at 900 ms) and of the interaction GROUP x WORD ($F = 14$; $p < 0.001$ at 250 ms and $F = 22$; $p < 0.001$ at 900 ms). Both HS and MCI answered more quickly for word than for non-word; non converters-MCI and converters-MCI were significantly slower than HS both for words ($p < 0.001$) that for non-words ($p < 0.001$); the answers time of converters-MCI were not significantly different for the response times of subjects with converters-MCI, both in the presence of words ($p = 0.166$) and in the presence of non-words ($p = 0.9$).

3.1.1. Priming Effect at SOA 250 ms

To evaluate the priming effect, we have considered only reaction times of word–word pairs, comparing semantically related to semantically unrelated pairs of words.

The ANOVA analysis (considering the whole group of MCIs) showed a significant effect of the GROUP factor ($F = 131.6$; $p < 0.001$) and 'Semantic Relation' Factor (REL) ($F = 20.9$; $p < 0.001$) but not of the interaction between the two ($F = 0.2$; $p < 0.678$). On Table 2 are reported the reaction times in the two conditions (pairs of correlated first-target or unrelated strings).

The post-hoc analysis showed that for both related pairs and unrelated words. HS answered more quickly than MCI (in both cases, $p < 0.001$). The response times for related words were lower than the response times for unrelated words in both in HS and MCI (see Table 2). The Cohen's d show only a little effect size in both groups.

In the comparison between non converters-MCI, converters-MCI and HS, ANOVA showed a significant effect of the GROUP factors ($F = 69.9$; $p < 0.001$) and REL ($F = 20.2$; $p < 0.001$) but not of the interaction between the two ($F = 0.4$; $p < 0.650$). On Table 2 is reported the reaction times in the two conditions (pairs of correlated first-target or unrelated strings) in the three groups (non converters-MCI, converters-MCI and HS).

Table 2. Priming Effect at SOAs 250 ms and 900 ms.

	HS		MCI		No Converters-MCI		Converters-MCI	
SOA 250 ms								
	Mean	**SD**	**Mean**	**SD**	**Mean**	**SD**	**Mean**	**SD**
Related words	778.27	187.428	944.01	248.428	969.00	229.787	923.58	261.521
Unrelated words	814.46	212.969	985.38	253.232	1029.33	246.156	949.46	253.915
p	0.015		0.003		0.038		0.321	
Cohen's d	0.18		0.17		**0.25**		0.10	
SOA 900 ms								
	Mean	**SD**	**Mean**	**SD**	**Mean**	**SD**	**Mean**	**SD**
Related words	776.68	214.317	922.60	234.317	930.11	220.048	913.64	250.716
Unrelated words	806.21	204.353	962.37	242.047	982.23	244.109	938.63	238.152
p	0.071		0.003		0.010		0.745	
Cohen's d	0.07		0.17		**0.22**		0.10	

In this condition, we observed a rather larger Cohen's d effect size in non converters-MCI than in converters-MCI. In particular, the effect size in the converters-MCI was similar to the HS group.

The post-hoc analysis showed that for both the related and the unrelated pairs of words, the HS answered more quickly than the subjects non converters-MCI or converters-MCI ($p < 0.001$ in all cases). Response times for related words were shorter than response times for unrelated words in HS and non converters-MCI, but not in converters-MCI (see Table 2). Although both non converters-MCI and HS show a similar priming effect, the Cohen's d is different between these two groups suggesting that the priming in non converters-MCI is preserved only at the cost a higher discrepancy between the two conditions (with related and unrelated words).

3.1.2. Priming Effect at 900 ms

ANOVA analysis showed a significant effect of the GROUP factors ($F = 115.6$; $p < 0.001$) and REL ($F = 17.2$; $p < 0.001$). No interaction between GROUP and REL was found ($F = 0.5$; $p = 0.488$). Table 2 (upper part) reports the mean values of reaction times in the two conditions in HS and MCI.

The post-hoc analysis showed that HS answered more quickly than MCI both for the related pairs and the unrelated words ($p < 0.001$). In HS, the response times for related words did not differ from response time for unrelated words, while MCI answered more quickly for related words that for unrelated words.

Comparing non converters-MCI, converters-MCI and HS, ANOVA showed a significant effect of the GROUP factors ($F = 53.4$; $p < 0.001$) and REL ($F = 16.0$; $p < 0.001$), but no interaction between the two ($F = 0.96$; $p < 0.383$). On Table 2 are reported the means of reaction times in the two conditions in the three groups.

The post-hoc analysis showed that HS had shorter reaction times than non converters-MCI and converters-MCI for both related and unrelated words ($p < 0.001$ in all cases).

Comparing response times for related words vs. unrelated words among the three group, non converters-MCI answered more quickly for related pairs than for unrelated ones, while HS and converters-MCI did not differ in reaction times among related and unrelated words. (see Table 2). The Cohen's d effect size shows that this effect was higher in non converters-MCI than in bot converters-MCI and HS.

4. Discussion

Our data seem to confirm the hypothesis of early degradation of the semantic system in MCI.

A first consideration regards times of reaction: in all tasks, MCI answered significantly slower than HC. These findings are in line with previous studies about priming [42–44,49]. Despite the slower time of reactions, in our sample, lexicality effect was equally represented in HC and MCI, even after splitting MCI in non converters-MCI and converters-MCI. Lexicality effect reflects a physiological learning mechanism: the repeated exposition to verbal stimulus encourages the creation of phonological, syntactic and semantic representations of stimuli. This phenomenon does not happen when stimuli are non words. Our data confirm general findings of the integrity of the phonological, orthographic and syntactic system in early AD. Furthermore, in our study, the presence of lexicality effect in the MCI group demonstrate a good lexical activation and lexical access, even if it happens slower than in HS.

Our data show that at the shorter interval, both HS and MCI had SP effect; nevertheless, when MCI group was divided according to progression to AD, the converters-MCI group lost SP effect, while non converters-MCI had same behavior that HS. At 900 ms, HS lost priming effect, because of the intervention of attentional, strategic and inhibitory mechanisms. Non converters-MCI still showed priming effect, probably because they experienced slower reaction time, and consequently a slower activation of the attentional system. In converters-MCI no priming effect was found, as in the 250 ms interstimulus condition.

In our study MCI group globally considered does not differ from HS, partly because of the intrinsic heterogeneity of MCI population, who belong to subjects with prodromal AD and subjects without progressive memory deficit.

Nevertheless, it is very interesting that the MCI group behaved differently according to disease progression: non converters-MCI had normal priming effect as HS, while converters-MCI lost priming effect. Further, non converters-MCI experienced a larger effect size than converters-MCI; this means that non converters-MCI carry out a greater effort to maintain a SP effect in a compensatory manner. Instead, converters-MCI does not experience any compensatory strategy. This phenomenon happens both at 250 ms and at 900 ms.

These results deserve several considerations: first, the loss of priming effect in converters-MCI—that can be considered as prodromal AD—suggests that semantic system is early impaired regardless of executive functions from the beginning in AD; according to the hypothesis of a semantic store degradation, even in MCI, the priming effect disappears in our converters-MCI because the relationship within semantically close words is lost, preventing the activation of the semantic system or making it ineffective to generate priming effect. This explanation is in line with previous reports about the linguistic features of words produced in the semantic fluency task, by meaning the tendency to generate words with higher typicality and early AoA [20–24]. A possible explanation is that the progressive reduction of the knowledge of the attributes of objects and the relations between similar entities can cause the loss of SP effect that is the counterpart of difficulties observed in the semantic fluency tasks. In general, our findings could be accounted by spread-activation models, or proximity class of diffuse network models, in accordance to previous evidence from studies on semantic fluency [31,36]. On the other hand, learning models are not supported by our findings, since we observed a loss of SP over a long SOA in HS [34].

Some characteristics of the semantic system can help to support our findings. In their study, Mulatti et al. described the cumulative semantic effect in healthy subjects and MCI [51]. The cumulative semantic interference effect refers to a linear increase in the picture naming reaction times which is a function of the already named pictures belonging to the same semantic category to which the named picture belongs. In the author's opinion, this phenomenon is due to the interaction between different cognitive processes involved in picture naming as shared activation, priming and competition: when a representation is activated in the lexicon upon the presentation of a picture, the lexical representations of semantically related items are also activated (shared activation); the activated no-target lexical representations compete with the target lexical representation in a mutually inhibitory way (competition), thus slowing down processing, while any retrieval of a lexical representation facilitates its subsequent retrieval (priming). Analogously, even if in a different experimental condition, in our experiment we observed lexicality effect, but not SP effect in our MCI patients that progress to AD. Our data support the evidence of a loss of cumulative semantic interference effect in MCI converters that could rely on the lack of the shared activation of the semantic features belonging to same categories of knowledge, while the lexical priming still works in the early stages of AD.

The study has several limitations, including the relatively small number of subjects included. MCI patients were diagnosed as MCI due to AD according to clinical and imaging data, but without biomarkers confirmation. However, the rather long follow-up period reduces the possibility of inaccurate identification of MCI individuals both at the baseline and at the follow-up. Furthermore, the number of MCI patients who progressed to dementia is rather low; thus, it is possible that we were not able to detect the SP effect in converters-MCI because of insufficient statistical power. Nevertheless, the number of non-converters MCI was comparable to the number of converters-MCI, yet we were able to detect a significant SP effect, with a Cohen's d higher than the one observed in HS. However, a cautious interpretation of our results is mandatory.

5. Conclusions

In conclusion, our data are of same interest from a theoretical and clinical point of view. As for the theoretical significance, the SP seems a good paradigm to detect subclinical deficit of the semantic system in the early stages of the AD pathology. From a clinical point of view, the different behavior between non converters-MCI and converters-MCI at the SP suggests that this paradigm could be a practical method for evaluating semantic memory in subjects with MCI. If confirmed in larger samples, these results may have significant prognostic and therapeutic implications.

Author Contributions: Concept and design: V.G., D.Q., I.M., C.M. Acquisition, analysis, or interpretation of data: All authors. Drafting of the manuscript: V.G.; D.Q., C.M. Critical revision of the manuscript for important intellectual content: All authors. Statistical analysis: D.Q. Supervision: C.M., D.Q. All authors have read and agreed to the published version of the manuscript.

Appendix A List of Items

TARGET WORD	RELATED PRIME	UNRELATED PRIME
vinegar	Salad	Hawk
student	Schoolchildren	Peacock
aerial	Cable	Walnut
banana	Gorilla	Die
mouth	Tongue	Species
orange	Peel	Sign
Dog	Peace	Owner
song	Voice	Point
horse	Animal	Example
colour	Red	Need
deluge	Thunder	Ram
dragon	fairy tales	Lip
grass	Lawn	People
summer	Sun	Land
river	Water	Game
giraffe	Height	Accent
Trip	Coach	Gasp
Ant	Bug	Candle
winter	Snow	Number
lake	Fish	Time
snail	Shell	Wax
mum	Sun	News

Sea	Island	Year
pencil	Case	Diamond
mule	Stable	Witch
nose	Face	Day
Ship	Voat	Arm
grandchild	Family	Answer
gandfather	Father	Bottom
track	Trace	Fear
vegetable garden	Vegetable	Loft
package	Courier	Bundle
planet	Heart	Minute
Rain	Weather	Type
spider	Venom	Steam
noise	Sound	Begin
classroom	School	Cold
seed	Grain	Injury
sister	Brother	Space
sauce	Tomato	Sheet
nest	Hibernation	Paint
roof	House	Name
cough	Sickness	Can
trumpet	Brass	Mill
coach	Binary	Steak
wind	Air	Part
worm	Maggot	Elf
volcano	Eruption	Reflex
Paw	Claw	Door
mosquito	Sting	Chest

References

1. Taylor, K.I.; Probst, A. Anatomic localization of the transentorhinal region of the perirhinal cortex. *Neurobiol. Aging* **2008**, *29*, 1591–1596. [CrossRef] [PubMed]
2. Bejanin, A.; Schonhaut, D.R.; La Joie, R.; Kramer, J.H.; Baker, S.L.; Sosa, N.; Ayakta, N.; Cantwell, A.; Janabi, M.; Lauriola, M.; et al. Tau pathology and neurodegeneration contribute to cognitive impairment in Alzheimer's disease. *Brain J. Neurol.* **2017**, *140*, 3286–3300. [CrossRef] [PubMed]
3. Martin, A.; Fedio, P. Word production and comprehension in Alzheimer's disease: The breakdown of semantic knowledge. *Brain Lang.* **1983**, *19*, 124–141. [CrossRef]
4. Huff, F.J.; Collins, C.; Corkin, S.; Rosen, T.J. Equivalent forms of the Boston Naming Test. *J. Clin. Exp. Neuropsychol.* **1986**, *8*, 556–562. [CrossRef]
5. Hodges, J.R.; Salmon, D.P.; Butters, N. Semantic memory impairment in Alzheimer's disease: Failure of access or degraded knowledge? *Neuropsychologia* **1992**, *30*, 301–314. [CrossRef]
6. Ober, B.A.; Dronkers, N.F.; Koss, E.; Delis, D.C.; Friedland, R.P. Retrieval from semantic memory in Alzheimer-type dementia. *J. Clin. Exp. Neuropsychol.* **1986**, *8*, 75–92. [CrossRef]
7. Tröster, A.I.; Salmon, D.P.; McCullough, D.; Butters, N. A comparison of the category fluency deficits associated with Alzheimer's and Huntington's disease. *Brain Lang.* **1989**, *37*, 500–513. [CrossRef]
8. Bayles, K.A.; Tomoeda, C.K.; Trosset, M.W. Naming and categorical knowledge in Alzheimer's disease: The process of semantic memory deterioration. *Brain Lang.* **1990**, *39*, 498–510. [CrossRef]
9. Hodges, J.R.; Patterson, K. Is semantic memory consistently impaired early in the course of Alzheimer's disease? Neuroanatomical and diagnostic implications. *Neuropsychologia* **1995**, *33*, 441–459. [CrossRef]
10. Monsch, A.U.; Bondi, M.W.; Butters, N.; Salmon, D.P.; Katzman, R.; Thal, L.J. Comparisons of verbal fluency tasks in the detection of dementia of the Alzheimer type. *Arch. Neurol.* **1992**, *49*, 1253–1258. [CrossRef] [PubMed]

11. Nutter-Upham, K.E.; Saykin, A.J.; Rabin, L.A.; Roth, R.M.; Wishart, H.A.; Pare, N.; Flashman, L.A. Verbal fluency performance in amnestic MCI and older adults with cognitive complaints. *Arch. Clin. Neuropsychol.* **2008**, *23*, 229–241. [CrossRef]
12. Adlam, A.L.; Bozeat, S.; Arnold, R.; Watson, P.; Hodges, J.R. Semantic knowledge in mild cognitive impairment and mild Alzheimer's disease. *Cortex* **2006**, *42*, 675–684. [CrossRef]
13. Murphy, K.J.; Rich, J.B.; Troyer, A.K. Verbal fluency patterns in amnestic mild cognitive impairment are characteristic of Alzheimer's type dementia. *J. Int. Neuropsychol. Soc.* **2006**, *12*, 570–574. [CrossRef] [PubMed]
14. Amieva, H.; Letenneur, L.; Dartigues, J.F.; Rouch-Leroyer, I.; Sourgen, C.; D'Alchee-Biree, F.; Dib, M.; Barberger-Gateau, P.; Orgogozo, J.M.; Fabrigoule, C. Annual rate and predictors of conversion to dementia in subjects presenting mild cognitive impairment criteria defined according to a population-based study. *Dement. Geriatr. Cogn. Disord.* **2004**, *18*, 87–93. [CrossRef] [PubMed]
15. Joubert, S.; Brambati, S.M.; Ansado, J.; Barbeau, E.J.; Felician, O.; Didic, M.; Lacombe, J.; Goldstein, R.; Chayer, C.; Kergoat, M.J. The cognitive and neural expression of semantic memory impairment in mild cognitive impairment and early Alzheimer's disease. *Neuropsychologia* **2010**, *48*, 978–988. [CrossRef]
16. Schilling, H.E.H.; Rayner, K.; Chumbley, J.I. Comparing naming, lexical decision, and eye fixation times: Word frequency effects and individual differences. *Mem. Cognit.* **1998**, *26*, 1270–1281. [CrossRef]
17. Juhasz, B.J. Age-of-acquisition effects in word and picture identification. *Psychol. Bull.* **2005**, *131*, 684–712. [CrossRef]
18. Holmes, S.J.; Jane Fitch, F.; Ellis, A.W. Age of acquisition affects object recognition and naming in patients with Alzheimer's disease. *J. Clin. Exp. Neuropsychol.* **2006**, *28*, 1010–1022. [CrossRef]
19. Garrard, P.; Maloney, L.M.; Hodges, J.R.; Patterson, K. The effects of very early Alzheimer's disease on the characteristics of writing by a renowned author. *Brain J. Neurol.* **2005**, *128*, 250–260. [CrossRef]
20. Forbes-McKay, K.E.; Ellis, A.W.; Shanks, M.F.; Venneri, A. The age of acquisition of words produced in a semantic fluency task can reliably differentiate normal from pathological age related cognitive decline. *Neuropsychologia* **2005**, *43*, 1625–1632. [CrossRef]
21. Sailor, K.M.; Zimmerman, M.E.; Sanders, A.E. Differential impacts of age of acquisition on letter and semantic fluency in Alzheimer's disease patients and healthy older adults. *Q. J. Exp. Psychol.* **2011**, *64*, 2383–2391. [CrossRef] [PubMed]
22. Venneri, A.; McGeown, W.J.; Hietanen, H.M.; Guerrini, C.; Ellis, A.W.; Shanks, M.F. The anatomical bases of semantic retrieval deficits in early Alzheimer's disease. *Neuropsychologia* **2008**, *46*, 497–510. [CrossRef] [PubMed]
23. Vita, M.G.; Marra, C.; Spinelli, P.; Caprara, A.; Scaricamazza, E.; Castelli, D.; Canulli, S.; Gainotti, G.; Quaranta, D. Typicality of words produced on a semantic fluency task in amnesic mild cognitive impairment: Linguistic analysis and risk of conversion to dementia. *J. Alzheimer's Dis.* **2014**, *42*, 1171–1178. [CrossRef] [PubMed]
24. Venneri, A.; Jahn-Carta, C.; de Marco, M.; Quaranta, D.; Marra, C. Diagnostic and prognostic role of semantic processing in preclinical Alzheimer's disease. *Biomark. Med.* **2018**, *12*, 637–651. [CrossRef] [PubMed]
25. Duong, A.; Whitehead, V.; Hanratty, K.; Chertkow, H. The nature of lexico-semantic processing deficits in mild cognitive impairment. *Neuropsychologia* **2006**, *44*, 1928–1935. [CrossRef]
26. Albert, M.S.; Moss, M.B.; Tanzi, R.; Jones, K. Preclinical prediction of AD using neuropsychological tests. *J. Int. Neuropsychol. Soc.* **2001**, *7*, 631–639. [CrossRef]
27. Chen, P.; Ratcliff, G.; Belle, S.H.; Cauley, J.A.; DeKosky, S.T.; Ganguli, M. Patterns of cognitive decline in presymptomatic Alzheimer disease: A prospective community study. *Arch. Gen. Psychiatry* **2001**, *58*, 853–858. [CrossRef]
28. Hodges, J.R.; Patterson, K.; Graham, N.; Dawson, K. Naming and knowing in dementia of Alzheimer's type. *Brain Lang.* **1996**, *54*, 302–325. [CrossRef] [PubMed]
29. Perry, R.J.; Watson, P.; Hodges, J.R. The nature and staging of attention dysfunction in early (minimal and mild) Alzheimer's disease: Relationship to episodic and semantic memory impairment. *Neuropsychologia* **2000**, *38*, 252–271. [CrossRef]
30. Rosser, A.; Hodges, J.R. Initial letter and semantic category fluency in Alzheimer's disease, Huntington's disease, and progressive supranuclear palsy. *J. Neurol. Neurosurg. Psychiatry* **1994**, *57*, 1389–1394. [CrossRef] [PubMed]

31. Quaranta, D.; Piccininni, C.; Caprara, A.; Malandrino, A.; Gainotti, G.; Marra, C. Semantic Relations in a Categorical Verbal Fluency Test: An Exploratory Investigation in Mild Cognitive Impairment. *Front. Psychol.* **2019**, *10*, 2797. [CrossRef]
32. Collins, A.M.; Loftus, E.F. A spreading-activation theory of semantic processing. *Psychol. Rev.* **1975**, *82*, 407–428. [CrossRef]
33. Neely, J.H. Semantic priming and retrieval from lexical memory: Roles of inhibitionless spreading activation and limited-capacity attention. *J. Exp. Psychol. Gen.* **1977**, *106*, 226–254. [CrossRef]
34. McNamara, P.; Holbrook, J.P. Semantic memory and priming. In *Handbook of Psychology*; Healy, A.F., Proctor, R.W., Eds.; John Wiley & Sons, Inc.: Hoboken, NJ, USA, 2003; Volume 4.
35. Plaut, D.C.; Booth, J.R. Individual and developmental differences in semantic priming: Empirical and computational support for a single-mechanism account of lexical processing. *Psychol. Rev.* **2000**, *107*, 786–823. [CrossRef] [PubMed]
36. Foster, P.S.; Drago, V.; Yung, R.C.; Pearson, J.; Stringer, K.; Giovannetti, T.; Libon, D.; Heilman, K.M. Differential lexical and semantic spreading activation in Alzheimer's disease. *Am. J. Alzheimer's Dis. Other Demen.* **2013**, *28*, 501–507. [CrossRef]
37. Bell, E.E.; Chenery, H.J.; Ingram, J.C. Semantic priming in Alzheimer's dementia: Evidence for dissociation of automatic and attentional processes. *Brain Lang.* **2001**, *76*, 130–144. [CrossRef]
38. Silveri, M.C.; Monteleone, D.; Burani, C.; Tabossi, P. Automatic semantic facilitation in Alzheimer's disease. *J. Clin. Exp. Neuropsychol.* **1996**, *18*, 371–382. [CrossRef] [PubMed]
39. Salmon, D.P.; Butters, N.; Chan, A.S. The deterioration of semantic memory in Alzheimer's disease. *Can. J. Exp. Psychol. Rev. Can. Psychol. Exp.* **1999**, *53*, 108–117. [CrossRef]
40. Perri, R.; Carlesimo, G.A.; Zannino, G.D.; Mauri, M.; Muolo, B.; Pettenati, C.; Caltagirone, C. Intentional and automatic measures of specific-category effect in the semantic impairment of patients with Alzheimer's disease. *Neuropsychologia* **2003**, *41*, 1509–1522. [CrossRef]
41. Ober, B.A.; Shenaut, G.K.; Jagust, W.J.; Stillman, R.C. Automatic semantic priming with various category relations in Alzheimer's disease and normal aging. *Psychol. Aging* **1991**, *6*, 647–660. [CrossRef]
42. Chertkow, H.; Bub, D.; Bergman, H.; Bruemmer, A.; Merling, A.; Rothfleisch, J. Increased semantic priming in patients with dementia of the Alzheimer's type. *J. Clin. Exp. Neuropsychol.* **1994**, *16*, 608–622. [CrossRef] [PubMed]
43. Chertkow, H.; Bub, D.; Seidenberg, M. Priming and semantic memory loss in Alzheimer's disease. *Brain Lang.* **1989**, *36*, 420–446. [CrossRef]
44. Nebes, R.D.; Brady, C.B.; Huff, F.J. Automatic and attentional mechanisms of semantic priming in Alzheimer's disease. *J. Clin. Exp. Neuropsychol.* **1989**, *11*, 219–230. [CrossRef] [PubMed]
45. Balota, D.A.; Watson, J.M.; Duchek, J.M.; Ferraro, F.R. Cross-modal semantic and homograph priming in healthy young, healthy old, and in Alzheimer's disease individuals. *J. Int. Neuropsychol. Soc.* **1999**, *5*, 626–640. [CrossRef]
46. Giffard, B.; Desgranges, B.; Nore-Mary, F.; Lalevée, C.; de la Sayette, V.; Pasquier, F.; Eustache, F. The nature of semantic memory deficits in Alzheimer's disease: New insights from hyperpriming effects. *Brain J. Neurol.* **2001**, *124*, 1522–1532. [CrossRef]
47. Perri, R.; Zannino, G.D.; Caltagirone, C.; Carlesimo, G.A. Semantic priming for coordinate distant concepts in Alzheimer's disease patients. *Neuropsychologia* **2011**, *49*, 839–847. [CrossRef]
48. Rogers, S.L.; Friedman, R.B. The underlying mechanisms of semantic memory loss in Alzheimer's disease and semantic dementia. *Neuropsychologia* **2008**, *46*, 12–21. [CrossRef]
49. Glosser, G.; Friedman, R.B.; Grugan, P.K.; Lee, J.H.; Grossman, M. Lexical semantic and associative priming in Alzheimer's disease. *Neuropsychology* **1998**, *12*, 218–224. [CrossRef]
50. Giffard, B.; Desgranges, B.; Nore-Mary, F.; Lalevée, C.; Beaunieux, H.; de la Sayette, V.; Pasquier, F.; Eustache, F. The dynamic time course of semantic memory impairment in Alzheimer's disease: Clues from hyperpriming and hypopriming effects. *Brain J. Neurol.* **2002**, *125*, 2044–2057. [CrossRef]
51. Mulatti, C.; Calia, C.; De Caro, M.F.; Della Sala, S. The cumulative semantic interference effect in normal and pathological ageing. *Neuropsychologia* **2014**, *65*, 125–130. [CrossRef]
52. Winblad, B.; Palmer, K.; Kivipelto, M.; Jelic, V.; Fratiglioni, L.; Wahlund, L.O.; Nordberg, A.; Backman, L.; Albert, M.; Almkvist, O.; et al. Mild cognitive impairment–beyond controversies, towards a consensus: Report of the International Working Group on Mild Cognitive Impairment. *J. Intern. Med.* **2004**, *256*, 240–246. [CrossRef] [PubMed]

53. McKhann, G.M.; Knopman, D.S.; Chertkow, H.; Hyman, B.T.; Jack, C.R.; Kawas, C.H.; Klunk, W.E.; Koroshetz, W.J.; Manly, J.J.; Mayeux, R.; et al. The diagnosis of dementia due to Alzheimer's disease: Recommendations from the National Institute on Aging-Alzheimer's Association workgroups on diagnostic guidelines for Alzheimer's disease. *Alzheimer's Dement.* **2011**, *7*, 263–269. [CrossRef] [PubMed]
54. Carlesimo, G.A.; Caltagirone, C.; Gainotti, G.; Fadda, L.; Gallassi, R.; Lorusso, S.; Marfia, G.; Marra, C.; Nocentini, U.; Parnetti, L. The mental deterioration battery: Normative data, diagnostic reliability and qualitative analyses of cognitive impairment. *Eur. Neurol.* **1996**, *36*, 378–384. [CrossRef]
55. Caffarra, P.; Vezzadini, G.; Dieci, F.; Zonato, F.; Venneri, A. Una versione abbreviata del test di Stroop: Dati normativi nella popolazione italiana. *Nuova Riv. Neurol.* **2002**, *12*, 111–115.
56. Marra, C.; Gainotti, G.; Scaricamazza, E.; Piccininni, C.; Ferraccioli, M.; Quaranta, D. The Multiple Features Target Cancellation (MFTC): An attentional visual conjunction search test. Normative values for the Italian population. *Neurol. Sci.* **2013**, *34*, 173–180. [CrossRef] [PubMed]
57. Monaco, M.; Costa, A.; Caltagirone, C.; Carlesimo, G.A. Forward and backward span for verbal and visuo-spatial data: Standardization and normative data from an Italian adult population. *Neurol. Sci.* **2013**, *34*, 749–754. [CrossRef]
58. Quaranta, D.; Caprara, A.; Piccininni, C.; Vita, M.G.; Gainotti, G.; Marra, C. Standardization, Clinical Validation, and Typicality Norms of a New Test Assessing Semantic Verbal Fluency. *Arch. Clin. Neuropsychol. Off. J. Natl. Acad. Neuropsychol.* **2016**, *31*, 434–445. [CrossRef]
59. Balota, D.A.; Chumbley, J.I. Are lexical decisions a good measure of lexical access? The role of word frequency in the neglected decision stage. *J. Exp. Psychol. Hum. Percept. Perform.* **1984**, *10*, 340–357. [CrossRef]

8

Development of Convenient System for Detecting Yeast Cell Stress, Including That of Amyloid Beta

Yen Nhi Luu and Ian Macreadie *

School of Science, RMIT University, Bundoora, VIC 3083, Australia; s3691025@student.rmit.edu.au
* Correspondence: ian.macreadie@rmit.edu.au

Abstract: (1) Background: As a model eukaryote, the study of stress responses in yeast can be employed for studying human health and disease, and the effects of various drugs that may impact health. "Reporting" of stress in yeast has frequently utilised enzymes like β-galactosidase that require laborious assays for quantitative results. The use of a stress reporter that can be measured quantitatively and with high sensitivity in living cells in a multi-well plate reader is a more desirable approach; (2) Methods: A multi-copy yeast-*Escherichia coli* shuttle plasmid containing the *HSP42* promoter upstream of the mCherry reporter, along with the *URA3* selectable marker was constructed and tested; (3) Results: Under certain stress conditions inducing the heat shock response, transformants containing the plasmid produced red fluorescence that could be readily quantitated in a microtitre plate reader. Stresses that produced red fluorescence included exposure to heat shock, copper ions, oligomeric amyloid beta ($A\beta_{42}$) and fibrillar $A\beta_{42}$; (4) Conclusions: Being able to conveniently and quantitatively monitor stresses in whole live populations of yeast offers great opportunities to screen compounds and conditions that cause stress, as well as conditions that alleviate stress. While freshly prepared oligomeric amyloid beta has previously been shown to exhibit high toxicity, fibrils have been generally considered to be non-toxic or of low toxicity. In this study, fibrillar amyloid beta has also been shown to induce stress.

Keywords: heat shock response; heat shock protein; Alzheimer's disease; beta amyloid; yeast

---

1. Introduction

Heat shock proteins (HSPs) are ubiquitously expressed and conserved in both yeast and humans [1]. Low level, constitutive expression of HSPs perform housekeeping functions, assisting in maintenance of proteostasis [2]. HSPs target up to 3% of the total number of genes in yeast, with some acting as molecular chaperones to assist in binding of and folding of proteins and sequester misfolded polypeptides towards proteolytic pathways, while others are involved in intracellular transport, cell wall maintenance, and oxidative stress mechanisms [3–5]. While HSPs are always present within cells, their expression may be upregulated during the heat shock response (HSR) in response to cellular stress which may include changes in environment, such as elevated temperature [6,7], misfolding or aggregation of proteins [2,3], and reactive oxygen species (ROS) production [8,9]. The HSR is mediated by activity of heat response factors (HRFs) that bind to a 5 bp heat shock element (HSE) in the promotor regions of heat shock genes to initiate transcription [4,10,11].

As a defense mechanism against misfolded and aggregated proteins, HSPs are vital in the response against the toxic Alzheimer's disease (AD) protein Aβ. Aβ is present in many forms in an AD-affected brain including monomers, toxic oligomeric intermediates and fibrils. The soluble oligomeric form, particularly $A\beta_{42}$, produces cytotoxic effects that initiate a cascade of events that contribute to the development of AD due to a higher propensity to aggregate [12–14]. HSPs are found at elevated levels in AD-affected brains, activating microglial phagocytosis and degradation, inhibiting Aβ formation,

and slowing down or inhibiting the rate of aggregation, thereby contributing to the clearance of Aβ [3,5,15,16].

β-galactosidase reporter assays have previously been used for measurement of the HSR towards Aβ, in which a yeast HSE was placed upstream of the *lacZ* gene and β-galactosidase levels were measured with and without the presence of Aβ [17]. The use of such an assay is somewhat inconvenient in that a preparation of cell lysate is required as well as several commercial reagents.

The aim of this study was to develop an alternative reporter assay for quick screening of the HSR using the mCherry fluorescence reporter, to measure cell stress in whole living cell populations without a need for any reagent addition. Development of this expression system could allow for quick, high throughput screening assays to determine conditions that may cause stress to cells. The demonstration of the use of this system is outlined as follows.

2. Results

2.1. Construction of the pYHSRed1 Plasmid

The schematic map of the pYHSRed1 plasmid is shown in Figure 1. It has a 2 μ *ori* for high copy replication in *S. cerevisiae*. The mCherry reporter is located downstream from the promotor of *HSP42*, the most abundant cytosolic HSP in yeast for suppression of aggregation [18]. It contains a *URA3* gene for selection in *S. cerevisiae* strains that have a *URA3* gene mutation or disruption and therefore require uracil supplementation. For propagation of the plasmid in *E. coli* it contains the pUC *ori* and an ampicillin resistance selection marker (encoding β-lactamase). Transformation of this plasmid into a *ura3* mutant *S. cerevisiae* BY4743 strain that requires uracil for growth produces a transformant that no longer requires uracil supplementation. The expression of mCherry expression and red fluorescence should be regulated by the *HSP42* promoter, so the intensity of red fluorescence should indicate the amount of the stress response in the recombinant yeast.

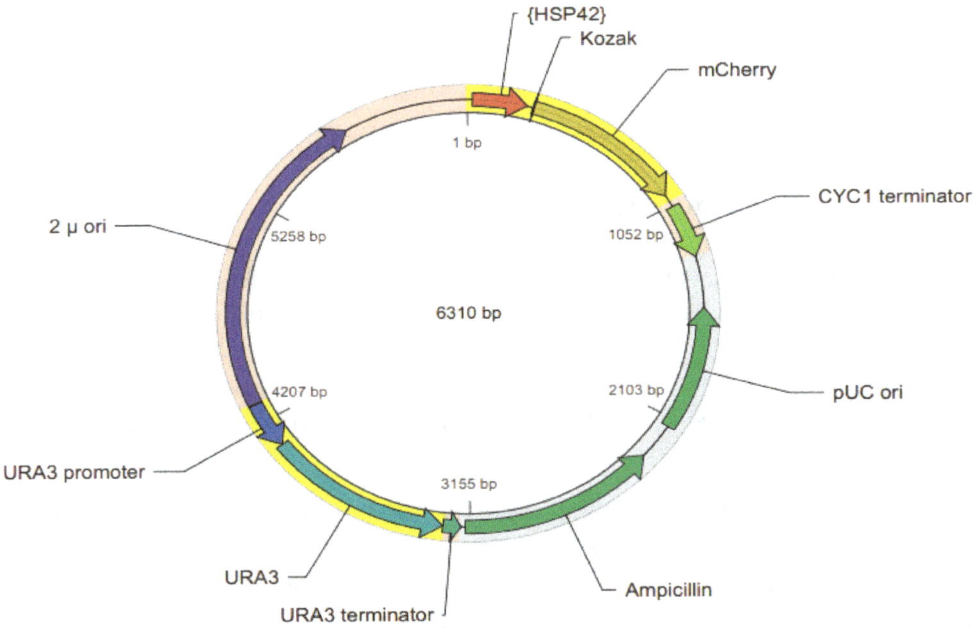

Figure 1. Schematic map of the pYHSRed1 plasmid.

2.2. Transformation of Yeast with pYHSRed1 and Basal Expression of mCherry

To examine the basal levels of red fluorescence afforded by pYHSRed1, a comparison was made between BY4743 and its transformant, BY4743 [pYHSRed1]. BY4743 and BY4743 [pYHSRed1] were grown to exponential phase in liquid minimal media with the appropriate supplementation required by each strain, incubated at 30 °C for two hours. Transformants had some production of mCherry, as indicated by the increased red fluorescence (Figure 2). This basal expression of mCherry fluorescence in BY4743 [pYHSRed1] was significantly higher ($p < 0.05$ for all comparisons at same cell density) than that of the untransformed parental BY4743 strain, indicative of the low level constitutive expression of HSPs in yeast cells when unstressed (Figure 2). The measurement of mCherry fluorescence in cultures of varying cell densities was also analysed to determine how the density of cell cultures affected fluorescence. Fluorescence was proportional to cell density, with cell cultures of larger OD_{600} readings producing higher mCherry fluorescence. Arbitrary measurements of higher mCherry fluorescence of the parental BY4743 strain were also observed at greater cell densities which may be attributed to high sensitivity of the spectrophotometer. For measurement of fluorescence in successive experiments, cell cultures of $OD_{600} \geq 0.6$ were utilised.

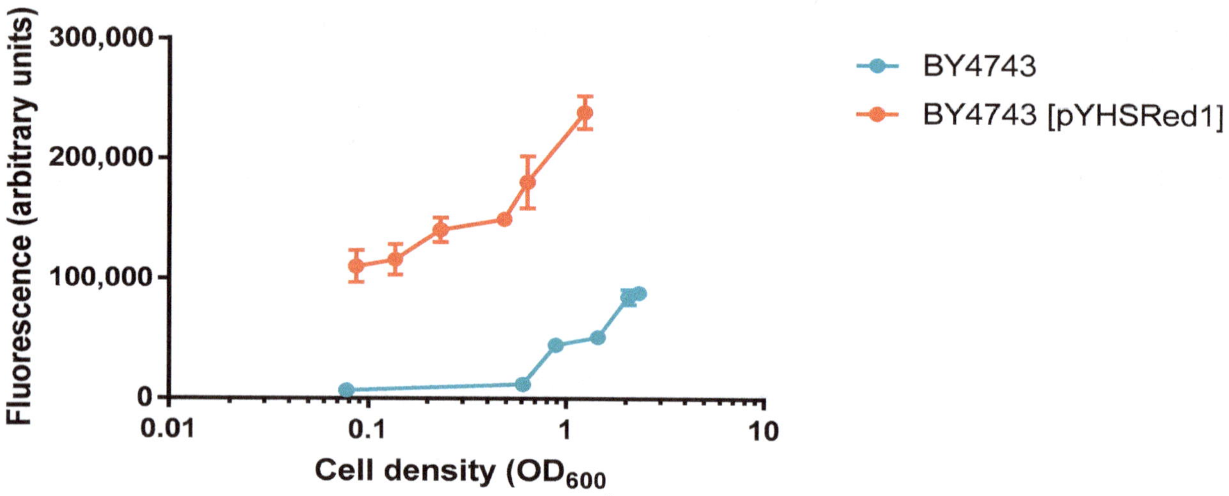

Figure 2. Comparison of basal levels of red fluorescence in BY4743 and BY4743 [pYHSRed1] in cultures of varying cell densities. Mean ±SEM of Data are shown as triplicate measurements.

2.3. Increased mCherry Fluorescence in Cells Exposed to Heat Shock and Copper Sulphate

The mCherry reporter was examined under conditions that induce HSR in cells: elevated temperatures and exposure to metal ions. BY4743 [pYHSRed1] cells were incubated at 42 °C for two hours, with control cells being incubated at 30 °C. Exposure to 42 °C resulted in a significant increase in mCherry fluorescence being measured, indicating a significant upregulation in heat shock response genes compared to the control (Figure 3a).

Yeast cells were also exposed to copper sulphate for two hours. Treatment with 0.1 and 0.3 mM $CuSO_4$ did not produce a significant increase in HSR but cells treated with 0.5 mM $CuSO_4$ produced a significant increase in mCherry fluorescence (Figure 3b).

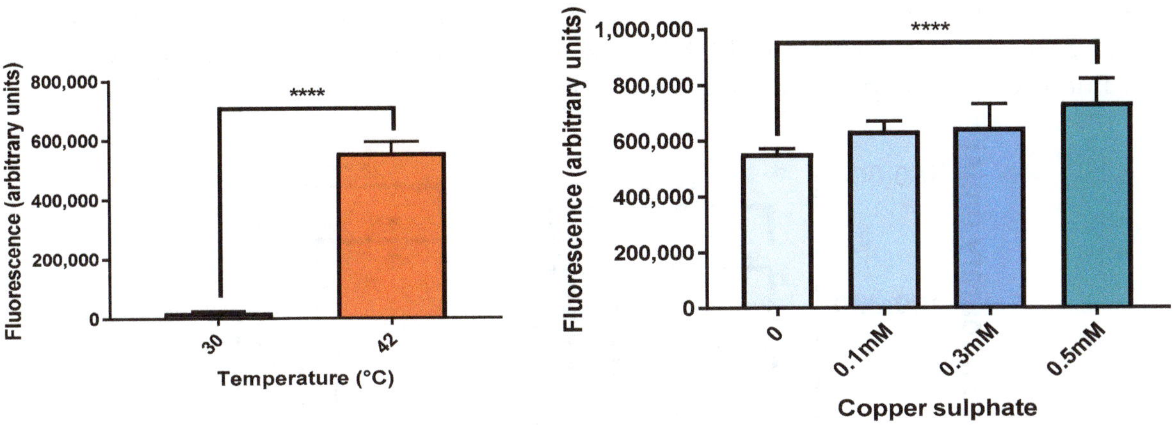

(a) (b)

Figure 3. mCherry fluorescence in BY4743 [pYHSRed1] under heat and copper stress. (**a**) Heat stress; (**b**) Stress due to copper sulphate. Data shown as mean ± SEM of triplicate measurements; **** $p < 0.0001$.

2.4. Stress Induced by Oligomeric and Fibrillar Aβ₄₂ Measured by mCherry Fluorescence

Elevated mCherry levels were measured when yeast cells were treated with both oligomeric and fibrillar $A\beta_{42}$. Cell responses of both exponential and stationary phase cells were measured due to the differing vulnerability of yeast cells in different growth phases to $A\beta_{42}$ toxicity [19].

Oligomeric $A\beta_{42}$ (Figure 4) induced a dose-dependent response in mCherry fluorescence in both stationary and exponential phase cells. A significant increase in mCherry fluorescence was observed in stationary phase yeast cells at 500 nM and 1 µM $A\beta_{42}$, but not with 50 nM $A\beta_{42}$. $A\beta_{42}$ also induced significant mCherry fluorescence at 50 nM in exponential phase yeast cells, but there was no significant effect at lower levels.

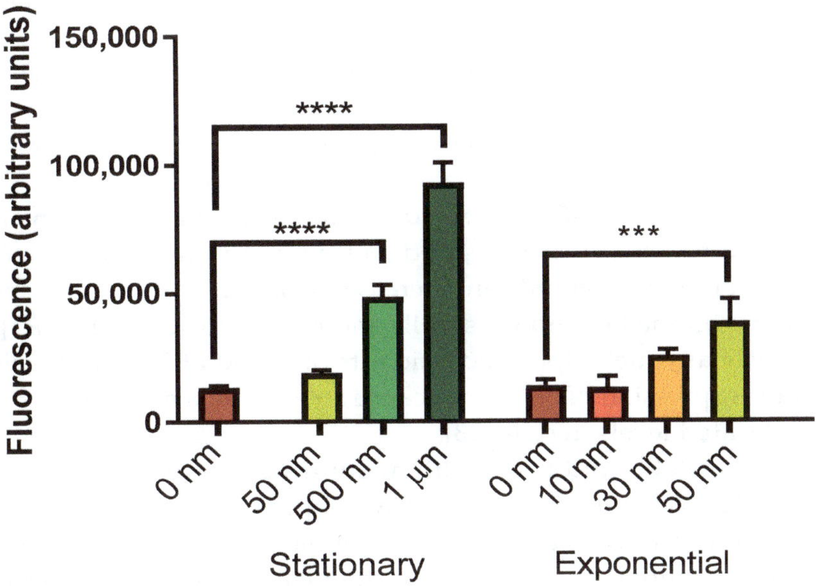

Figure 4. Measurement of mCherry fluorescence of BY4743 [pYHSRed1] cells in stationary and exponential phase growth treated with oligomeric $A\beta_{42}$. Data are shown as mean ± SEM of triplicate measurements; *** $p > 0.001$, **** $p < 0.0001$.

Fibrillar Aβ_{42} (Figure 5) induced a significant elevation in mCherry fluorescence in stationary phase yeast cells at 50, 500 nM and 1 μM Aβ_{42}. Levels of 30 and 50 nM Aβ_{42} also induced significant mCherry fluorescence in exponential phase yeast cells.

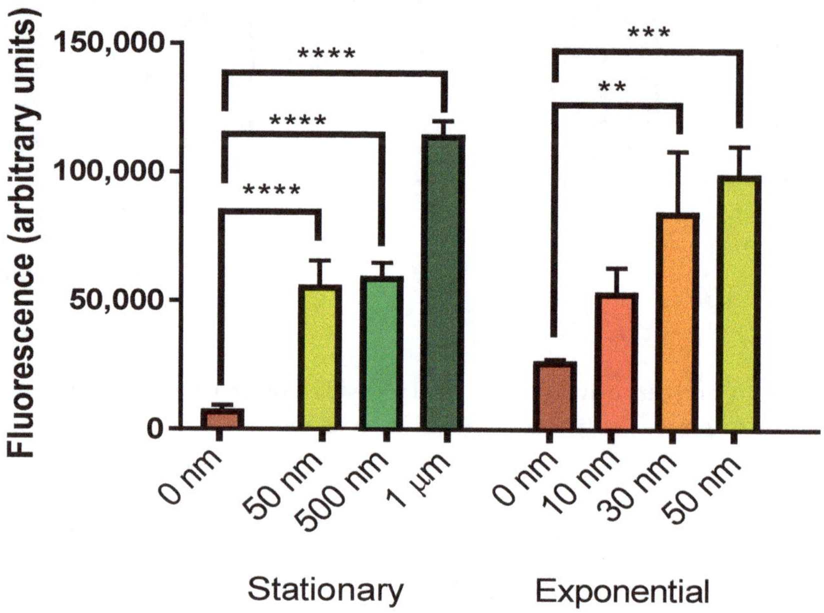

Figure 5. Measurement of mCherry fluorescence of BY4743 [pYHSRed1] cells in stationary and exponential phase growth treated with fibrillar Aβ_{42}. Data are shown as mean ± SEM of triplicate measurements; ** $p > 0.01$, *** $p > 0.001$, **** $p < 0.0001$.

3. Discussion

This study aimed to develop a convenient yeast reporter system to measure cell stress correlated with induction of the heat shock response by measuring fluorescence of the mCherry reporter, induced from the HSE of *HSP42*.

Significant basal mCherry expression of the transformant compared to the wildtype was observed, confirming functionality of pYHSRed1 in transformed yeast. Basal expression of HSPs is expected, as in unstressed conditions, HSPs perform housekeeping functions for proteostasis and regulation of protein quality control [9,20].

mCherry fluorescence in BY4743 [pYHSRed1] transformants after exposure to some known inducers of the heat shock response was measured and significant increases in red fluorescence were observed. For example, there was a significant increase in HSR at 42 °C, as this temperature is a heat shock condition in both mammalian and yeast cells and known to activate HSFs [4,21]. Likewise the HSR is also induced by heavy metal ions and oxidants [22], and at 0.5 mM levels it induced highly significant red mCherry expression. Copper can cause stress as it is a heavy metal and may promote oxidative damage at elevated levels in cells [23].

Oligomeric Aβ_{42} is unstable and toxic, with many studies showing its effect in killing of both yeast cells and neurons [24–26]. Effects of externally supplemented Aβ_{42} cells may differ based on growth stages, as non-quiescent cells are more susceptible to Aβ_{42} toxicity compared to quiescent cells in the first 24 h of exposure [19]. There is reduced viability of cells exposed to Aβ_{42} oligomers compared to fibrils [24], therefore, lower concentrations of oligomers were applied for treatment. The lower levels of mCherry fluorescence observed compared to fibrillar Aβ_{42} treatment may be due to this cell killing, reducing the number of cells able to emit fluorescence.

In contrast to oligomers, fibrils are generally viewed as harmless and benign, contributing to the non-toxic plaques found in the brain [14]. Though HSPs can sequester oligomer aggregates, they do not cause significant changes to fibrillar Aβ, possibly accumulating on the fibrils due to their inability to process them [3,27]. However, insoluble fibrils may induce oxidative stress from fibrillization [28,29]. Ladiwala et al. [30] also found fibrils formed at elevated concentrations of Aβ were toxic. Fibrils prepared with both HFIP and NH_4OH pretreatment caused toxicity to *S. cerevisiae* [19]. It is possible that, while not cytotoxic like oligomers, the fibrils cause stress and HSR induction in cells through production of ROS and mild cell killing.

Further work needs to be performed to gain greater understanding of this new attribute of fibrillar $A\beta_{42}$.

4. Materials and Methods

4.1. pYHSRed1, Yeast Strain and Transformation

The pYHSRed1 was custom designed and produced by VectorBuilder (Cyagen, Santa Clara, CA, USA). It utilises a *URA3* multi-copy VectorBuilder plasmid with 238 nt of the *HSP42* promoter sequences inserted immediately upstream of the mCherry reporter.

The *Saccharomyces cerevisiae* yeast strain BY4743 (*MATa/α his3Δ1/his3Δ1, leu2Δ0/leu2Δ0 LYS2/lys2Δ0 met15Δ0/MET15 ura3Δ0/ura3Δ0*) was the host strain used in this study. The plasmid pYHSRed1 was transformed into the host strain as described by Porzoor and Macreadie [31].

4.2. Yeast Culture Protocol

Minimal media was used for growth of the BY4743 transformants. The media composition is as follows: Yeast nitrogen base without amino acids (0.67%) and dextrose (2%). For solidification of media agar (1.5%) was added. Supplementation of auxotrophic requirements of BY4743 [pYHSRed1] was performed by adding 20 mg/L histidine and 30 mg/L leucine.

Overnight fresh cultures of the transformants were obtained by inoculating one colony into 10 mL fresh selective minimal media in a 50 mL tube. The tubes were incubated at 30 °C at 250 rpm. Overnight stationary cultures were further grown to exponential phase by transferring 100 μL aliquot to fresh selective minimal media in 15 mL tubes and incubating at 30 °C at 250 rpm for a further two hours.

4.3. Preparation of $A\beta_{42}$

$A\beta_{42}$ was pretreated with NH_4OH as described by [19]. To obtain oligomers, $A\beta_{42}$ was solubilized in water and used immediately. To obtain fibrils, the $A\beta_{42}$ was solubilised in water and incubated at 37 °C for 24 h.

4.4. Exposure of Yeast Cells to Heat Shock

Yeast cells were analysed for the effect of exposure to heat shock conditions on mCherry levels. Yeast cells from exponential phase cultures were aliquoted into wells in 96-well microtiter plates. Cells were incubated for a further two hours at 30 and 42 °C.

4.5. Exposure of Yeast Cells to Copper Ions

Yeast cells were analysed for the effect of exposure to copper sulphate on mCherry levels. Cells from overnight cultures and exponential phase cultures were suspended in water and then were aliquoted into wells in 96-well microtiter plates. Copper sulphate was added to the diluted cell suspension to required concentrations. The final volume of each well was made up to 200 μL. The microtiter plate was incubated at 30 °C for two hours.

4.6. Effect of Exposure to Oligomeric and Fibrillar Aβ on Yeast Cells

Yeast cells were analysed for the effect of exposure to fibrillar and oligomeric $A\beta_{42}$ on mCherry levels. Cells from overnight cultures and exponential phase cultures were pelleted by centrifugation and resuspended in water and aliquoted into wells in 96-well microtiter plates. Oligomeric and fibrillar

Aβ_{42} were added to the diluted cell suspension to required concentrations. The final volume of each well was made up to 200 µL. The microtiter plate was incubated at 30 °C for two hours.

4.7. Spectrophotometry

Cell density and mCherry fluorescence was measured with the POLARstar omega microplate reader and analysed with BMG Labtech Mars Data Analysis Software (Ortenberg, Germany). Cell density was measured in Corning 96 Well TC-Treated microplates at 600 nm. mCherry fluorescence was measured from a Nunclon Surface black F96 microtiter plate with top optics using an Ex584 excitation filter and 600–680 emission filter.

Raw data was blank corrected, subtracting the mCherry fluorescence reading of the liquid the cell culture was suspended in, to remove background fluorescence. This figure was then divided by the cell density (OD_{600}) reading for the culture.

5. Conclusions

The heat shock response is vital in both yeast and human cells for defense against various cell stressors, including misfolded and aggregated proteins associated with neurodegenerative diseases such as Alzheimer's disease. A novel outcome in this study was development of pYHSRed1, a plasmid reporting on stress, especially the HSR, in yeast cells. Coupled with measurement of mCherry fluorescence by a spectrophotometer, the level of stress in live yeast cells may be determined.

Yeast cells containing the pYHSRed1 plasmid were exposed to several conditions known to induce the heat shock response. Elevated temperatures, exposure to metal ions and the subsequent ROS production, and oligomeric and fibrillar Aβ_{42} all induced significant increases in mCherry production, indicative of the upregulation of transcription of heat shock genes. The significant upregulation of mCherry observed after exposure to fibrillar Aβ, considered to be of low or no toxicity, implicates fibrils as a contributor to cellular stress by induction of the HSR.

Transformation of this plasmid into yeast provides an improved method of stress and HSR detection and may be useful for high throughput analysis of therapeutic compounds that may reduce stress caused by Aβ. Future studies could also determine the stress of mutant versions of Aβ on yeast cells and to identify therapeutic compounds that may alleviate the effects of other deleterious proteins, biochemicals or cellular states that cause cellular stress.

Author Contributions: Y.N.L. conceived, designed, and performed the experiments and wrote the paper. I.M. conceived, designed, and supervised the study.

Abbreviations

AD	Alzheimer's disease
Aβ	Beta-amyloid
HSE	Heat shock element
HSF	Heat shock factor
HSP	Heat shock protein
HSR	Heat shock response
ROS	Reactive oxygen species

References

1. Lindquist, S. The heat-shock proteins. *Annu. Rev. Genet.* **1988**, *22*, 631–677. [CrossRef] [PubMed]
2. Fink, A.L. Chaperone-mediated protein folding. *Physiol. Rev.* **1999**, *79*, 425–449. [CrossRef] [PubMed]
3. Evans, C.G.; Wisen, S.; Gestwicki, J.E. Heat shock proteins 70 and 90 inhibit early stages of amyloid β-(1-42) aggregation in vitro. *J. Biol. Chem.* **2006**, *281*, 33182–33191. [CrossRef] [PubMed]

4. Hahn, J.S.; Hu, Z.; Thiele, D.J.; Iyer, V.R. Genome-wide analysis of the biology of stress responses through heat shock transcription factor. *Mol. Cell. Biol.* **2004**, *24*, 5249–5256. [CrossRef] [PubMed]
5. Ou, J.R.; Tan, M.S.; Xie, A.M.; Yu, J.T.; Tan, L. Heat shock protein 90 in Alzheimer's disease. *BioMed Res. Int.* **2014**, *2014*, 1–8. [CrossRef] [PubMed]
6. Nisamedtinov, I.; Lindsey, G.G.; Karreman, R.; Orumets, K.; Koplimaa, M.; Kevvai, K.; Paalme, T. The response of the yeast *Saccharomyces cerevisiae* to sudden vs. gradual changes in environmental stress monitored by expression of the stress response protein hsp12p. *FEMS Yeast Res.* **2008**, *8*, 829–838. [CrossRef] [PubMed]
7. Sanchez, Y.; Lindquist, S. Hsp104 required for induced thermotolerance. *Science* **1990**, *248*, 1112–1115. [CrossRef] [PubMed]
8. Dubey, A.K.; Bharadwaj, P.R.; Varghese, J.N.; Macreadie, I.G. Alzheimer's amyloid-β rescues yeast from hydroxide toxicity. *J. Alzheimer's Dis.* **2009**, *18*, 31–33. [CrossRef] [PubMed]
9. Kalmar, B.; Greensmith, L. Induction of heat shock proteins for protection against oxidative stress. *Adv. Drug Deliv. Rev.* **2009**, *61*, 310–318. [CrossRef] [PubMed]
10. Liu, X.D.; Liu, P.C.; Santoro, N.; Thiele, D.J. Conservation of a stress response: Human heat shock transcription factors functionally substitute for yeast hsf. *EMBO J.* **1997**, *16*, 6466–6477. [CrossRef] [PubMed]
11. Wu, C. Heat shock transcription factors: Structure and regulation. *Annu. Rev. Cell Dev. Biol.* **1995**, *11*, 441–469. [CrossRef] [PubMed]
12. Thirumalai, D.; Reddy, G.; Straub, J.E. Role of water in protein aggregation and amyloid polymorphism. *Acc. Chem. Res.* **2012**, *45*, 83–92. [CrossRef] [PubMed]
13. Hartley, D.M.; Walsh, D.M.; Ye, C.P.; Diehl, T.; Vasquez, S.; Vassilev, P.M.; Teplow, D.B.; Selkoe, D.J. Protofibrillar intermediates of amyloid β-protein induce acute electrophysiological changes and progressive neurotoxicity in cortical neurons. *J. Neurosci.* **1999**, *19*, 8876–8884. [CrossRef] [PubMed]
14. Hardy, J.; Selkoe, D.J. The amyloid hypothesis of Alzheimer's disease: Progress and problems on the road to therapeutics. *Science* **2002**, *297*, 353–356. [CrossRef] [PubMed]
15. Kakimura, J.; Kitamura, Y.; Takata, K.; Umeki, M.; Suzuki, S.; Shibagaki, K.; Taniguchi, T.; Nomura, Y.; Smith, M.A.; Gebicke-Haerter, P.J.; et al. Microglial activation and amyloid-β clearance induced by exogenous heat-shock proteins. *FASEB J.* **2002**, *16*, 601–603. [CrossRef] [PubMed]
16. Smith, R.C.; Rosen, K.M.; Pola, R.; Magrane, J. Stress proteins in Alzheimer's disease. *Int. J. Hyperther.* **2005**, *21*, 421–431. [CrossRef] [PubMed]
17. Caine, J.; Sankovich, S.; Antony, H.; Waddington, L.; Macreadie, P.; Varghese, J.; Macreadie, I. Alzheimer's Aβ fused to green fluorescent protein induces growth stress and a heat shock response. *FEMS Yeast Res.* **2007**, *7*, 1230–1236. [CrossRef] [PubMed]
18. Haslbeck, M.; Braun, N.; Stromer, T.; Richter, B.; Model, N.; Weinkauf, S.; Buchner, J. Hsp42 is the general small heat shock protein in the cytosol of *Saccharomyces cerevisiae*. *EMBO J.* **2004**, *23*, 638–649. [CrossRef] [PubMed]
19. Porzoor, A.; Caine, J.M.; Macreadie, I.G. Pretreatment of chemically-synthesized $A\beta_{42}$ affects its biological activity in yeast. *Prion* **2014**, *8*, 404–410. [CrossRef] [PubMed]
20. Jakobsen, B.K.; Pelham, H.R. Constitutive binding of yeast heat shock factor to DNA in vivo. *Mol. Cell. Biol.* **1988**, *8*, 5040–5042. [CrossRef] [PubMed]
21. Mager, W.H.; De Kruijff, A.J. Stress-induced transcriptional activation. *Microbiol. Rev.* **1995**, *59*, 506–531. [PubMed]
22. Ananthan, J.; Goldberg, A.L.; Voellmy, R. Abnormal proteins serve as eukaryotic stress signals and trigger the activation of heat shock genes. *Science* **1986**, *232*, 522–524. [CrossRef] [PubMed]
23. Avery, S.V.; Howlett, N.G.; Radice, S. Copper toxicity towards *Saccharomyces cerevisiae*: Dependence on plasma membrane fatty acid composition. *Appl. Environ. Microbiol.* **1996**, *62*, 3960–3966. [PubMed]
24. Bharadwaj, P.; Waddington, L.; Varghese, J.; Macreadie, I.G. A new method to measure cellular toxicity of non-fibrillar and fibrillar Alzheimer's Aβ using yeast. *J. Alzheimer's Dis.* **2008**, *13*, 147–150. [CrossRef]
25. Dahlgren, K.N.; Manelli, A.M.; Stine, W.B., Jr.; Baker, L.K.; Krafft, G.A.; LaDu, M.J. Oligomeric and fibrillar species of amyloid-ß peptides differentially affect neuronal viability. *J. Biol. Chem.* **2002**, *277*, 32046–32053. [CrossRef] [PubMed]
26. Stefani, M. Biochemical and biophysical features of both oligomer/fibril and cell membrane in amyloid cytotoxicity. *FEBS J.* **2010**, *277*, 4602–4613. [CrossRef] [PubMed]

27. Lee, S.; Carson, K.; Rice-Ficht, A.; Good, T. Small heat shock proteins differentially affect Aβ aggregation and toxicity. *Biochem. Biophys. Res. Commun.* **2006**, *347*, 527–533. [CrossRef] [PubMed]
28. Chauhan, V.; Chauhan, A. Oxidative stress in Alzheimer's disease. *Pathophysiology* **2006**, *13*, 195–208. [CrossRef] [PubMed]
29. Varadarajan, S.; Yatin, S.; Aksenova, M.; Butterfield, D.A. Alzheimer's amyloid β-peptide-associated free radical oxidative stress and neurotoxicity. *J. Struct. Biol.* **2000**, *130*, 184–208. [CrossRef] [PubMed]
30. Ladiwala, A.R.; Litt, J.; Kane, R.S.; Aucoin, D.S.; Smith, S.O.; Ranjan, S.; Davis, J.; Van Nostrand, W.E.; Tessier, P.M. Conformational differences between two amyloid β oligomers of similar size and dissimilar toxicity. *J. Biol. Chem.* **2012**, *287*, 24765–24773. [CrossRef] [PubMed]
31. Porzoor, A.; Macreadie, I. Yeast as a model for studies on abeta aggregation toxicity in Alzheimer's disease, autophagic responses, and drug screening. *Methods Mol. Biol.* **2016**, *1303*, 217–226. [PubMed]

9

Flotillin: A Promising Biomarker for Alzheimer's Disease

Efthalia Angelopoulou [1], Yam Nath Paudel [2], Mohd. Farooq Shaikh [2,*] and Christina Piperi [1,*]

1 Department of Biological Chemistry, Medical School, National and Kapodistrian University of Athens, 11527 Athens, Greece; angelthal@med.uoa.gr
2 Neuropharmacology Research Strength, Jeffrey Cheah School of Medicine and Health Sciences, Monash University Malaysia, Bandar Sunway 47500, Selangor, Malaysia; yam.paudel@monash.edu
* Correspondence: farooq.shaikh@monash.edu (M.F.S.); cpiperi@med.uoa.gr (C.P.)

Abstract: Alzheimer's disease (AD) is characterized by the accumulation of beta amyloid (Aβ) in extracellular senile plaques and intracellular neurofibrillary tangles (NFTs) mainly consisting of tau protein. Although the exact etiology of the disease remains elusive, accumulating evidence highlights the key role of lipid rafts, as well as the endocytic pathways in amyloidogenic amyloid precursor protein (APP) processing and AD pathogenesis. The combination of reduced Aβ42 levels and increased phosphorylated tau protein levels in the cerebrospinal fluid (CSF) is the most well established biomarker, along with Pittsburgh compound B and positron emission tomography (PiB-PET) for amyloid imaging. However, their invasive nature, the cost, and their availability often limit their use. In this context, an easily detectable marker for AD diagnosis even at preclinical stages is highly needed. Flotillins, being hydrophobic proteins located in lipid rafts of intra- and extracellular vesicles, are mainly involved in signal transduction and membrane–protein interactions. Accumulating evidence highlights the emerging implication of flotillins in AD pathogenesis, by affecting APP endocytosis and processing, Ca^{2+} homeostasis, mitochondrial dysfunction, neuronal apoptosis, Aβ-induced neurotoxicity, and prion-like spreading of Aβ. Importantly, there is also clinical evidence supporting their potential use as biomarker candidates for AD, due to reduced serum and CSF levels that correlate with amyloid burden in AD patients compared with controls. This review focuses on the emerging preclinical and clinical evidence on the role of flotillins in AD pathogenesis, further addressing their potential usage as disease biomarkers.

Keywords: flotillin; Alzheimer's disease; biomarker; exosomes; beta-amyloid; Tau

---

1. Introduction

Alzheimer's disease (AD) is pathologically characterized by the accumulation of beta amyloid (Aβ), a peptide of 40 or 42 amino acids, in extracellular senile plaques, as well as intracellular neurofibrillary tangles (NFTs) mainly consisting of tau protein [1,2]. Aβ is generated by the sequential cleavage of the transmembrane amyloid-β precursor protein (APP) via β- and γ-secretases [1]. It has been shown that amyloidogenic APP processing mainly occurs in lipid rafts, which are caveolae-like membrane microdomains enriched in sphingolipids, glycolipids, and cholesterol, serving as dynamic platforms for signal transduction, protein trafficking, and clathrin-independent endocytosis [3,4]. Most AD cases are sporadic, whereas a small percentage (1%–5%) of them are caused by mutations in genes including *APP*, *presenilin-1*, and *presenilin-2* [5]. Although the exact etiology and pathophysiological mechanisms of AD remain elusive, growing preclinical and clinical evidence highlights the key role of the homeostasis of lipid rafts and both intra- and extracellular vesicles in AD pathogenesis, even at early stages of the disease [6].

Currently, there is no easy and objective method available for early AD diagnosis. The combined estimation of reduced Aβ_{42} levels and increased phosphorylated tau protein levels in the cerebrospinal fluid (CSF) is the most well established biomarker for the diagnosis of the disease, along with Pittsburgh compound B and positron emission tomography (PiB-PET) for amyloid imaging [7–9]. Although both methods can relatively reliably detect AD at prosymptomatic stages [8,9], the lumbar puncture required for CSF collection is an invasive procedure demanding specialized staff technical skills and cannot be carried out in primary care settings [10]. On the other hand, PiB-PET is quite expensive and not available worldwide. Specific patterns of various sets of plasma proteins or phospholipids have been proposed as promising AD biomarkers by several studies, usually involving specialized experimental procedures, such as mass spectrometry, or necessitating the measurement of multiple factors [7]. In this context, an easily accessible and detectable marker with high sensitivity and specificity for AD diagnosis, reflecting Aβ burden or underlying AD pathophysiological mechanisms even at preclinical stages, is highly needed.

Flotillins are highly conserved hydrophobic myristoylated and palmitoylated proteins that belong to the prohibitin (PHB) family [3]. They are located in the inner part of the plasma membrane and play an essential role in the formation of lipid rafts [3,4]. Moreover, intracellular and extracellular vesicles are enriched in flotillins, whose subcellular localization is constantly changing [3,4]. Flotillins were first detected in the lung plasma membrane of mice, described as "float like a flotilla of ships in the Triton-insoluble, buoyant fraction" [3], and since then they have been widely utilized as markers of lipid rafts and exosomes for many years. In metazoans, there are two flotillin paralogues, termed as flotillin-1/reggie-2 and flotillin-2/reggie-1. Within cells, flotillins form flotillin-1/flotillin-2 hetero-oligomers mediated by C-terminal interactions [11]. Their expression is particularly high in cell types lacking caveolin, including neurons. Functionally, flotillins are implicated in various cellular processes, including membrane–cytoskeletal interaction, membrane and vesicular trafficking, signal transduction, axonal regeneration, cell migration, and clathrin-independent endocytosis. It has been demonstrated that flotillins (mainly flotillin-1) are abundantly expressed in pyramidal neurons in the cortex, as well as in the astrocytes of the white matter of normal human brain tissue [12]. Notably, their levels have been shown to be higher in brain samples from non-demented patients with amyloid plaques, subjects with Down syndrome (who overexpress APP), and AD patients compared with non-demented individuals without amyloid plaques [12], suggesting a key role in AD pathogenesis. Since then, several preclinical and human studies have investigated the implication of flotillins in AD pathophysiology, also highlighting their potential as promising molecular biomarkers.

In this mini review, we summarize the emerging preclinical and clinical evidence on the role of flotillins in AD pathogenesis, and discuss their potential usage as biomarker candidates (Figure 1) for AD along with possible limitations.

2. The Role of Endocytic Pathway and Exosome Release in AD Pathogenesis

Abnormal APP processing, trafficking, and turnover are considered to play a major role in AD pathogenesis [1]. Several studies indicate that amyloidogenic APP processing is predominantly carried out in lipid rafts, since APP, Aβ, presenilin-1, β-secretase, and specific components of the γ-secretase complex have been located in the membrane microdomains of neurons [13–17]. On the contrary, non-amyloidogenic APP processing usually occurs in areas of the plasma membrane that are enriched in phospholipids [18]. However, there is also evidence suggesting that amyloidogenic APP cleavage may occur outside lipid rafts. In particular, membrane cholesterol reduction in hippocampal neuronal cells from AD patients has been associated with enhanced β-site APP-cleaving enzyme 1 (BACE1)–APP colocalization and increased Aβ load, implying that amyloidogenic APP processing may be carried out in more fluid membrane domains [19]. In addition, depletion of the cholesterol-synthesizing enzyme seladin-1 in mice has been shown to be related to decreased cholesterol levels, disrupted cholesterol-rich detergent-resistant membrane domains (DRMs), displacement of BACE1 from DRMs to membrane fractions containing APP, enhanced APP cleavage, and increased Aβ load [20]. It has been proposed that BACE1 in cholesterol-rich membrane domains could represent a relatively inactive pool of the enzyme, which may be transferred to APP-containing domains under specific conditions. Based on these contradictory findings, more studies are needed in order to clarify this issue. Aβ can be produced by proteolytic cleavage of APP in the endoplasmic reticulum (ER) and *trans*-Golgi network, resulting in the formation of secretory vesicles. Alternatively, after APP internalization it can be directed from the plasma membrane into the endosomal system and subsequently targeted to lysosomes [21,22]. Early endosomes are the first vesicles of endocytic pathway responsible for APP endocytosis [23]. Internalization of APP into endosomes has been required for its cleavage by BACE1 [24], which proteolyzes APP [25]. Aβ generated in early endosomes has been also shown to be transported into late endosomes in a retrograde manner, leading to their fusion with cellular membrane and subsequent extracellular secretion as exosomes [26]. Impaired APP endocytosis has been associated with reduction in the secretion of Aβ in vitro [27], while abnormally enlarged endosomes have been identified in early stages of sporadic AD [23]. Therefore, dysregulation of the endocytic pathway has been implicated in AD pathophysiology, mainly by affecting APP processing and trafficking.

Exosomes are small membrane vesicles (20–120 nm in diameter) derived from endosomes through the formation of multivesicular bodies, being able to transport their internalized content into recipient cells, thus mainly contributing to cell-to-cell communication [28]. Exosomes can be secreted by various cell types, including neurons, astrocytes, oligodendrocytes, and microglia in the extracellular space and subsequently CSF, containing several kinds of cargos, including RNAs, micro-RNAs, and proteins [29,30]. It has been suggested that exosomes may be involved in AD pathogenesis by affecting Aβ metabolism and aggregation, as well as through tau-related molecular mechanisms [31]. More specifically, in vitro evidence has indicated that neuron-derived exosomes can bind to and promote conformational alterations in extracellular Aβ, leading to the formation of nontoxic amyloid fibrils. They can also enhance Aβ clearance by microglia through the facilitation of Aβ transportation to lysosomes for degradation [31]. Exosome secretion by neurons has been shown to be regulated by enzymes involved in the metabolism of sphingolipids, such as sphingomyelin synthase 2 (SMS2) and neutral sphingomyelinase 2 (nSMase2) [31]. Upregulation of exosome release with SMS2 siRNA use has been associated with increased Aβ uptake by microglia and reduced levels of extracellular Aβ in vitro [31]. In vivo evidence has revealed that exogenous intracerebral injection of neuroblastoma-derived exosomes into APP transgenic mice led to decreased Aβ depositions and Aβ-induced synaptotoxicity in their hippocampus [32]. In this study, glycosphingolipids (GSLs) enriched with glycans, which are essential components of exosome membrane, have exerted a contributing role in Aβ binding and internalization by the exosomes [32]. Notably, apart from Aβ exosomes also contain β- and γ-secretase complexes, full-length APP, as well as APP C-terminal fragments (CTFs) in APP transgenic mice, highlighting their potential contribution to Aβ metabolism in the brain [33]. Apart from their role in Aβ pathology, secretion of phosphorylated tau proteins has been shown to be at least partially exosome-mediated in tauopathy models in vitro [34]. Moreover, exosome-associated phosphorylated tau has been found released in the cerebrospinal fluid of AD patients [34], further confirming the significant implication of exosomes in tau-related pathophysiology in human AD. It has been also demonstrated that exosomes can attenuate the Aβ-mediated disruption of synaptic plasticity in vivo [35]. Another study has shown that $A\beta_{1-42}$ treatment inhibited exosome release from astrocytes, as demonstrated by decreased flotillin levels in vitro, by inducing c-Jun N-terminal kinase (JNK) signaling pathway [29]. Furthermore, exosomes, as Aβ carriers, have been proposed to contribute to the prion-like spreading of Aβ aggregates in AD [5]. Collectively, these findings reveal the key role of exosomes in AD pathogenesis by affecting Aβ pathology, tau-related mechanisms, and Aβ-mediated neurotoxicity.

3. The Role of Flotillin in AD Pathogenesis

3.1. Evidence from Human Studies

Several human studies support the potential implication of flotillin in AD pathogenesis. In this regard, it has been indicated that flotillin accumulates in the endosomes of neurons of AD patients' brains [36], possibly playing a key role in neuronal endosomal pathway. More specifically, flotillin-1 immunoreactivity has been shown to be higher in neurons bearing NFTs in the amygdala, hippocampus, and isocortex of AD patients compared with controls [36], and flotillin-1 was found to be co-localized with cathepsin-D, a lysosomal protease, indicating its contribution to lysosomal degradation [36]. Of note, some neurons bearing NFTs did not contain flotillin-1, implying a possible secondary reduction in synthesis of flotillin-1 in these cells [36]. Flotillin-1 has been also demonstrated to be highly enriched in extracellular Aβ plaques and neurons bearing NFTs in brain specimens of AD patients compared with PD patients and controls [4]. Furthermore, it has been reported that flotillin-positive extracellular vesicles (EVs) isolated from the CSF and plasma of sporadic, late-onset AD patients contained an increased amounts of Aβ42 in their external surface compared with age-matched neurologically healthy controls, which could be internalized by cortical neurons and acted in a neurotoxic manner, by impairing Ca^{2+} homeostasis, causing mitochondrial dysfunction, increasing the vulnerability of neurons to excitotoxicity, and triggering neuronal apoptosis [37]. On the contrary, the EVs derived from controls displayed no neurotoxic effects [37]. These effects were also observed in vivo in transgenic APP and presenilin-1 mice, as well *as* in vitro in neural cells expressing presenilin-1 mutations of familial AD [37]. It was also reported that impaired autophagy could enhance the release of EVs [37]. Of note, these flotillin-positive EV-mediated effects have been shown to be prevented via Aβ antibody treatment, highlighting the essential role of Aβ in the EV-induced neurotoxicity [37]. Furthermore, another study has demonstrated that flotillin-1-positive exosomes isolated from postmortem brain sections of AD patients were highly enriched in toxic Aβ oligomers compared with healthy controls, which could be transferred into recipient's cultured neurons [38]. Disruption of the production, release, or uptake of these exosomes was shown to attenuate the spreading of Aβ oligomers and Aβ-induced neurotoxicity [38]. Furthermore, a neuropathological study in brain tissues from AD patients has also reported that flotillins are also present in granulovacuolar degeneration (GVD) bodies [39], which are basophilic perinuclear vacuoles accumulating in neurons of AD patients [40]. Moreover, it has been indicated that levels of flotillin-2, along with other endocytic-associated proteins, were increased in brain sections of older non-demented humans [41]. Given the fact that age is a significant risk factor for AD development, these data further strengthen the potential contribution of flotillins in the pathophysiology of AD. These findings suggest that flotillin-positive exosomes may play a key role in AD pathogenesis and particularly, be implicated in the prion-like propagation of Aβ pathology in AD.

3.2. Evidence from In Vivo Models

In addition to human studies, a growing body of preclinical evidence demonstrates the key role of flotillin in the pathogenesis of AD, shedding more light into the underlying molecular mechanisms (Table 1).

Table 1. In vitro and in vivo evidence about the role of flotillin in Alzheimer's disease (AD).

S.N.	Type of Study	Main Findings	Reference
1	*In vitro*	• Flotillin-1 directly interacted with the intracellular domain of APP (AICD), and the residues 189-282 of flotillin-1 were essential for this interaction	[42]
2	*In vitro*	• FKBP12 overexpression enhanced the amyloidogenic APP processing, possibly by affecting the affinity of AICD to flotillin-1	[43]
3	*In vitro*	• Flotillin-1 could stabilize LGI3, and LGI3/Flo1 complex downregulation could directly affect APP trafficking via the disruption of exosome formation	[44]
4	*In vitro*	• si-RNA-mediated flotillin-2 knockdown impaired APP endocytosis in primary cultures of hippocampal neurons, and reduced Aβ production in tissue cell cultures • Flotillin-2 acted as a scaffold protein and enhanced APP clustering at the plasma membrane and subsequent APP endocytosis in a clathrin-dependent manner	[45]
5	*In vitro*	• Flotillin-1 bound to BACE1, whereas flotillin-1 overexpression was associated with increased recruitment into rafts and reduced activity of BACE1	[46]
6	*In vitro*	• Flotillin-1 could directly interact with the dileucine motif in the cytoplasmic domain of BACE1, thus affecting its endosomal sorting • Flotillin-2-BACE1 interaction was at least partially mediated by flotillin-1 • Depletion of flotillin-1 and -2 led to increased accumulation of overexpressed BACE1 into late endosomes in shRNA-mediated flotillin knockdown HeLa cells • Flotillin-1 knockdown resulted in overexpression of BACE1 • Flotillin-2 knockdown increased amyloidogenic processing of APP	[47]
7	*In vitro*	• Neuroblastoma cells transfected with mutant *DNM 2* gene displayed higher flotillin levels, and APP was mainly localized in the lipid rafts	[48]
8	*In vivo & in vitro*	• Copper inhibited the association of flotillin-2 with lipid rafts via its redistribution into non-raft fractions, resulting in the reduction of endocytosis and processing of APP in membrane microdomains both in vitro and in mutant APP transgenic mice	[49]
9	*In vivo*	• Endosomes of neurons in the amygdala, hippocampus, and isocortex of APP and presenilin-1 transgenic mice contained flotillin-1	[21]
10	*In vivo*	• Intracellular Aβ was accumulated in early and late endosomes positive for flotillin-1 in transgenic ArcAβ mice	[4]

Table 1. *Cont.*

S.N.	Type of Study	Main Findings	Reference
11	*In vivo*	• Knockout of *flotillin-1* gene (with or without additional knockout of flotillin-2 gene) in APP and presenilin-1 transgenic mice was correlated with reduced Aβ accumulation and plaque formation • No differences on APP clustering or endocytosis were indicated in mouse embryonic fibroblasts with flotillin-1 depletion	[50]
12	*In vivo*	• Treadmill exercise inhibited amyloidogenic APP cleavage and Aβ production in APP and presenilin-1 transgenic mice by inhibiting flotillin-1 levels and lipid raft formation	[51]
13	*In vivo*	• Treatment of senescence-accelerated mouse prone 8 mice with Yizhijiannao granule reduced flotillin-1 levels	[52]
14	*In vivo*	• Flotillin levels were not altered in mutant APP transgenic mice, compared with proteins associated with clathrin-dependent pathways	[53]

AD, Alzheimer's disease; APP, amyloid precursor protein; Aβ, amyloid β; LGI3, leucine-rich glioma inactivated 3; BACE1, beta-site APP cleaving enzyme 1; DNM, dynamin; FKBP12, FK506-binding protein; shRNAs, short hairpin RNAs; siRNAs, small interfering RNAs.

More specifically, flotillin-1 was present in endosomes of neurons in the amygdala, hippocampus, and isocortex of transgenic mice expressing human mutant APP and presenilin-1 [21]. Furthermore, intracellular Aβ has been shown to accumulate in early and late endosomes of the endocytic pathway that is positive for flotillin-1 in transgenic ArcAβ mice [4], overexpressing human APP 695 (and containing the Swedish and Arctic mutations in a single construct). Another study demonstrated that knockout of *flotillin-1* gene (with or without additional knockout of *flotillin-2* gene) in transgenic mice overexpressing APP and mutant presenilin-1 was associated with reduced Aβ accumulation and plaque deposition [50]. However, no significant differences in APP clustering or endocytosis were observed in mouse embryonic fibroblasts with no flotillin-1 expression [50]. Another study has indicated that treadmill exercise could inhibit amyloidogenic APP cleavage and subsequent Aβ production in the brain of APP and presenilin-1 transgenic mouse models, by suppressing lipid raft formation and flotillin-1 levels [51]. Furthermore, it has been reported that treatment of senescence-accelerated mouse prone 8 mice with *Yizhijiannao* granule, a Chinese medicinal compound, could downregulate flotillin-1 levels in the temporal lobes of the animals [52]. Interestingly, it has been demonstrated that copper could inhibit the association of flotillin-2 with lipid rafts by redistributing it into non-raft fractions, thus decreasing the endocytosis and processing of APP in membrane microdomains both in vitro and in mutant APP transgenic mice [49]. Previous works have shown that copper can attenuate Aβ production [54], and suppression of flotillin-2-mediated APP processing in rafts may represent one potential underlying mechanism. On the other hand, there is also evidence indicating that clathrin-independent endocytic pathways may not play a significant role in APP processing, since flotillin levels have been shown to remain unchanged in mutant APP transgenic mice, compared with proteins associated with clathrin-dependent pathways [53]. Nevertheless, these findings highlight the important implication of flotillins in the pathogenesis of AD, however, further studies are needed for deeper understanding of the underlying molecular mechanisms.

3.3. Evidence from In Vitro Studies

There is also a growing amount of in vitro evidence investigating the role of flotillins at a molecular level. Specifically, flotillin-1 was shown to directly interact with the intracellular domain of APP

(AICD), the C-terminus of APP consisting of 57–59 amino acids, while the residues 189–282 of flotillin-1 were found essential for this interaction. [42]. In this context, it has been demonstrated that the overexpression of FKBP12, a protein interacting with AICD, could trigger the amyloidogenic APP processing pathway in vitro, possibly by altering the affinity of AICD to flotillin-1 [43]. AICD has been demonstrated to play an important role in signal transduction via the interaction with specific PTB domain-containing proteins, including X11 and Fe65 [55]. Flotillin-1 has been also found to interact with leucine-rich glioma inactivated 3 (LGI3), a protein that is implicated in the internalization of APP in neurons [44]. More specifically, flotillin-1 was indicated to stabilize LGI3, and downregulation of the LGI3/Flo1 complex directly affected APP trafficking, by disrupting the formation of exosomes [44]. Another study has revealed that knockdown of flotillin-2 by small interfering RNA (siRNA) could impair APP endocytosis in primary cultures of hippocampal neuronal cells, resulting in reduced Aβ production in tissue cell cultures [45]. In addition, this study has demonstrated that flotillin-2 was able to act as a scaffold protein and enhance APP clustering at the surface of the plasma membrane, leading to APP endocytosis via a clathrin-dependent pathway [45]. Moreover, it has been indicated that flotillin-1 could bind to BACE1, whereas flotillin-1 overexpression was associated with increased recruitment of BACE1 into rafts and reduced activity of β-secretase in vitro [46]. Another study showed that flotillin-1 was able to directly interact with the dileucine motif in the cytoplasmic domain of BACE1, thus affecting its endosomal sorting. The flotillin-2–BACE1 interaction was shown to be indirect at least partially via flotillin-1 [47]. Depletion of both flotillins was also indicated to be associated with more prominent perinuclear localization and accumulation of overexpressed BACE1 into late endosomes in HeLa cells in which the expression of flotillin expression was knocked down via lentiviral shRNAs, suggesting that flotillins may affect its subcellular localization [47]. Additionally, flotillin-1 knockdown was demonstrated to result in overexpression of BACE1, and flotillin-2 knockdown led to increased amyloidogenic processing of endogenous APP in the same cellular system, possibly by affecting BACE1 trafficking [47]. Therefore, flotillins play a major role in BACE1 trafficking and expression, thus affecting APP cleavage. Moreover, neuroblastoma cells that were transfected with mutant *dynamin (DNM) 2* gene, in which a specific polymorphism has been associated with late-onset AD in non-carriers of the apolipoprotein E-ε4 allele [56], displayed higher levels of flotillin, and APP was predominantly localized in the lipid rafts [48].

Taken together, flotillins have been shown to affect APP endocytosis and processing, Ca^{2+} homeostasis, mitochondrial dysfunction, neuronal apoptosis, Aβ-induced neurotoxicity, and prion-like spreading of Aβ, thus playing an emerging role in AD pathogenesis.

4. Flotillin as a Novel Biomarker Candidate for AD: Clinical Evidence

CSF analysis is considered as the most reliable biofluid for detection of biomarkers of the central nervous system (CNS) disorders since it allows a more accurate elucidation of the underlying molecular processes in the brain. However, its acquisition requires lumbar puncture, which is an invasive procedure. Alternatively, blood biomarkers present a more optimal approach, and enormous research efforts are made towards this direction. However, the abundance of proteins in the plasma compared with the CSF limits the efficacy of this strategy for several molecules including $A\beta_{42}$, and the results of respective clinical studies are often inconsistent [57]. In this regard, plasma neuron-derived exosomes obtained from AD patients have been shown to contain higher levels of Aβ42 and phosphorylated tau protein compared with controls, highlighting their potential usage as AD biomarkers [57]. Several methodological concerns remain to be clarified for the estimation of exosomes per se in AD, since their detection in blood or CSF may be affected by conditions of sample storage, temperature, and the use of anticoagulants [57]. Although various techniques for the isolation of exosomes from biofluids have been developed, there is still no established validated reference method for their effective purification [57].

Flotillin, as one of the main components of exosomes, has been recently proposed as an alternative single molecule that could be used as an AD biomarker. Proteomic analyses have already indicated that flotillins are constituents of CSF-derived exosomes [58,59]. Importantly, flotillin levels can be relatively easily measured by ELISA method and/or immunoblot analysis [10], providing a significant advantage compared with other biomarker candidates that may require more expensive and specialized equipment.

Interestingly, a recent clinical study has indicated that flotillin levels were lower not only in the CSF, but also in the serum of AD patients, compared with subjects with mild cognitive impairment (MCI) or age-matched non-AD controls [10]. Additionally, CSF and serum flotillin levels have been shown to be reduced in patients with AD-related MCI, compared with non-AD-related MCI (determined by PiB-PET) [10]. Investigation of postmortem brain tissues further revealed that flotillin levels were also lower in the cerebroventricular fluid (CVF) samples obtained from AD patients compared with subjects with vascular dementia [10]. Furthermore, flotillin levels have been found to be negatively correlated with amyloid burden, as shown by the mean cortical PiB retention levels in PiB-PET [10]. However, flotillin-2 levels were shown elevated in brain sections of older non-demented humans compared with younger individuals [41], as well as levels of plasma neuron-derived exosomes were lower in aged HIV-infected individuals compared with controls [60], raising concerns regarding the efficacy of flotillin levels to effectively discriminate between AD and normal ageing. In this regard, flotillin levels were found to remain stable with advancing age in healthy controls in the abovementioned study [10], highlighting the possibility that their levels may not be affected by ageing process itself.

Although clinical evidence on the diagnostic utility of flotillins in AD is limited and the subject is still in its infancy, these findings strongly support the promising role of flotillin as a novel early CSF and serum diagnostic biomarker for AD (Figure 1). Future studies with larger sample size are therefore required for the validation of these results.

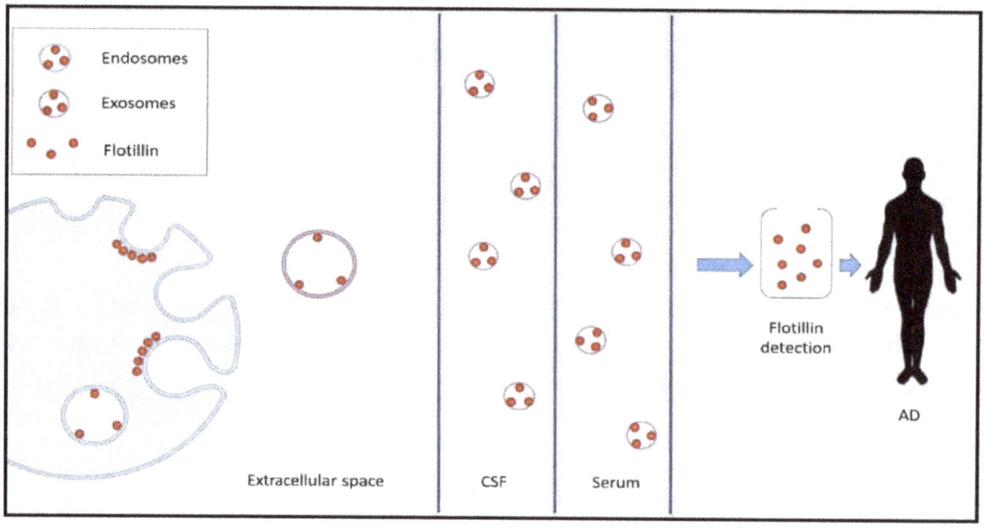

Flotillin can be detected in the CSF and serum of AD patients, and it has been demonstrated that its levels are lower in AD patients compared with controls, suggesting their use as potential AD biomarkers. AD, Alzheimer's disease; CSF: Cerebrospinal fluid.

Figure 1. Lipid rafts, endosomes, and exosomes are enriched in flotillin.

5. Discussion and Future Perspectives

Accumulating evidence highlights the emerging implication of flotillins in AD pathogenesis, through their implication in APP endocytosis and processing, Ca^{2+} homeostasis, mitochondrial dysfunction, neuronal apoptosis, Aβ-induced neurotoxicity, and prion-like spreading of Aβ. Importantly, there is also clinical evidence suggesting their potential use as biomarker candidates for AD, based on the reduced serum and CSF levels observed in AD patients compared with controls that correlated with amyloid burden.

On the other hand, there are specific challenges related to the development of flotillins as valid AD biomarkers. Firstly, it is important to note that flotillins are universally expressed by all cell types, and consist as a component of all subtypes of extracellular vesicles, independently to their density or size [61]. In addition, it has been indicated that the concentration of plasma neuron-derived exosomes was lower in neurocognitively impaired individuals (regardless of the cause) in comparison with controls [60]. Furthermore, flotillin-1 has been reported to be enriched in exosomes from CSF samples obtained from patients at early stage of severe traumatic brain injury, although no comparisons with control subjects were made in this study [62]. Moreover, levels of CSF exosomal α-synuclein have been shown to distinguish patients with Parkinson's disease, dementia with Lewy bodies, and controls with other neurological disorders, and correlate well with cognitive impairment [63]. However, flotillin-1 levels were shown to be higher in neurons bearing NFTs in brain specimens of AD compared with PD patients [4]. Nevertheless, these findings raise important concerns about the specificity of flotillin detection in AD, and highlight the need for future comparative studies in age-matched patients with other neurological disorders.

Notably, accumulating evidence reveals the potential role of tissue flotillin levels as prognostic biomarkers in various types of solid tumors, including breast cancer and lung carcinoma [64]. Although data about plasma flotillin levels in cancer patients are lacking, other comorbidities including tumors should be also considered for the evaluation of flotillin levels in AD patients. Furthermore, preclinical evidence has demonstrated that several types of statins may alter the expression of flotillins in brain plasma membrane [65], implying that treatment with statins may affect flotillin levels in AD patients. In addition, the potential effects of anti-cholinesterase inhibitors, currently prescribed for AD patients, on flotillin levels should be also considered.

Another issue that should be mentioned is the selective detection of flotillin-1 and -2 levels in the CSF. In this context, it has been indicated that flotillin-2 levels were positively correlated with flotillin-1 levels in the CSF obtained from patients after severe traumatic brain injury [62]. Nevertheless, further research is required regarding the differential role of both types of flotillins in the serum and CSF of AD patients.

Apart from flotillins, another mechanism of clathrin-independent endocytosis involves caveolins, which have been also implicated in Aβ production [66]. Caveolin-1 levels have been increased in the cortex and hippocampus of brain specimens from AD patients compared with age-matched controls [67], indicating another potential endocytosis-associated biomarker candidate for AD that could be further investigated.

Importantly, it has been shown that specific gene polymorphisms of the *neuronal sortilin-related receptor* (*SORL1*), which is highly implicated in the APP endosomal trafficking, may affect the susceptibility to AD development [68]. It has been shown that specific polymorphisms of *flotillin-2* gene may be associated with coronary artery disease in the Chinese population. Given the connection of hypercholesterolemia with AD development [18,69], further research is needed for the potential link between these *flotillin-2* polymorphisms and AD risk.

6. Conclusions

Collectively, flotillin may serve as a single CSF or blood biomarker, or be used supplementary to CSF Aβ42 and tau levels, as well as PET neuroimaging findings for more efficient and earlier AD diagnosis. However, additional larger comparative studies with age-matched controls and patients with other neurodegenerative disorders are needed for the validation of their usage as biomarkers for AD in clinical settings.

Author Contributions: E.A. carried out the literature review, conceptualized, and prepared the initial draft. Y.N.P. and M.F.S. edited and contributed in the final manuscript. C.P. provided critical inputs, edited and contributed to the final version of the manuscript. All authors have read and agreed to the published version of the manuscript.

Acknowledgments: Y.N.P. would like to acknowledge Monash University Malaysia for supporting with HDR Scholarship.

Abbreviations

AD: Alzheimer's disease; APP, Amyloid precursor protein; Aβ, Amyloid β; NFTs, neurofibrillary tangles;LGI3, Leucine-rich glioma inactivated 3; BACE1, Beta-site APP cleaving enzyme 1; DNM, Dynamin; FKBP12, FK506-binding protein; shRNAs, Short hairpin RNAs; siRNAs, Small-interfering RNAs; PiB-PET; Pittsburgh compound B and positron emission tomography; PHB, Prohibitin; ER, Endoplasmic reticulum;SMS2, Sphingomyelin synthase 2;GSLs, Glycosphingolipids; CTFs, C-terminal fragments; EVs, Extracellular vesicles; GVD, Granulovacuolar degeneration; CNS, Central nervous system; CVF, Cerebroventricular fluid; SORL1, sortilin-related receptor 1; JNK, C-jun N-terminal kinases.

References

1. Tiwari, S.; Atluri, V.; Kaushik, A.; Yndart, A.; Nair, M. Alzheimer's disease: Pathogenesis, diagnostics, and therapeutics. *Int. J. Nanomed.* **2019**, *14*, 5541–5554. [CrossRef] [PubMed]
2. Paudel, Y.N.; Angelopoulou, E.; Piperi, C.; Othman, I.; Aamir, K.; Shaikh, M. Impact of HMGB1, RAGE, and TLR4 in Alzheimer's Disease (AD): From Risk Factors to Therapeutic Targeting. *Cells* **2020**, *9*, 383. [CrossRef] [PubMed]
3. Bickel, P.E.; Scherer, P.E.; Schnitzer, J.E.; Oh, P.; Lisanti, M.P.; Lodish, H.F. Flotillin and epidermal surface antigen define a new family of caveolae-associated integral membrane proteins. *J. Biol. Chem.* **1997**, *272*, 13793–13802. [CrossRef] [PubMed]
4. Rajendran, L.; Knobloch, M.; Geiger, K.D.; Dienel, S.; Nitsch, R.; Simons, K.; Konietzko, U. Increased Abeta production leads to intracellular accumulation of Abeta in flotillin-1-positive endosomes. *Neurodegener. Dis.* **2007**, *4*, 164–170. [CrossRef]
5. Xiao, T.; Zhang, W.; Jiao, B.; Pan, C.Z.; Liu, X.; Shen, L. The role of exosomes in the pathogenesis of Alzheimer' disease. *Transl. Neurodegener.* **2017**, *6*, 3. [CrossRef]
6. Tate, B.A.; Mathews, P.M. Targeting the role of the endosome in the pathophysiology of Alzheimer's disease: A strategy for treatment. *Sci. Aging Knowl. Environ.* **2006**, *2006*, re2. [CrossRef]
7. Irizarry, M.C. Biomarkers of Alzheimer disease in plasma. *NeuroRx J. Am. Soc. Exp. Neurother.* **2004**, *1*, 226–234. [CrossRef]
8. Racine, A.M.; Koscik, R.L.; Nicholas, C.R.; Clark, L.R.; Okonkwo, O.C.; Oh, J.M.; Hillmer, A.T.; Murali, D.; Barnhart, T.E.; Betthauser, T.J.; et al. Cerebrospinal fluid ratios with Abeta42 predict preclinical brain beta-amyloid accumulation. *Alzheimer's Dement.* **2016**, *2*, 27–38. [CrossRef]
9. Vlassenko, A.G.; Benzinger, T.L.; Morris, J.C. PET amyloid-beta imaging in preclinical Alzheimer's disease. *Biochim. Biophys. Acta* **2012**, *1822*, 370–379. [CrossRef]
10. Abdullah, M.; Kimura, N.; Akatsu, H.; Hashizume, Y.; Ferdous, T.; Tachita, T.; Iida, S.; Zou, K.; Matsubara, E.; Michikawa, M. Flotillin is a Novel Diagnostic Blood Marker of Alzheimer's Disease. *J. Alzheimer's Dis.* **2019**, *72*, 1165–1176. [CrossRef]
11. Neumann-Giesen, C.; Falkenbach, B.; Beicht, P.; Claasen, S.; Luers, G.; Stuermer, C.A.; Herzog, V.; Tikkanen, R. Membrane and raft association of reggie-1/flotillin-2: Role of myristoylation, palmitoylation and oligomerization and induction of filopodia by overexpression. *Biochem. J.* **2004**, *378*, 509–518. [CrossRef] [PubMed]
12. Kokubo, H.; Lemere, C.A.; Yamaguchi, H. Localization of flotillins in human brain and their accumulation with the progression of Alzheimer's disease pathology. *Neurosci. Lett.* **2000**, *290*, 93–96. [CrossRef]
13. Bouillot, C.; Prochiantz, A.; Rougon, G.; Allinquant, B. Axonal amyloid precursor protein expressed by neurons in vitro is present in a membrane fraction with caveolae-like properties. *J. Biol. Chem.* **1996**, *271*, 7640–7644. [CrossRef] [PubMed]
14. Lee, S.J.; Liyanage, U.; Bickel, P.E.; Xia, W.; Lansbury, P.T., Jr.; Kosik, K.S. A detergent-insoluble membrane compartment contains A beta in vivo. *Nat. Med.* **1998**, *4*, 730–734. [CrossRef] [PubMed]
15. Riddell, D.R.; Christie, G.; Hussain, I.; Dingwall, C. Compartmentalization of beta-secretase (Asp2) into low-buoyant density, noncaveolar lipid rafts. *Curr. Biol.* **2001**, *11*, 1288–1293. [CrossRef]
16. Vetrivel, K.S.; Cheng, H.; Lin, W.; Sakurai, T.; Li, T.; Nukina, N.; Wong, P.C.; Xu, H.; Thinakaran, G. Association of gamma-secretase with lipid rafts in post-Golgi and endosome membranes. *J. Biol. Chem.* **2004**, *279*, 44945–44954. [CrossRef]

17. Kokubo, H.; Kayed, R.; Glabe, C.G.; Yamaguchi, H. Soluble Abeta oligomers ultrastructurally localize to cell processes and might be related to synaptic dysfunction in Alzheimer's disease brain. *Brain Res.* **2005**, *1031*, 222–228. [CrossRef]
18. Vetrivel, K.S.; Thinakaran, G. Membrane rafts in Alzheimer's disease beta-amyloid production. *Biochim. Biophys. Acta* **2010**, *1801*, 860–867. [CrossRef]
19. Abad-Rodriguez, J.; Ledesma, M.D.; Craessaerts, K.; Perga, S.; Medina, M.; Delacourte, A.; Dingwall, C.; De Strooper, B.; Dotti, C.G. Neuronal membrane cholesterol loss enhances amyloid peptide generation. *J. Cell Biol.* **2004**, *167*, 953–960. [CrossRef]
20. Crameri, A.; Biondi, E.; Kuehnle, K.; Lutjohann, D.; Thelen, K.M.; Perga, S.; Dotti, C.G.; Nitsch, R.M.; Ledesma, M.D.; Mohajeri, M.H. The role of seladin-1/DHCR24 in cholesterol biosynthesis, APP processing and Abeta generation in vivo. *EMBO J.* **2006**, *25*, 432–443. [CrossRef]
21. Langui, D.; Girardot, N.; El Hachimi, K.H.; Allinquant, B.; Blanchard, V.; Pradier, L.; Duyckaerts, C. Subcellular topography of neuronal Abeta peptide in APPxPS1 transgenic mice. *Am. J. Pathol.* **2004**, *165*, 1465–1477. [CrossRef]
22. Yamazaki, T.; Koo, E.H.; Selkoe, D.J. Trafficking of cell-surface amyloid beta-protein precursor. II. Endocytosis, recycling and lysosomal targeting detected by immunolocalization. *J. Cell Sci.* **1996**, *109*, 999–1008. [PubMed]
23. Cataldo, A.M.; Barnett, J.L.; Pieroni, C.; Nixon, R.A. Increased neuronal endocytosis and protease delivery to early endosomes in sporadic Alzheimer's disease: Neuropathologic evidence for a mechanism of increased beta-amyloidogenesis. *J. Neurosci. Off. J. Soc. Neurosci.* **1997**, *17*, 6142–6151. [CrossRef]
24. Vetrivel, K.S.; Thinakaran, G. Amyloidogenic processing of beta-amyloid precursor protein in intracellular compartments. *Neurology* **2006**, *66*, S69–S73. [CrossRef]
25. Refolo, L.M.; Sambamurti, K.; Efthimiopoulos, S.; Pappolla, M.A.; Robakis, N.K. Evidence that secretase cleavage of cell surface Alzheimer amyloid precursor occurs after normal endocytic internalization. *J. Neurosci. Res.* **1995**, *40*, 694–706. [CrossRef]
26. Rajendran, L.; Honsho, M.; Zahn, T.R.; Keller, P.; Geiger, K.D.; Verkade, P.; Simons, K. Alzheimer's disease beta-amyloid peptides are released in association with exosomes. *Proc. Natl. Acad. Sci. USA* **2006**, *103*, 11172–11177. [CrossRef]
27. Perez, R.G.; Soriano, S.; Hayes, J.D.; Ostaszewski, B.; Xia, W.; Selkoe, D.J.; Chen, X.; Stokin, G.B.; Koo, E.H. Mutagenesis identifies new signals for beta-amyloid precursor protein endocytosis, turnover, and the generation of secreted fragments, including Abeta42. *J. Biol. Chem.* **1999**, *274*, 18851–18856. [CrossRef]
28. Elkin, S.R.; Lakoduk, A.M.; Schmid, S.L. Endocytic pathways and endosomal trafficking: A primer. *Wien. Med. Wochenschr.* **2016**, *166*, 196–204. [CrossRef]
29. Abdullah, M.; Takase, H.; Nunome, M.; Enomoto, H.; Ito, J.; Gong, J.S.; Michikawa, M. Amyloid-beta Reduces Exosome Release from Astrocytes by Enhancing JNK Phosphorylation. *J. Alzheimer's Dis.* **2016**, *53*, 1433–1441. [CrossRef]
30. Paolicelli, R.C.; Bergamini, G.; Rajendran, L. Cell-to-cell Communication by Extracellular Vesicles: Focus on Microglia. *Neuroscience* **2019**, *405*, 148–157. [CrossRef]
31. Yuyama, K.; Sun, H.; Mitsutake, S.; Igarashi, Y. Sphingolipid-modulated exosome secretion promotes clearance of amyloid-beta by microglia. *J. Biol. Chem.* **2012**, *287*, 10977–10989. [CrossRef] [PubMed]
32. Yuyama, K.; Sun, H.; Sakai, S.; Mitsutake, S.; Okada, M.; Tahara, H.; Furukawa, J.; Fujitani, N.; Shinohara, Y.; Igarashi, Y. Decreased amyloid-beta pathologies by intracerebral loading of glycosphingolipid-enriched exosomes in Alzheimer model mice. *J. Biol. Chem.* **2014**, *289*, 24488–24498. [CrossRef] [PubMed]
33. Perez-Gonzalez, R.; Gauthier, S.A.; Kumar, A.; Levy, E. The exosome secretory pathway transports amyloid precursor protein carboxyl-terminal fragments from the cell into the brain extracellular space. *J. Biol. Chem.* **2012**, *287*, 43108–43115. [CrossRef] [PubMed]
34. Saman, S.; Kim, W.; Raya, M.; Visnick, Y.; Miro, S.; Saman, S.; Jackson, B.; McKee, A.C.; Alvarez, V.E.; Lee, N.C.; et al. Exosome-associated tau is secreted in tauopathy models and is selectively phosphorylated in cerebrospinal fluid in early Alzheimer disease. *J. Biol. Chem.* **2012**, *287*, 3842–3849. [CrossRef] [PubMed]
35. An, K.; Klyubin, I.; Kim, Y.; Jung, J.H.; Mably, A.J.; O'Dowd, S.T.; Lynch, T.; Kanmert, D.; Lemere, C.A.; Finan, G.M.; et al. Exosomes neutralize synaptic-plasticity-disrupting activity of Abeta assemblies in vivo. *Mol. Brain* **2013**, *6*, 47. [CrossRef] [PubMed]

36. Girardot, N.; Allinquant, B.; Langui, D.; Laquerriere, A.; Dubois, B.; Hauw, J.J.; Duyckaerts, C. Accumulation of flotillin-1 in tangle-bearing neurones of Alzheimer's disease. *Neuropathol. Appl. Neurobiol.* **2003**, *29*, 451–461. [CrossRef]
37. Eitan, E.; Hutchison, E.R.; Marosi, K.; Comotto, J.; Mustapic, M.; Nigam, S.M.; Suire, C.; Maharana, C.; Jicha, G.A.; Liu, D.; et al. Extracellular Vesicle-Associated Abeta Mediates Trans-Neuronal Bioenergetic and Ca(2+)-Handling Deficits in Alzheimer's Disease Models. *NPJ Aging Mech. Dis.* **2016**, *2*. [CrossRef]
38. Sardar Sinha, M.; Ansell-Schultz, A.; Civitelli, L.; Hildesjo, C.; Larsson, M.; Lannfelt, L.; Ingelsson, M.; Hallbeck, M. Alzheimer's disease pathology propagation by exosomes containing toxic amyloid-beta oligomers. *Acta Neuropathol.* **2018**, *136*, 41–56. [CrossRef]
39. Nishikawa, T.; Takahashi, T.; Nakamori, M.; Yamazaki, Y.; Kurashige, T.; Nagano, Y.; Nishida, Y.; Izumi, Y.; Matsumoto, M. Phosphatidylinositol-4,5-bisphosphate is enriched in granulovacuolar degeneration bodies and neurofibrillary tangles. *Neuropathol. Appl. Neurobiol.* **2014**, *40*, 489–501. [CrossRef]
40. Woodard, J.S. Clinicopathologic significance of granulovacuolar degeneration in Alzheimer's disease. *J. Neuropathol. Exp. Neurol.* **1962**, *21*, 85–91. [CrossRef]
41. Alsaqati, M.; Thomas, R.S.; Kidd, E.J. Proteins Involved in Endocytosis Are Upregulated by Ageing in the Normal Human Brain: Implications for the Development of Alzheimer's Disease. *J. Gerontol. Ser. A Biol. Sci. Med Sci.* **2018**, *73*, 289–298. [CrossRef] [PubMed]
42. Chen, T.Y.; Liu, P.H.; Ruan, C.T.; Chiu, L.; Kung, F.L. The intracellular domain of amyloid precursor protein interacts with flotillin-1, a lipid raft protein. *Biochem. Biophys. Res. Commun.* **2006**, *342*, 266–272. [CrossRef] [PubMed]
43. Liu, F.L.; Liu, T.Y.; Kung, F.L. FKBP12 regulates the localization and processing of amyloid precursor protein in human cell lines. *J. Biosci.* **2014**, *39*, 85–95. [CrossRef] [PubMed]
44. Okabayashi, S.; Kimura, N. LGI3 interacts with flotillin-1 to mediate APP trafficking and exosome formation. *Neuroreport* **2010**, *21*, 606–610. [CrossRef] [PubMed]
45. Schneider, A.; Rajendran, L.; Honsho, M.; Gralle, M.; Donnert, G.; Wouters, F.; Hell, S.W.; Simons, M. Flotillin-dependent clustering of the amyloid precursor protein regulates its endocytosis and amyloidogenic processing in neurons. *J. Neurosci. Off. J. Soc. Neurosci.* **2008**, *28*, 2874–2882. [CrossRef] [PubMed]
46. Hattori, C.; Asai, M.; Onishi, H.; Sasagawa, N.; Hashimoto, Y.; Saido, T.C.; Maruyama, K.; Mizutani, S.; Ishiura, S. BACE1 interacts with lipid raft proteins. *J. Neurosci. Res.* **2006**, *84*, 912–917. [CrossRef]
47. John, B.A.; Meister, M.; Banning, A.; Tikkanen, R. Flotillins bind to the dileucine sorting motif of beta-site amyloid precursor protein-cleaving enzyme 1 and influence its endosomal sorting. *FEBS J.* **2014**, *281*, 2074–2087. [CrossRef]
48. Kamagata, E.; Kudo, T.; Kimura, R.; Tanimukai, H.; Morihara, T.; Sadik, M.G.; Kamino, K.; Takeda, M. Decrease of dynamin 2 levels in late-onset Alzheimer's disease alters Abeta metabolism. *Biochem. Biophys. Res. Commun.* **2009**, *379*, 691–695. [CrossRef]
49. Hung, Y.H.; Robb, E.L.; Volitakis, I.; Ho, M.; Evin, G.; Li, Q.X.; Culvenor, J.G.; Masters, C.L.; Cherny, R.A.; Bush, A.I. Paradoxical condensation of copper with elevated beta-amyloid in lipid rafts under cellular copper deficiency conditions: Implications for Alzheimer disease. *J. Biol. Chem.* **2009**, *284*, 21899–21907. [CrossRef]
50. Bitsikas, V.; Riento, K.; Howe, J.D.; Barry, N.P.; Nichols, B.J. The role of flotillins in regulating abeta production, investigated using flotillin 1-/-, flotillin 2-/- double knockout mice. *PLoS ONE* **2014**, *9*, e85217. [CrossRef]
51. Zhang, X.L.; Zhao, N.; Xu, B.; Chen, X.H.; Li, T.J. Treadmill exercise inhibits amyloid-beta generation in the hippocampus of APP/PS1 transgenic mice by reducing cholesterol-mediated lipid raft formation. *Neuroreport* **2019**, *30*, 498–503. [CrossRef] [PubMed]
52. Zhu, H.; Luo, L.; Hu, S.; Dong, K.; Li, G.; Zhang, T. Treating Alzheimer's disease with Yizhijiannao granules by regulating expression of multiple proteins in temporal lobe. *Neural Regen. Res.* **2014**, *9*, 1283–1287. [CrossRef] [PubMed]
53. Thomas, R.S.; Lelos, M.J.; Good, M.A.; Kidd, E.J. Clathrin-mediated endocytic proteins are upregulated in the cortex of the Tg2576 mouse model of Alzheimer's disease-like amyloid pathology. *Biochem. Biophys. Res. Commun.* **2011**, *415*, 656–661. [CrossRef] [PubMed]
54. Kong, G.K.; Miles, L.A.; Crespi, G.A.; Morton, C.J.; Ng, H.L.; Barnham, K.J.; McKinstry, W.J.; Cappai, R.; Parker, M.W. Copper binding to the Alzheimer's disease amyloid precursor protein. *Eur. Biophys. J.* **2008**, *37*, 269–279. [CrossRef]

55. Guenette, S.; Strecker, P.; Kins, S. APP Protein Family Signaling at the Synapse: Insights from Intracellular APP-Binding Proteins. *Front. Mol. Neurosci.* **2017**, *10*, 87. [CrossRef]
56. Aidaralieva, N.J.; Kamino, K.; Kimura, R.; Yamamoto, M.; Morihara, T.; Kazui, H.; Hashimoto, R.; Tanaka, T.; Kudo, T.; Kida, T.; et al. Dynamin 2 gene is a novel susceptibility gene for late-onset Alzheimer disease in non-APOE-epsilon4 carriers. *J. Hum. Genet.* **2008**, *53*, 296–302. [CrossRef]
57. Lee, S.; Mankhong, S.; Kang, J.H. Extracellular Vesicle as a Source of Alzheimer's Biomarkers: Opportunities and Challenges. *Int. J. Mol. Sci.* **2019**, *20*, 1728. [CrossRef]
58. Chiasserini, D.; van Weering, J.R.; Piersma, S.R.; Pham, T.V.; Malekzadeh, A.; Teunissen, C.E.; de Wit, H.; Jimenez, C.R. Proteomic analysis of cerebrospinal fluid extracellular vesicles: A comprehensive dataset. *J. Proteom.* **2014**, *106*, 191–204. [CrossRef]
59. Street, J.M.; Barran, P.E.; Mackay, C.L.; Weidt, S.; Balmforth, C.; Walsh, T.S.; Chalmers, R.T.; Webb, D.J.; Dear, J.W. Identification and proteomic profiling of exosomes in human cerebrospinal fluid. *J. Transl. Med.* **2012**, *10*, 5. [CrossRef]
60. Sun, B.; Dalvi, P.; Abadjian, L.; Tang, N.; Pulliam, L. Blood neuron-derived exosomes as biomarkers of cognitive impairment in HIV. *Aids* **2017**, *31*, F9–F17. [CrossRef]
61. Kowal, J.; Arras, G.; Colombo, M.; Jouve, M.; Morath, J.P.; Primdal-Bengtson, B.; Dingli, F.; Loew, D.; Tkach, M.; Thery, C. Proteomic comparison defines novel markers to characterize heterogeneous populations of extracellular vesicle subtypes. *Proc. Natl. Acad. Sci. USA* **2016**, *113*, E968–E977. [CrossRef] [PubMed]
62. Kuharic, J.; Grabusic, K.; Tokmadzic, V.S.; Stifter, S.; Tulic, K.; Shevchuk, O.; Lucin, P.; Sustic, A. Severe Traumatic Brain Injury Induces Early Changes in the Physical Properties and Protein Composition of Intracranial Extracellular Vesicles. *J. Neurotrauma* **2019**, *36*, 190–200. [CrossRef]
63. Stuendl, A.; Kunadt, M.; Kruse, N.; Bartels, C.; Moebius, W.; Danzer, K.M.; Mollenhauer, B.; Schneider, A. Induction of alpha-synuclein aggregate formation by CSF exosomes from patients with Parkinson's disease and dementia with Lewy bodies. *Brain J. Neurol.* **2016**, *139*, 481–494. [CrossRef] [PubMed]
64. Ou, Y.X.; Liu, F.T.; Chen, F.Y.; Zhu, Z.M. Prognostic value of Flotillin-1 expression in patients with solid tumors. *Oncotarget* **2017**, *8*, 52665–52677. [CrossRef] [PubMed]
65. Kirsch, C.; Eckert, G.P.; Mueller, W.E. Statin effects on cholesterol micro-domains in brain plasma membranes. *Biochem. Pharmacol.* **2003**, *65*, 843–856. [CrossRef]
66. Dominguez-Prieto, M.; Velasco, A.; Tabernero, A.; Medina, J.M. Endocytosis and Transcytosis of Amyloid-beta Peptides by Astrocytes: A Possible Mechanism for Amyloid-beta Clearance in Alzheimer's Disease. *J. Alzheimer's Dis.* **2018**, *65*, 1109–1124. [CrossRef]
67. Gaudreault, S.B.; Dea, D.; Poirier, J. Increased caveolin-1 expression in Alzheimer's disease brain. *Neurobiol. Aging* **2004**, *25*, 753–759. [CrossRef]
68. Cong, L.; Kong, X.; Wang, J.; Du, J.; Xu, Z.; Xu, Y.; Zhao, Q. Association between SORL1 polymorphisms and the risk of Alzheimer's disease. *J. Integr. Neurosci.* **2018**, *17*, 185–192. [CrossRef]
69. Reitz, C. Dyslipidemia and the risk of Alzheimer's disease. *Curr. Atheroscler. Rep.* **2013**, *15*, 307. [CrossRef]

10

Significance of Blood and Cerebrospinal Fluid Biomarkers for Alzheimer's Disease: Sensitivity, Specificity and Potential for Clinical Use

Cristina d'Abramo [1], Luciano D'Adamio [2] and Luca Giliberto [1,3,4,*]

[1] The Litwin-Zucker Center for Alzheimer's Disease & Memory Disorders, Institute of Molecular Medicine, Feinstein Institutes for Medical Research, Northwell Health System, Manhasset, NY 11030, USA; cdabramo@northwell.edu

[2] Rutgers Alzheimer's Disease & Dementia Research Center (RUADRC), Rutgers Brain Health Institute, Rutgers University, Piscataway, NJ 08854, USA; luciano.dadamio@rutgers.edu

[3] Northwell Health Neuroscience Institute, Northwell Health System, Manhasset, NY 11030, USA

[4] Donald and Barbara Zucker School of Medicine, Hofstra University, Hempstead, NY 11549, USA

* Correspondence: lgiliberto@northwell.edu

Abstract: Alzheimer's disease (AD) is the most common type of dementia, affecting more than 5 million Americans, with steadily increasing mortality and incredible socio-economic burden. Not only have therapeutic efforts so far failed to reach significant efficacy, but the real pathogenesis of the disease is still obscure. The current theories are based on pathological findings of amyloid plaques and tau neurofibrillary tangles that accumulate in the brain parenchyma of affected patients. These findings have defined, together with the extensive neurodegeneration, the diagnostic criteria of the disease. The ability to detect changes in the levels of amyloid and tau in cerebrospinal fluid (CSF) first, and more recently in blood, has allowed us to use these biomarkers for the specific in-vivo diagnosis of AD in humans. Furthermore, other pathological elements of AD, such as the loss of neurons, inflammation and metabolic derangement, have translated to the definition of other CSF and blood biomarkers, which are not specific of the disease but, when combined with amyloid and tau, correlate with the progression from mild cognitive impairment to AD dementia, or identify patients who will develop AD pathology. In this review, we discuss the role of current and hypothetical biomarkers of Alzheimer's disease, their specificity, and the caveats of current high-sensitivity platforms for their peripheral detection.

Keywords: Alzheimer's disease; biomarkers; cerebrospinal fluid; blood; amyloid; tau; soluble TREM2; NfL; Multiplex; SiMoA

---

1. Introduction

1.1. Clinicopathological Definition of Alzheimer's Disease

Alzheimer's disease (AD) is a neurodegenerative disorder, characterized by progressive cognitive impairment, affecting the domains of memory, speech, praxis, awareness and executive function, representing a decline from the prior functional state, with a relentless course [1]. It is the most common cause of dementia. Along with the destructive nature of the disease, which affects patients and their families, AD represents an enormous burden on public health. An estimated of 5+ million Americans have AD, and the prevalence worldwide reaches almost 60 million; the diseases hits the elderly population the most, with 11% of individuals 65 and older affected by the disease [2,3]. Two thirds of AD patients are women, implying hormonal, lifestyle and genetic factors as co-causative elements [2,4–15]. AD is the sixth leading cause of death in the US [16] and mortality due to AD has steadily increased in the last 20 years, in contrast to opposite trends for other chronic diseases, such as cardiovascular, cancer, HIV and more. The socio-economic burden of the disease, on patients, families and caregivers at large, and on society, is unparalleled; AD is the disease that contributes most to disability and poor health in the US, reducing life expectancy and productivity of the affected individuals and the wellbeing of caregivers, who often have to give up jobs and careers to care for their loved ones [17–19]; this is often disproportionally affecting women too [20–22]. Finally, AD has a tremendous economic impact: the sole health care costs, variably covered by insurances (including Medicare and Medicaid) or out of pocket, to care for this disease, is in excess of 230 billion [23]. Age-matched comparisons show that individuals affected by dementia had 3–4x the annual health care expenses than those not affected. It is estimated that these costs will reach, in 2050, 1 trillion dollars (2020 Alzheimer's Disease Facts and Figures. Available online: https://www.alz.org/media/Documents/alzheimers-facts-and-figures.pdf. Accessed on 29 July 2020), a figure comparable to the US budget deficit in 2020. Interestingly, these numbers should probably be corrected upward, as the disease is often under-recognized and under-reported. This is particularly relevant to our discussion, given current limitations in performing early and accurate diagnosis.

The pathological diagnosis of AD relies on the assessment of specific brain features [24–27], based on the presence, morphology and density of lesions and their topographic distribution, in the appropriate clinical setting. Alzheimer's brains are characterized by a spatiotemporally defined accumulation of amyloid beta (Aβ) plaques, neurofibrillary tangles (NFT), of hyperphosphorylated and aggregated tau and neuronal loss [25,28,29]. Aβ accumulates mostly as the Aβ peptide ending at residue 42, which is considered the most toxic and most prone to aggregation [30]; tau accumulates as a hyperphosphorylated and conformationally altered form, in both its 3- and 4-repeats variants [31]. The trajectory of protein accumulation is relevant. It is speculated that Aβ accumulates first; this is followed by the hyperphosphorylation, conformational changes and aggregation of tau; finally, neuronal loss ensues.

The link between these three features is, to some degree, still loose. Both Aβ [30,32] and tau [33,34] are per se neurotoxic; Aβ accumulation can trigger tau accumulation [35] but, in several models, tau can independently aggregate and cause neurodegeneration [36]. Furthermore, amyloid deposition, by pathological and imaging staging (amyloid positron emission tomography—PET), does not topographically and functionally correlate with the clinical cognitive decline seen in our patients, while tau does, and there are cases of aged individuals who have amyloid deposition in their brain, but no tau and no clinical dementia [25,37,38].

A significant degree of co-pathology, not strictly specific of AD, is common in these brains [39]. This includes the presence of activated microglia and reactive astrocytes, which appear initially around neuritic plaques, and increase in density and activation in proportion to the neuronal damage and the presence of tau pathology [40–42]; vascular alterations, in the form of amyloid deposition in the blood vessels (CAA: cerebral amyloid angiopathy); accumulation of other structural proteins in neurons, such as actin and actin-associated proteins in the form of Hirano bodies [43]; granulovacuolar degeneration (GVD), a feature often associated with the initial hyperphosphorylation and aggregation of tau in the hippocampus [44]. Argyrophilic grains of 4-repeat tau can also be found in neuronal dendrites, near oligodendrocytes inclusions and seems to be relevant to disease progression [45].

In some AD cases, specific neuronal populations are vulnerable to develop Lewy body pathology of α-synuclein [43,46], which is a signature of Parkinson's disease (PD), mostly at the axonal level, in cortico-limbic regions, olfactory bulbs and substantia nigra. Finally, TAR DNA-binding protein 43 (TDP-43) pathology, more commonly found in cases of frontotemporal lobe degeneration (FTD), can be present in AD, in the amygdala, hippocampus and eventually in the neocortex and more diffusely [47,48], being not specific of AD, but underlying the vast array of cellular dysfunction present in this disease, which can affect RNA-related metabolism as well [49]. The common path, which is likely consequent to all the above changes, is the dramatic loss of synapses, which precedes neuronal loss, and mostly follows the distribution of tau pathology [43,50–52].

The routine clinical diagnosis of possible or probable AD is currently based on the identification of symptoms by the clinician, mostly Neurologists, Geriatricians, Psychiatrists and Primary Care Physicians, followed by more in-depth assessment by Neuropsychology testing and using the tools available in clinical practice, e.g., Magnetic Resonance Imaging (MRI) of the brain and common blood works. Once AD is suspected, these tools allow to rule out secondary dementia and other, different pattern of primary dementia. On a more sophisticated level, the analysis of the cerebrospinal fluid (CSF), the use of PET imaging and genetics (in familial cases) may allow us to obtain a definitive diagnosis of AD in vivo: due to cost and perception of invasiveness, this is often limited to Academic centers or in the context of clinical trials.

Ideally, we should diagnose AD, and every dementia, as early as possible. Mild cognitive impairment (MCI) is a prodromal phase of dementia, where the patient shows symptoms of cognitive changes but maintains good functionality. This is a moment where the application of biomarkers is paramount and significant therapeutic intervention may still possible. Unfortunately, there is a significant underappreciation of the disease, which is missed in more than 20% of the cases. On the other hand, lack of familiarity with alternative diagnoses, leads to overdiagnosis of AD in more than 25% of the cases, where potentially curable conditions are instead the underlying cause of the cognitive and functional decline [53–56].

1.2. Pathogenesis

The majority of our understanding of the pathogenesis of AD derives from the identification of key genes involved in the etiology and pathology of the disease. In a small percentage of the cases, the disease is inherited as autosomal dominant (FAD: familial AD), with an early age of onset, as early as the 40s, and a faster progression [57]. FAD is caused by mutations of one of three genes, Amyloid Precursor Protein (APP), Presenilin 1 (PS1) or Presenilin 2 (PS2). APP is the precursor of the amyloid peptide, Aβ, which is generated from APP by two sequential cleavages: first, the beta-secretase activity of BACE1 (beta-site amyloid precursor protein cleaving enzyme 1) generates a peptide of ~99 amino acids (C99); subsequently, the activity of the gamma-secretase, a multi-peptide protease, progressively cleaves C99 to generate the Aβ peptide ending at residues 40 or 42. The gamma secretase complex is composed of PS1 or PS2 and three other proteins, nicastrin, Aph1 and Pen2 [58]. Mutations in APP mostly lead to increase affinity of APP itself for BACE1, with increased generation of C99. Mutations of PS1 and PS2, which result in an actual loss of function mutations of gamma-secretase [59–62], lead to increased generation of the Aβ peptide ending in residue 42. This is recognized as the most toxic of the Aβ peptides [63]. About 95% of AD cases are sporadic (SAD) and have a later onset (after 65 years of age): although SAD cases lack a Mendelian cause, variants of genes such as Apolipoprotein E (*APOE*) [64,65], and triggering receptors expressed on myeloid cells 2 (TREM2) [66] are known to increase the risk of developing SAD. It is not clear what the initial trigger to Aβ and tau accumulation is in the sporadic disease. At the subcellular and molecular level, the complexity of Aβ and tau accumulation and their specific contribution to pathology has been extensively studied, and is beyond the scope of the current publication. The general understanding is that both amyloid and tau oligomers have the ability to disrupt several of the essential functions of neurons, and possibly other brain cells, i.e., metabolic and mitochondrial activity [67,68], synaptic communication [69,70], membrane integrity [71], membrane pore formation with ions leakage [72,73], protein trafficking and degradation [74,75]. Both Aβ and tau possess the ability to trigger a cascade of functional changes in neurons, microglia, astrocytes and oligodendrocytes, which results in neuronal dysfunction, synaptic loss, innate immune system activation, inflammation, blood-brain barrier impairment and neurodegeneration [39,76]. Relevant to our discussion, the immune system is activated (early) in AD, and may contribute, by means of ineffective clearance of Aβ and tau by the microglia, to the diffusion of such pathology to neighboring or connected areas [77,78], and inflammation per se is a trigger to further production of Aβ and activation of kinases to hyper-phosphorylate tau [79], cascading more neuropathology.

1.3. The (Amyloid, Tau, Neurodegeneration) ATN System

Stemming from the above definitions, pathological correlates and pathogenic theories, AD can be viewed as the combination of specific brain pathology, Aβ and tau, and neurodegeneration, which eventually results in the clinical presentation. Recent advances in brain imaging and more sensitive and specific means to detect Aβ and tau in biological fluids, associated with our ability to detect loss of brain matter, metabolism or function, have allowed for development of a classification and staging system for AD, the ATN system [80], which is routinely revised [81], to include the everchanging horizon of new biomarkers available. Patients are classified by positivity to markers of amyloid deposition (A), tau load (T) and neurodegeneration (N). Amyloid markers include the positivity to Amyloid PET (several tracers are now available) or reduced levels of cerebrospinal fluid (CSF) Aβ42, Aβ40 or of the Aβ42/40 ratio (see below). T is defined by the high levels of total or phosphorylated tau in the CSF (see below), although the new available tau PET tracers may soon be included in the criteria. Finally, N is related to the neurodegenerative aspect, and can be defined by loss of volume/activity in specific areas of the brain by magnetic resonance imaging (MRI, e.g., NeuroQuant, [82,83]), fluorodeoxyglucose (FDG)-PET or by the presence of CSF biomarkers of synaptic or neuronal loss, e.g., Neurofilament Light chain (NfL).

This system has been a useful tool for many biomarkers studies, both in biological fluids and imaging, remaining the "benchmark" for AD diagnosis and prognosis determination. Importantly, the ATN system can be extremely useful to identify and correctly classify individuals who may have amyloid deposition but no neurodegeneration (A+T-N-) and vice versa (A-T-N+); this is extremely important when studying pathophysiological correlates and in longitudinal assessments. As hinted above, a good proportion of the ageing population will show deposition of amyloid in their brain, but no clinical dementia; we know that this amyloid may not be the same amyloid that accumulates in AD proper [84], hence not cause the disease, but also other factors may not be present in these individuals that predispose to tau accumulation and neurodegeneration. On the other hand, neurodegeneration and dementia may occur because of pathology other than Alzheimer's, e.g., vascular, TDP43, alpha-synuclein, etc. If rigorously determined and applied to our studies, the ATN system will be invaluable, as it prescinds from the subjective interpretation of the clinical status of the patients, and is purely descriptive of their biomarkers status.

It must be noted, though, that not all the pathophysiological events and biomarkers in AD can be inscribed in the ATN definition, hence we will be presenting a wider paradigm, that includes, for example, inflammation.

1.4. Treatment Options

No disease-modifying treatment is available as of today, despite decades of efforts aimed to curb the pathological changes of the disease [85–87]. The widest attempts to tackle the disease have been directed against the production/accumulation of Aβ and have overall been underwhelming [85]. Reducing its production via inhibition of BACE or gamma-secretase has not been effective, resulting in potential side effects, included hastening the cognitive decline [86]; active vaccination efforts against Aβ has also not been successful, mostly due to cases of dramatic adverse events, in the form of hemorrhagic encephalitis [88], despite some cognitive benefits in the survivors [89]. Alternative active vaccinations strategies, aimed at inducing a wide reactivity to Aβ without the excessive inflammatory response, have been tested [90,91] with scarce success. Passive immunization against Aβ was also tainted by questionable clinical efficacy and concerns of serious side effects [92–95], but efforts are well under way: at the moment that we write this review, a monoclonal antibody against amyloid has been submitted for U.S. Food and Drug Administration (FDA) expedited approval as a modifying drug against AD, with some skepticism among the scientific community in respect to the available efficacy data [95] (NCT02477800). Tau has been the other logical therapeutic target. Current strategies are directed to target total tau, which is thought to accumulate intra- and extracellularly, and may spread from cell to cell, aggregating and getting hyperphosphorylated, contributing to neurodegeneration.

Antibodies targeting extracellular tau have been in clinical trial now for some time, and we are all bracing for the upcoming results. Of note, this strategy has so far failed in progressive supranuclear palsy (PSP) cases with tau pathology (NCT03068468). An active immunization approach against tau is currently under way as well [96,97].

What clinicians are left with is the use of symptomatic treatments. Acetylcholine deficits are well recognized in AD [98], and are the basis for acetylcholine esterase inhibitors, which can ameliorate quality of life. Memantine, a noncompetitive N-methyl-D-aspartate-receptor antagonist, has also shown some benefit in maintaining cognitive function, alone and in association with acetylcholine esterase inhibitors. In all, unfortunately, the enthusiasm for these agents is very low, due to low efficacy and possible adverse events, such as behavioral changes, heart arrhythmias, loss of appetite and weight, which in the elderly population are a major concern.

The neuropathological changes described above are projected to begin decades before the presentation of symptoms. This makes any medical intervention, even in the prodromal stages, a "too little-too late" approach, with few chances of being meaningful. The challenges in AD are, in our opinion, 2-fold; first, defining the actual pathogenesis of the disease, by far not yet clear; second, be able to identify the risk to develop the disease early enough so that disease-modifying intervention can be effective.

1.5. Definition of AD Biomarkers and Diagnostic Challenges

What is a biomarker? What is an adequate and useful diagnostic biomarker for Alzheimer's disease? While it is fairly easy to respond to the first question, it is very difficult to answer the second. The reason for the latter is that, save for the genetically determined cases of AD (a minority of the cases), in the absence of a univocal and comprehensive pathogenic pathway, it is unlikely to be able to diagnose AD with certainty in the living adult in a time frame that would be useful for significant intervention.

A biomarker is a "defined characteristic that is measured as an indicator of normal biological processes, pathogenic processes, or responses to an exposure or intervention, including therapeutic interventions" (FDA-NIH Biomarker Working Group. BEST (Biomarkers, EndpointS, and other Tools). Available online: https://www.ncbi.nlm.nih.gov/books/NBK326791/. Accessed on 29 July 2020). This definition includes both a diagnostic and prognostic element. The current literature about AD biomarkers is extensive and rich of analyses and reviews. The popular website, Alzforum, has its own dedicated meta-analysis page (Alzforum. Available online: https://www.alzforum.org/alzbiomarker. Accessed on 29 July 2020).

AD biomarkers are quite reliable indicators of disease presence, topographical extension and stage. Levels of Aβ, total tau (t-tau), and phosphorylated tau (p-tau) are concurrent with AD pathology [99,100] and indicate its presence; at this stage amyloid [101] and tau PET imaging [102] define the topographical extension of such pathology, while MRI [103] and FDG-PET [104] define the topographical severity of the neurodegenerative process; finally, markers such as p-tau, NfL [105] and YKL40 [106] can be useful, and early, peripheral indicators of disease stage.

We can use a combination of fluid and imaging biomarkers to complement the clinical investigation in our patients, and fulfill the current diagnostic criteria [107–110] with ease. One caveat is that while these criteria can work well in research settings [111,112], the reality of clinical practice is tainted by the reluctance of patients to have invasive testing done (CSF) and by the lack or insurance support for the more "fancy" imaging [113]. Fortunately, as described below, the rapid evolution of detection techniques is allowing to reach remarkable results from blood biomarkers, which would improve access for patients.

Another element must be taken in consideration when defining a useful biomarker: time. The concept of early diagnosis has become crucial in neurodegeneration, since protein aggregation and accumulation might only reflect the last stage of the pathogenic cascade, a point of no return in the clinical manifestation and progression of the diseases, where therapeutic interventions have so far been ineffective. As mentioned above, the exact succession of pathogenic events in AD is still unclear;

Aβ and tau may be causative, but subtler prior changes in neuronal connectivity, metabolic patterns and inflammation could represent an early disruption of neuronal function, leading to secondary accumulation of Aβ and tau [36]. In this context, an early diagnosis should go beyond Aβ and tau. A "late" biomarker' profile may also be tainted by ongoing and long-standing pathology, and by other factors related to ageing, e.g., brain trauma, infections, microvascular disease/strokes, and co-morbidity with other frequent neurodegenerative conditions such as PD [114]. The clinical presentation of FAD and SAD is similar, except for the age of onset. For FAD mutations carriers, preclinical diagnosis is possible by genetic analysis; the more common SAD cases, instead, remain elusive until clinically evident. Hence, the challenge of procuring an early preclinical diagnosis of disease or susceptibility to it.

With these limitations in mind, the science of AD biomarkers has evolved tremendously in the last decade, and we are looking now at the possibility to have reliable peripheral non-invasive, scalable and affordable biomarkers of AD pathology and disease stage.

We will review below the current, most promising fluid (blood and CSF) biomarkers available, discuss the pathophysiologic correlate of each, their clinical significance, their general applicability in the clinical and research setting. We will then take tau as an example of biomarker detection complexity, with blessings and caveats, stemming from the need to accurately validate data emerging from new ultra-sensitive platforms, in light of their biochemical limitations.

Importantly, we have divided the below presentation in biomarkers that are specific of AD, where their appropriate combination in biological fluids defines the disease, from biomarkers that are representative of neurodegeneration or associated pathology, such as synaptic and neuronal loss, inflammation, vascular disease and others. The latter biomarkers may be present in neurodegenerative diseases different from AD, in head trauma, in stroke and infections, hence they are not specific for AD. They are, though, extremely useful to follow, and at time predict, AD progression and presentation. Their precise causative role in the neurodegenerative process is still unknown, hence we will present the current known hypotheses in descriptive fashion.

2. Biomarkers of AD Pathology

2.1. Aβ

Given its pathophysiological role, Aβ has revealed itself as the major biomarker of the disease, in addition to being one of main therapeutic targets so far. Over the last 30+ years, exponential efforts have demonstrated that CSF (and more recently blood) levels of Aβ (1) are reduced in AD compared to non-demented controls [115], (2) are decreased in mild cognitive impairment (MCI) patients compared to normal controls [116], (3) the trend of Aβ decrease is predictive of the clinical progression of MCI to AD and preclinical AD [117,118] to MCI. Similarly, and (4) the Aβ42/40 ratio is reduced in MCI and AD, with better clinical correlations to than total Aβ [119,120].

What is the pathogenic significance of Aβ reduction in biological fluids? Why is the Aβ42/40 ratio going down as the disease progresses? Is there ever a time, in the preclinical phases of the disease, when Aβ is instead increased in biological fluids, possibly marking a pivotal moment where a therapeutic intervention would still be effective?

In FAD, APP mutations lead to an increased overall production of Aβ, since the amyloidogenic cleavage of APP is favored. Mutations in PS1 or PS2 result instead in a preferential cleavage of C99 to form the Aβ42, while in reality the overall amount of Aβ may be reduced, since these are loss of function mutations [121]. In either case, there is an absolute or relative abundance of Aβ42 released in the brain parenchyma, which has a high tendency to aggregate and deposit as oligomers, fibrils and plaques in a process of nucleation [122]. Furthermore, BACE cleavage is seldom limited to residue #1 of Aβ; the amyloid peptide often starts at residue #3 or #11, a glutamate residue (E), which tends to be cyclized [123,124] as pyro-glutamate (pE). The resulting AβN3(pE) and AβN11(pE) peptides also have high tendency to aggregation, adding to the stickiness of Aβ42, and have been considered one of the first seeding species of Aβ [125]. In this context, it is easy to understand how the parenchymal sequestration of Aβ results in lower level of the soluble molecule available to diffuse to the interstitial fluid, CSF and blood, hence the low levels thereof. Further decrease of Aβ in the periphery may also be related to the progressive and massive loss of neuronal cells along the progression of the disease, as neurons are the highest manufacturers of the peptide [126]. Finally, other factors such as inflammation, infection or perturbation of Aβ clearance mechanism may affect its peripheral levels, though unlikely to have a chronic effect [127].

Other conditions show the opposite; in traumatic brain injury (TBI), for example, CSF and plasma levels of Aβ1-42 increase steadily after the acute event, and normalize with recovery in weeks [127–129]; in some cases, an increase of APP itself was noted when sampling intraventricular CSF [130]. These data tend to correlate with other markers of neuronal damage, i.e., the release of total tau, neuronal specific enolase (NSE) and APOE, but the actual mechanism of shedding is unclear. Notably, axonal injury after TBI is associated with redistribution of APP towards the axons and increased processing to generate Aβ, explaining part of the CSF levels [131,132].

Interestingly, whereas Aβ accumulation in the brain results in a reduction in the periphery, tau accumulation in the brain parallels its peripheral abundance [115] (discussed below). Tau accumulation follows, in time, Aβ accumulation. Can this time difference (maybe decades) explain the dichotomy? If so, is there a moment in time in AD pathogenesis when Aβ levels are actually increased or normal in the periphery? The current data on autosomal dominant AD show initial amyloid-PET abnormalities ca. 22 years prior the expected symptom onset (EYO-22) and CSF Aβ reduction (and tau increase) a few years later (EYO-19 to -14) [133]. This series of events signifies that (1) sensible Aβ deposition in the brain happens quite early in the pathogenesis, (2) current CSF (and blood) biomarkers follow brain changes by several years, and (3) measures of neuronal damage (peripheral tau, etc.) do not fall far behind peripheral Aβ changes. This leaves open the question of what happens even earlier to peripheral Aβ, is it ever elevated? Is that the ideal moment where anti-Aβ therapeutic strategies would be most effective? Only longitudinal studies with a very early CSF and blood sampling will be able to answer these questions.

A recent study in a Down syndrome (DS) cohort [134], with CSF sampling from age 30 to 61, showed Aβ42 reductions which was proportional to age and cognitive decline (from cognitive stable, to MCI to AD), with higher levels than those reported in corresponding older non-DS controls, MCI and AD [135], but did not have a non-DS age-matched control group. In another study [136], CSF levels of Aβ peptide were found to be elevated from 8 to 54 months of age in DS children, while tau was low, likely due to Aβ overproduction in the absence of significant parenchymal sequestration and neuronal loss at that age.

<u>CSF</u>. Sampling CSF by lumbar puncture (LP) is the most direct way to obtain biomarkers that reflect what happens in the brain. Being invasive, most patients do not feel comfortable undergoing a spinal tap, although the rate of complications, i.e., post-LP headache, bleeds or infections is very low [137]. CSF levels and variations of Aβ have long been the hallmark features of AD-type dementia. The literature on the matter is extremely extensive and will not be reviewed here. We will limit our discussion to the clinicopathological relevance of Aβ in CSF. The first attempts at measuring soluble APP-derived fragment in the CSF of AD patients were carried out by D. Selkoe and S. Younkin [138] and B. Frangione [139] labs, determining the reduction of soluble APP (sAPP) fragments in the CSF of AD patients. Soon after, scientists were able to map the Aβ region and retrieve the peptide in the CSF [140]. This led to the first studies looking at differences between AD and control subjects in soluble APP and Aβ peptides [141–145], with notable differences likely due to detection methods and populations [146,147].

CSF levels of Aβ 42 are generally lower in AD compared to control subjects, and have been seen to decline with disease progression [135,147–150]. Aβ1-42 levels can be reduced as much as 50% in patients with AD compared to control subjects [151]. There seems to be, though, significant overlap of total Aβ1-42 levels between AD and non-AD dementia, such as vascular dementia, Parkinson's disease dementia (PDD), Lewy body disease (LBD), frontotemporal lobe degeneration (FTD) and even amyotrophic lateral sclerosis (ALS), and this may be due to population selection, stage of disease or overlap of pathogenic events in advanced disease [152–158].

In the pre-dementia stages, both amnestic MCI (aMCI), the most frequent precursor of AD, and non-amnestic MCI, showed low levels of Aβ1-42 [154,159–162] compared to control subjects, also with significant overlap.

In all, the use of Aβ1-42 alone does not seem to be too promising for differentiating AD from non-AD dementia and less so at the MCI stage, due to heterogeneity and overlap. As mentioned above, the pathophysiology of APP processing in AD is characterized by an imbalance of the 1-42 over the 1-40 species of Aβ, with preferential deposition of the former in the brain. Additionally, the gamma-secretase complex cleaves APP in a sequential fashion, generating progressively shorter fragments, like the Aβ1-38. These fragments have been identified in CSF, and may be useful biomarkers as well [162]. Thus, measuring the CSF ratio of Aβ42/40 (and other 42/X peptides ratios, e.g., 42/38, etc.) has been attempted. Indeed, the CSF ratio of Aβ42/40 has proven to be a reliable marker of AD, both at the dementia and MCI stage, as well as of the risk of progression from MCI to AD [163–166]. Furthermore, this ratio was also useful to differentiate AD from other non-AD cognitive changes, such as subcortical deficits of vascular disease. Such correlations were validated by both amyloid PET and extensive clinical and conventional MRI approaches. CSF Aβ42/40 correlates almost completely with amyloid PET, and when there is discordance, longitudinal studies have shown that PET imaging turns positive within a few years [117,119,150]. Finally, it was shown that different assay platforms resulted in similar results [167].

Blood. Serum or plasma measurement of Aβ has become possible and reliable thanks to the increased sensitivity and specificity of the available diagnostic platforms. Initial testing was based on ELISA (enzyme-linked immunosorbent assay), but results have been equivocal at best [148,168]. Interference by plasma proteins was likely significant in these early attempts. ELISA have been progressively improved to reach higher sensitivity, and other platforms have been developed, including SiMoA (Single Molecule Array) [169–171], immunomagnetic reduction [172], multiplex assays (e.g., xMAP- [173]), MSD [174] and more. As discussed in more detail below, in order to overcome the complexity of the blood and the interference by blood proteins and heterophilic antibodies and low concentrations of the target biomarker [113], the more modern platforms work with very high dilution of the sample and amplification of the specific signal, allowing for detection of picomolar/mL (or less) concentrations of the target protein [175,176]. Thanks to these advances, we can now reliably measure the Aβ42/40 ratio in plasma.

Studies using SiMoA have, first of all, confirmed a significant correlation between CSF and plasma [170,177] Aβ42, Aβ40 and their ratio, and further confirmed the CSF data on AD and MCI vs. control patients; AD and MCI patients show reduced levels of Aβ42 and Aβ42/40 ratio compared to cognitively intact control subjects, confirmed by amyloid PET.

High-precision assays for plasma Aβ42/40, using immunoprecipitation followed by liquid chromatography-mass spectroscopy (IP–MS) [178], are strongly predictive of brain amyloidosis as validated by benchmark amyloid-β-PET, and reach 90% accuracy [175,179,180]. In one study, a novel fragment ratio to Aβ42 (APP669–711/Aβ42) was also used to predict amyloid-β-PET positivity [175].

Interestingly, in the case of Aβ, another factor that interferes with the accurate plasma measurement is its extra-cerebral production (e.g., platelets, [181]), which is difficult to control. Hence, while it is possible to detect a reduction of the Aβ42/40 ratio in plasma in AD vs. control subjects, plasma reduction only totals about 15%, while in CSF we can see as much as 50% reduction [115,176]. When analyzing the overall trajectory of Aβ variation in plasma vs. CSF, in parallel with Aβ deposition in the brain by PET, by a variety of modern assays, plasma Aβ does not perform as well as CSF [182], showing a narrower range, making it still a less sensitive tool.

2.2. *Tau*

In AD, tau undergoes significant conformational change and abnormal phosphorylation, leading to the formation of inclusions throughout the brain, that start in the entorhinal cortex (EC) and, as the disease evolves, spread progressively throughout the brain, leading to synapse loss and neuronal death, which correlate well with the clinical onset and progression of symptoms [25,183,184]. High levels of tau, both total (t-tau) and phosphorylated (p-tau), have consistently been detected in CSF of AD patients compared to healthy controls [115,185–192]. Studies in FAD and SAD suggest that the tau-PET signal associated with neurofibrillary tangle pathology increases at symptom onset and appears about one decade after CSF soluble tau increase [193–196]. Other studies suggest that, while neurodegeneration progresses, the rate of increase of p-tau and t-tau levels may actually be reduced [118,133,197], likely in relation to the massive neuronal loss. In this dynamic scenario, where the rate of p-tau accumulation changes, and Aβ may show fluctuations in time, as discussed previously, an ideal biomarker should be specific enough for an adequate pre-clinical detection of AD and to track the disease progression.

As previously reported by Augustinack et al. [183], distinct tau phosphorylation sites correlate with severity of neuronal cytopathology in AD. Pre-tangle state, intra- and extra- neuronal neurofibrillary tangles were used to characterize different stages of pathology. More specifically, p-T231, p-S262, and p-T153 (T: Threonine, S: Serine) were shown to stain non fibrillar tau and were identified as early phosphorylation markers; p-T175/181, p-S262/p-S356, p-S422, p-S46 and p-S214 co-localized with intra-neuronal fibrillar tau structures, and increase as disease progresses; p-S199/p-S202/p-T205, p-T212/p-S214 and p-S396/p-S404 identified instead extracellular tangles composed of substantial filamentous tau structures, seen in later stages of the disease.

In addition to focusing on crucial site-specific phosphorylation, it has been shown, by cryo-EM analysis in AD as well as in other tauopathies, that the most disease-specific change is a tridimensional folding of the tau filaments, which is a signature of the particular disease examined; these tau molecular conformers can in fact differentiate between AD, Pick's disease and corticobasal degeneration (CBD) [198–201]. Moreover, an AD-specific epitope formed by two discontinuous portions of tau, $_7$EFE$_9$ and $_{313}$VDLSKVTSKC$_{322}$ and recognized by the MC1 antibody [198,202,203], represents an early aberrant conformation of tau present both in a soluble form of the protein and in paired helical filaments (PHF) assemblies [204]. Interestingly, the level of MC1 reactivity correlates with the severity and progression of AD. To our knowledge, no assay has been developed to detect this early marker of pathology in biofluids, likely due to the possibility that tau truncated species [205–208] could prevent the identification of a conformational tau epitope using the currently available immunoassays, which are-based primarily on mid-region-directed antibodies. We believe that, although this pathological feature is not per se easily "translatable", it should be kept in consideration when designing and developing new tau biomarkers platforms.

In summary, the identification of precise phosphorylated tau species and conformers in the biological fluids will contribute not only to early preclinical diagnosis of AD, but will also allow for a "personalized" approach by staging the disease in its progression and possibly monitoring the effect of therapeutic interventions. Here below is a review of the classic and novel approaches to detect tau and its phosphorylated modifications in CSF and blood.

CSF. Increased phosphorylation and axonal degeneration are believed to induce passive release of tau from the microtubules into the extracellular space, possibly as a neuronal response to Aβ toxicity [209,210]. This process results in augmented levels of t-tau and p-tau in the interstitial fluid and consequently in the CSF. From a neuropathological perspective, analysis of postmortem brains has shown a certain degree of correlation between the neocortical tau burden and CSF p-tau [190,211]. Tau phosphorylated at Threonine 181 (p-T181), t-tau and Aβ42 have been extensively validated in the CSF as biomarkers of AD and are currently widely used as diagnostic benchmarks in clinical and research studies [54,109,212]. CSF p-T181 tau has also proven useful in differential diagnosis of dementia [213–215] and to predict cognitive decline in preclinical and prodromal disease stages [213,216,217], with specificity for AD.

An ongoing effort focuses on standardizing protocols and developing criteria for the appropriate use of CSF tau assessment in the diagnosis of AD, with the intent of integrating CSF biomarkers into clinical practice [218–220]. In this respect, the distinctive value of the CSF p-T181 tau level has still to be thoroughly demonstrated. In one comparison study, p-T181, tau phosphorylated at Serine 199 (p-S199), and tau phosphorylated at Threonine 231 (p-T231) showed similar diagnostic accuracies for AD [221]. On the other hand, Spiegel et al. [222] reported that CSF p-T231 tau levels are superior to p-T181 in clustering AD subjects from normal control, suggesting the potential for CSF p-T231 assay to be employed in early AD diagnosis. These data are in line with the AD neuropathological picture where p-tau231 shows greater sensitivity for neurofibrillary tangles than p-T181 [211,223], with propensity to accumulate in layer II of the entorhinal cortex [183], known to be the first limbic area in AD consistently targeted by neurofibrillary pathology [224].

Together with p-T181 and p-T231, other phospho-epitopes are under investigation with the hope to find even better AD diagnostics. Barthélemy et al. [225] reported that CSF tau phosphorylated at Threonine 217 (p-T217) is specifically associated with amyloid-β pathology, suggesting a strong interplay between AD amyloidosis and hyperphosphorylation of tau on p-T217; moreover, p-T217 outperforms p-T181 as a biomarker for detecting both the preclinical and advanced forms of Alzheimer's disease. In a second study, Barthelemy et al. [226] suggested a pattern of tau staging linking CSF site-specific phosphorylation to three different phases of the disease progression. By analyzing FAD, SAD and patients with unaffected cognition but at risk of disease (based on the presence of abnormal Aβ pathology); the authors identified an array of tau phosphorylation uniquely associated with structural, metabolic, neurodegenerative and clinical markers of disease. The study shows that (1) p-T217 and p-T181 rise in parallel to aggregated Aβ as early as 20 years before the development of neurofibrillary tangles, (2) p-T205 correlates with hypometabolism and atrophy closer to symptom onset, and (3) t-tau spikes when cognitive decline manifests. All of these data are in line with another study where the associations of p-T217 with tau PET, CSF and PET measures of amyloid pathology were tested in comparison to p-T181 [220]; the authors found that CSF p-T217 correlates better than p-T181 with PET measures of tau and amyloid pathologies in AD, and more accurately distinguishes AD from non-AD neurodegenerative disorders, suggesting the benefit of employing CSF p-T217 as a biomarker of AD in clinical practice.

Furthermore, investigating tau fragments in CSF, Chen et al. [227] developed a set of tau immunoassays able to detect different populations of tau fragments in CSF and blood. The authors were able to demonstrate that mid-region- and N-terminal-containing fragments increase with disease, while full-length tau is just a small fraction of the tau present in both normal and AD CSF. A recent study has also shown that the ratio between C-terminally truncated tau368 and t-tau is significantly decreased in patients with Alzheimer's disease, with a strong correlation with ^{18}F-GTP1 retention in brain [207] (a measure of tangle pathology in vivo); these data suggest that tau fragment may preferentially accumulate in tangles, and the CSF ratio tau368/t-tau reflects tangle pathology in brain and can be used as an additional tau biomarker to stage and improve the diagnosis of Alzheimer's disease.

Several studies indicate that TBI can be classified as an independent risk factor for developing Alzheimer's disease. As previously discussed for Aβ, the axonal injury resulting from the trauma drives the development of both Aβ plaques and NFT [228–232]. Interestingly, not only do tau levels increase in the CSF of the concussed patients undergoing repetitive trauma (i.e., sports players), but serum t-tau levels have been reported to increase in the acute stage following the concussion, while decreasing during rehabilitation [230,233,234]. Similarly, serum p-tau (p-T231 and p-S202) levels, though reduced, were shown to be still higher compared to the control levels even at six months post-injury [235].

When considering tauopathies different from AD with significant NFT pathology and neurodegeneration, CSF p-T181 and t-tau levels do not necessarily increase; this is the case for progressive supranuclear palsy (PSP) and some forms of FTD [221,236–238]. Why increased CSF t-tau and p-tau are specific to AD can be explained by considering that (1) the pattern of tau phosphorylation occurring in these disorders is disease-specific, (2) tangle pathology and neurodegeneration in AD may be consequent to Aβ accumulation, with disease-specific molecular cascades, such as kinases and proteases activation, (3) disease-specific tau truncation could prevent detection by currently available assays, and (4) specific pathological changes can be more severe in AD than in other tauopathies.

Blood. Until recently, AD biomarkers' quantification was limited to the CSF. However, while combining CSF biomarker analyses and PET scans have the potential to improve diagnostic accuracy, these methodologies show limitations, impeding their use as first-line diagnostics [113]. Developing an accurate and standardized blood test will be more cost effective than PET imaging [239,240], less invasive than CSF testing [241] and faster. Hence, blood-based biomarkers represent next-generation diagnostics for AD and other CNS diseases. One matter of concern is that blood tau has the potential to derive from other sources in addition to neuronal tau [242,243]. In this respect, novel ultrasensitive detection technologies have been developed to facilitate the detection of very low concentrations and variations of tau in the blood [186,244,245] using very high dilutions of the biological fluid: employing these technologies has pushed forward the potential for plasma tau to serve as a biomarker for neurodegeneration in AD, avoiding the interference of non-neuronal tau.

Longitudinal studies originally showed that higher levels of plasma t-tau are associated with greater cognitive decline and risk of MCI [246–248], with no correlation with elevated brain Aβ [247]. As discussed, plasma t-tau assays can identify neuronal injury in acute brain disorders, such as TBI, but work relatively poorly for AD diagnosis, and the correlation with CSF t-tau is weak [249]. In this context, t-tau could be intended as a non-specific prognostic marker for dementia and related endophenotypes [248]. Despite the lack of correlation between plasma and CSF t-tau, Fossati et al. [186] have recently demonstrated that by combining plasma t-tau with CSF t-tau or CSF p-T181 tau, the accuracy for the differentiation of AD versus cognitively normal controls increases, suggesting that plasma tau may be a useful biomarker to increase diagnostic power and determine therapeutic efficacy in clinical studies.

Analysis of phosphorylated tau in blood has so far been focused on the development and validation of assays for p-T181 [182,246,250–253], demonstrating that increased plasma p-T181 (1) correlates with amyloid and tau PET measures [250,254,255], allowing the identification of individuals with Aβ pathology but tau PET-negative measurements [253], (2) goes in parallel with CSF p-T181 [182,255], and (3) can help in the differential diagnosis of non-AD types of dementias [253–255].

While writing this review, two groups published strong data in support of the use of a blood-based assay detecting p-T217 tau. First, Barthelemy et al. [256] developed a protocol of purification and enrichment of tau from plasma, followed by liquid chromatography (LC-MS); this system (1) allows reliable detection of p-T217 showing high correlation with the CSF measurements, and (2) confirms the ability of this biomarker in clustering amyloid positive and negative patients. The limitation of this strategy is the high volume of blood needed to purify and extract tau and the elaborate methodology, not compatible with the idea of developing a fast and easy-to- use assay. In the second study, Palmqvist et al. [256] employed the Meso Scale Discovery (MSD)/Lilly platform (described below) and validated the value of p-T217 in plasma to discriminate Aβ+ MCI and AD patients from other neurodegenerative disorders and controls, including sensitive discrimination of autosomal-dominant pre-symptomatic Aβ+ patients. In all, given the high potential of measuring CSF p-T217 previously described, it will be of great interest to follow the development and validation of novel ultrasensitive platforms aimed at detecting p-T217 in blood, employing fully automated platforms to integrate this biomarker in clinical practice. Similarly, setting up sensitive and specific assays able to detect p-T231 (early phosphorylated epitope) and p-S396/404 (late phosphorylated epitope) in blood will also be relevant to stage the AD pathology and to monitor future therapeutic interventions.

Finally, an ultra-sensitive assay was developed in blood, to detect an N-terminal tau fragment (NT1) [227], showing that N-terminal fragments of tau mapping in the 6–198 sequence are increased in AD and MCI patients and may be useful as a screening blood-based test for AD. This approach is extremely significant due to the possible generation of disease-specific tau fragments (as for APP and Aβ), and will need further investigation.

Immunoassays and ultrasensitive platforms to detect tau in biological fluids. Several assays have been tested and extensively validated in CSF and plasma. In Table 1 we select and catalogue the most used assays in the tau biomarker field at the moment, with emphasis on their specificity, fluid samples' applicability and limit of detection. The list of assays includes (1) standard and second generation ELISAs (INNOTEST, EUROIMMUN, Elecsys), (2) MSD platforms (3) Single-Molecule enzyme-linked immunosorbent assay (SiMoA), (4) Mass spectrometry analysis, (5) superconducting-quantum-interference-device Immunomagnetic reduction (SQUID-IMR). The detection range spans from few pg/mL to fg/mL according to the sensitivity of the assay. EUROIMMUN and Elecsys are automated second-generation immune assays that have demonstrated good analytical performance with clinically relevant measuring ranges, supporting their use in clinical trials and practice [257,258]. MSD technology with electrochemiluminescence detection comes with several advantages compared to standard immunoassays, including high sensitivity, low background and wide dynamic range of detection [174]. Notably, Palmqvist et al. [182] recently ran a comparative analysis of Aβ and tau CSF assays from five different manufacturers: Elecsys (Aβ42, Aβ42/40, t-tau, p-tau181) EUROIMMUN (Aβ42, Aβ42/40, t-tau, p-tau181), INNOTEST (Aβ42, Aβ42/40, t-tau, p-tau181), MSD (Aβ42, Aβ42/40, t-tau) and Lilly (p-tau181, p-tau217): Aβ42, Aβ42/40, p-tau and t-tau had very similar trajectories between assays.

Moving to ultra-sensitive platforms, Rissn et al. previously developed [169,259] a Single-Molecule enzyme-linked immunosorbent assay (SiMoA) that detects serum proteins at sub-femtomolar concentrations, restricting the fluorophores produced by individual enzymes to considerably small volumes, hence capturing the fluorescence of each single molecule. This methodology has been extensively used to improve t-tau and p-tau detection in CSF and plasma (Quanterix).

SiMoA and INNOTEST ELISA have been also demonstrated to strongly correlate in CSF t-tau in a comparison study [186]. Moreover, in a recent study, Karikari et al. [253] validated a blood-based immunoassay measuring p-T181 using a sandwich immunoassay format on SiMoA technology.

To further quantify tau at high sensitivity, Barthelemy et al. has developed a protocol to detect tau and p-tau in CSF and plasma employing targeted high-resolution mass spectrometry (MS) [225,226,256,260,261]. Additionally, superconducting-quantum-interference-device Immunomagnetic reduction (SQUID-IMR) has proven efficient at quantifying t-tau and p-T181 in plasma in early stages of AD [172,252].

Table 1. Immunoassays and ultrasensitive platforms to detect tau in biological fluids.

Type of Assay	Platform/ Manufacturer	t-tau	p-tau	Fluid Sample	LOD pg/mL	References (PMID/link)
Standard ELISA	INNOTEST Fujirebio	Total tau Antibodies: Capture HT7/AT120 Detector BT2		CSF	34	8748926
	INNOTEST Fujirebio		p-T181 Antibodies: Capture HT7 Detector AT270	CSF	13	10788705
	Applied Neurosolutions (Dr. Peter Davies)		p-T231 Antibodies: Capture CP27 Detector CP9	CSF	9	26444757
Automated ELISA	Elecsys	Total tau Antibodies: Not available		CSF	63	31129184
	Elecsys		p-T181 Antibodies: N.A.	CSF	4	31129184
	EUROIMMUN	Total tau Antibodies: Capture ADx201 Detector ADx215		CSF	44.2	27447425
	EUROIMMUN		p-T181 Antibodies: N.A.	CSF	N.A.	27447425
MSD-ECL	MSD		p-T181 Antibodies: Capture biotinylated AT270 Detector SULFO-TAG-LRL (anti-tau, Lilly)	Plasma	N.A.	29626426
	MSD/Lilly		p-T181 Antibodies: Capture biotinylated AT270 Detector SULFO-TAG-LRL (anti-tau)	CSF	N.A.	31709776
	MSD/Lilly		p-T217 Antibodies: Capture biotinylated IBA413 Detector SULFO-TAG-LRL (anti-tau)	CSF	N.A.	31709776
	MSD/Lilly		p-T217 Antibodies: Capture Biotinylated-IBA493 Detector SULFO-TAG-4G10-E2 (anti-tau)	Plasma	N.A.	31709776

Table 1. *Cont.*

Type of Assay	Platform/ Manufacturer	t-tau	p-tau	Fluid Sample	LOD pg/mL	References (PMID/link)
SiMoA	Simoa™ Tau 2.0 kit HD-1 platform (Quanterix)	Total tau Antibodies: Capture sequence AA16–AA24 Detector sequence AA218–AA222		CSF	0.019	101444
	Janssen R&D Simoa technology HD-1 platform (Quanterix)	Total tau Antibodies: Capture HT7 Detector PT82		CSF	N.A.	32246036
	Modiefied version of Simoa™ Tau 2.0 kit HD-1 platform (Quanterix)		p-T181 Antibodies: Capture sequence AA16–AA24 Detector AT270	Plasma	0.0090	28866979
	Sandwich immunoassay format on Simoa technology (Quanterix)		p-T181 Antibodies: Capture AT270 Detector Tau12	Plasma Serum	N.A.	32333900
	Simoa™ p-181 kit HD-1 platform (Quanterix) NEW		p-T181 Antibodies: N/A	CSDF Plasma Serum		Alzheimer Association International Conference, 2020. Available online: https://alz.confex.com/alz/20amsterdam/meetingapp.cgi/Paper/41238. Accessed on 29 July 2020.
	Janssen R&D Simoa technology (Quanterix)		p-T217 Antibodies: Capture PT3 Detector PT82	CSF	N.A.	32246036
	Simoa® pTau-231 Advantage Kit HD-1 platform (Quanterix)		p-T231 Antibodies: Capture AT270 Detector Tau12	CSF	0.621	Quanterix.com. Available online: https://www.quanterix.com/sites/default/files/assays/Simoa_pTau-231_Data_Sheet_HD-1_HD-X_Rev02.pdf. Accessed on 29 July 2020.
	NT1 assay Simoa technology HD-1 platform (Quanterix)	N-terminal tau Antibodies: Capture Tau12 Detector BT2		CSF Plasma	0.2-0.7	30419228
Nano liquid chromatography-HRMS		Total tau	p-T181 p-S202 p-T205 p-T217	CSF	N.A.	26742856 32161412
(IP)-LC-MS			p-T217 p-T181	Plasma	p-T217:0.05 p-T181:0.2	32725127
SQUID-IMR		Total tau	p-T181	Plasma	N.A.	29376870

A detailed list of the original and the more updated assays used in the tau biomarker field is provided, with emphasis on total, phosphorylated or truncated tau. Type of assays and platforms: ELISA (Enzyme-linked immunosorbent assay); Meso Scale Discovery (MSD) technology with electrochemiluminescence; SiMoA: Single-Molecule enzyme-linked immunosorbent assay; Nano liquid chromatography–HRMMSD-ECLS: Nano liquid chromatography–high resolution mass spectrometry; (IP)-LC-MS: immunoprecipitation coupled with liquid chromatography-spectrometry; SQUID-IMR: superconducting-quantum-interference-device Immunomagnetic reduction. Fluid samples are specified (CSF, plasma, serum). Limit of detection (LOD) of the assay is provided where available, if not it is marked as N.A. References are listed as PMID or hyperlink.

3. Biomarkers of Synaptic and Neuronal Loss

Synaptic loss first and overt neuronal demise later are fundamental aspect of AD pathology and are, together with tau deposition, the real correlate of the manifestation of symptoms. Neurodegeneration is the "N" in the ATN system, and is a fundamental correlate of the functional disability of AD patients. When patients present to their doctors with memory loss or other cognitive changes, due to AD, it is estimated that a large number of neurons have already been lost to neurodegeneration, but recent models are looking at the effect of more subtle synaptic loss as an inciting event responsible for symptoms [70]. In this context, several markers of synaptic disruption have been proposed as indicators of disease onset and progression.

3.1. Neurofilament Light Chain (NfL)

NfL belongs to the type IV intermediate filaments, which make up the neuronal axoskeleton, maintain neuronal caliber and play a role in intracellular transport to axons and dendrites. With the neurodegenerative process, in AD as in other disease [262], NfL is released in the extracellular space. NfL has been detected in both CSF and blood, and appears to be extremely sensitive to AD onset and progression, predicting Aβ PET positivity as well; furthermore, longitudinal studies in familial AD, have shown accurate prediction of disease onset, as far as 10 years prior to symptoms [263–266]. The tight correlation between CSF and blood values [267] make NfL one of the most reliable blood biomarkers to predict onset and course of neurodegeneration.

3.2. Neurogranin

Neurogranin (Ng) is a neural-specific postsynaptic protein, concentrated on dendritic spines, in the hippocampus and basal forebrain. Given its localization at the epicenter of the pathogenic events in AD, it is not surprising that it would be released in the extracellular space and be detected in CSF. In AD, CSF levels of Ng grow quite rapidly prior to the presentation of cognitive deficits, before NfL does, in an Aβ-dependent way [268]. Plasma levels do not seem to be as reliable as CSF, possibly due to peripheral production [269]. Importantly, and contrarily to NfL, other neurodegenerative disease do not show an increase of Ng, raising the possibility of an AD-specific synaptic effect [185].

Other biomarkers in this category are being investigated, such as NSE and SNAP-25, and are the subject of extensive analysis, but are mostly used in complex and integrated predictive models [133,270] and will not be reviewed here.

4. Biomarkers of Inflammation and Microglia "Dysfunction"

Inflammation, microglia and astrocytes activation are well-recognized features of AD pathology, as for other neurodegenerative diseases. It is unclear if they are integral part of the original pathogenesis or are reactive features to the deposition of amyloid and tau. To really understand this aspect, we should investigate, with an unbiased approach, the very early features of patients with a predisposition to develop AD pathology, for example in large autosomal dominant cohorts, in prospective longitudinal studies, and some effort is under way in this context. For the time being, we will focus on the data available from the earliest detectable stages of AD pathology, the prodromal AD cases.

4.1. Soluble TREM2

The Triggering Receptor Expressed on Myeloid Cells 2 (TREM2) is a transmembrane receptor, belonging to the family of cell surface transmembrane glycoproteins [271] which mediates signaling and cell activation following ligand binding. It is expressed and functions in subsets of myeloid cells, e.g., granulocytes, dendritic cells, macrophages, and microglia in the brain [272–275]. Among its complex and protean roles, its function is to regulate immune cells' activation upon binding of a variety of ligands [66], including APOE and Aβ. In the brain, where it may be expressed preferentially in some regions, such as the hippocampus, and differentially in response to the pro/anti-inflammatory environment, it mediates microglia activation, proliferation, migration, apoptosis and expression of pro-inflammatory cytokines, in particular after binding with aggregated proteins such as Aβ, and facilitates the phagocytosis of apoptotic neurons [276]. TREM2 expression is increased in many neurodegenerative conditions, stroke, trauma and even ageing. Rare variants of TREM2, discovered by GWAS studies [277,278], have been associated with the risk of developing AD, in the range of the risk conferred by APOE4, of 2- to 4-fold (heterozygous). The most common AD-associated variant recognized in populations of Europeans descent, but not in Chinese and African-Americans, is the R47H [277,279]. This TREM2 mutant is associated with earlier onset of disease and higher CSF tau levels [280] and seems to demonstrate reduced activity in ligands-binding and hence signal transduction, with a net result of reduced microglia activation and, in AD models, less clearance of Aβ [274]. Given this premise, it is only natural to look at TREM2 as a possible biomarker for AD. The soluble form of TREM2 (sTREM2) is found in both CSF and blood [281,282]. In CSF, sTREM2 is elevated in AD patients vs. controls, with positive association with t-tau levels [212,283]. In familial AD, sTREM2 CSF levels increase prior to clinical onset, but after detectable changes of Aβ and tau in CSF [284]; this is a moment in time where the brain is already at an advanced stage of pathology, in particular tau, with significant neuronal loss and when patients are soon going to lose their cognitive reserve and show symptoms. From a clinical perspective, this is relatively late to be useful as early prediction of disease or point of intervention, but from a pathogenic point of view, it may signify a "breaking point" of the Aβ and tau pathology containment system, where microglia cannot keep up with plaques and tangles any more. This is extremely important to consider in the development of therapeutic strategies in the future. More work is needed to create more sensitive assays in order to detect sTREM2 blood changes, as early as possible. Additionally, since the degree of inflammation and microglia activation differs from patient to patient, and secondary to treatment (e.g., anti-amyloid strategies), a sensitive blood sTREM2 assay may be a very useful tool to monitor phenotypic variants and adverse events form upcoming treatments.

4.2. YKL-40

YKL-40 is a glycoprotein expressed in both astrocytes and microglia, and is the protein product of the CHI3L1 gene, a.k.a., Chitinase 3 Like 1. YKL-40 actually lacks chitinase activity and is secreted by activated macrophages, chondrocytes, neutrophils and synovial cells, and plays a role in inflammation and tissue remodeling [285–288]. The first indication that YKL-40 may be relevant for AD came from an aprioristic evaluation of potential novel AD biomarkers [289]. Since then, several studies have now looked at the both CSF and plasma levels of this protein. YKL-40 is elevated in AD vs. control subjects [106,289,290], although it was also significantly elevated in patients with FTD [291]. Similarly, in MCI, baseline higher levels of YKL-40 were associated with significant more risk to progress to AD [106,289] with a tendency to continue to raise with disease progression [182]. The CSF ratio of YKL-40/Aβ42 was shown to be predictive of the onset of cognitive symptoms [289]. Plasma levels of YKL-40 have shown similar trends, but further validation may be needed to confirm reliable use [292]. In all, YKL-40, with its trend toward increase with disease progression, can be an associated marker for progression and prognosis.

4.3. Other Biomarkers of Inflammation and Glial Activation

Several pro- and anti-inflammatory factors have been looked at in both CSF and blood, including IL1, IL6, TNFα, VILIP-1, sTNFR and IP-10 [293–295], with some correlation to AD and MCI. Their significant is still unclear, and some are now part of multiplex panes, used in association with specific AD markers, arguably as prognostic indicators of disease progression.

GFAP (glial fibrillary acidic protein) is one of the major intermediate filament proteins of mature astrocytes, and it is released by astrocytes during neurodegeneration [296]. It is not properly a marker of inflammation, but it is a sign of a reactive brain milieu, as astrocytes tend to proliferate in response to tissue injury, and eventually release large amounts of GFAP in the interstitial fluid. Recently, the astrocytic response to brain damage and the inflammatory microglia has been characterized [297–299], and is very relevant in the context of AD pathology. The currently available CSF GFAP data show a correlation between increased levels and Aβ and tau evidence of AD [115,300], and recent data on plasma GFAP showed increased concentrations in late and early onset AD patients compared with cognitively normal controls [301]. Given the non-specific nature of GFAP, its use may be in the future confined to monitoring disease onset and progression, and possible response to treatment.

In all, given both the convergent and divergent nature of the inflammatory response, which involves a myriad of molecules and pathways, leading to a fine balance between protective and deleterious inflammation, and the fact that inflammation is an unavoidable element of ageing, any single marker would not be useful in isolation. Rather, a comprehensive approach using combinations of such factors, associated with specific marker of AD and markers of synaptic/neuronal loss (see below), has the best chance to be useful in clinical practice and research.

5. Biomarkers of Other Associated Pathology

5.1. TAR DNA-Binding Protein 43 (TDP-43)

TDP-43 can be present as co-pathology in AD (up to 50% of cases), and is the main feature of other neurodegenerative diseases, such as FTD and ALS. Its role is that of a transcriptional repressor, which regulates genes' alternate splicing. An extensive study [302] was able to link the presence of TDP-43 in AD brains with the likelihood of clinical AD presentation; but to date, a reliable CSF or blood marker is not available, although notable attempts and data are present for ALS [303,304]. Part of the issue is the non-specificity of TDP-43 accumulation, as the concept of a spectrum of TDP-43 neurodegenerative presentation is becoming more evident [305]. In this context, TDP-43 may be useful as a biomarker in the future to predict course of disease or variants of AD presentation.

5.2. Alpha-Synuclein

Alpha-synuclein is the key component of Lewy bodies, and is classically found in Parkinson's pathology, LBD, multi-system atrophy (MSA) and AD (also 50% of cases) variants. It is involved in presynaptic signaling, inhibiting phospholipases and moderating vesicles transport at the terminals [306]. As for TDP-43, despite the feasible measurement of α-synuclein in CSF and blood, no significant correlation has been made to date, likely due to the non-specific nature. What is different here is the possibility to harness α-synuclein's specific tendency to aggregate in a "prion-like" fashion [307,308], for example by CSF RT-QuIC (real-time quaking-induced conversion), likely in virtue of its conformational changes [309]. Further studies will have to determine the sensitivity of the test for AD, as being able to detect synucleinopathy in AD cases would be highly significant for prognostic, therapeutic and research purposes.

6. Vascular Damage and the Blood Brain Barrier

Vascular damage is an increasingly recognized pathological component of AD, both as an independent consequence of the toxicity of Aβ and tau [310,311], and as a frequent co-morbidity [312,313] with microvascular disease. The diagnosis if "mixed dementia" is ever more frequent, as we scan more patients in our clinical practice. Although the real significance of the interplay between amyloid/tau pathology and the microvascular damage is still unclear, as the basic pathological mechanisms are quite complex, we have been able to detect vascular damage and blood-brain barrier (BBB) leak [314,315] in vivo. Modern magnetic resonance imaging (MRI) techniques, such as dynamic contrast-enhanced (DCE)-MRI, can show BBB permeability in specific regions, i.e., the hippocampus [315,316]. This abnormal permeability seems to be proportional to ageing [317], and is more frequent in MCI and AD patients compared to unimpaired control subjects [315,318,319]. An interesting correlate of MRI studies is the use of a marker of brain capillary damage, the soluble platelet-derived growth factor receptor-β (sPDGFRβ), which is highly expressed in brain capillary pericytes and vascular smooth muscle cells [315], and is shed in the CSF after brain injury, possibly in relation of the activation of proteases such as ADAM10 [320]. Emerging data show that ageing and cognitive decline, independently of AD pathology, are associated with increased CSF levels of sPDGFRβ, which correlate with MRI permeability [317]. Although the use of BBB permeability diagnostics is still in its infancy, and the specificity for AD pathology is unclear, it would certainly be a precious prognostic tool in the hands of clinicians. In this context, and somehow beyond the scope of the current manuscript, the use of gadolinium-free MRI techniques to assess BBB permeability (K-trans) would be extremely welcome.

7. Multi-Target Platforms

With so many biomarkers coming onto the scene, and in order to advance both the diagnostic and prognostic assessments, a new generation of assays is under development with the goal to simultaneously catch multiple targets within the same fluid sample. Using such types of assays will be extremely informative in order to identify AD co-pathologies, characterize disease progression and monitor treatment response. Table 2 contains a list of the more popular, commercially available, multi-target platforms.

Table 2. Multi-target platforms.

Type of Assay	Platform/ Manufacturer	Targets	Fluid Sample	LOD pg/mL	References (PMID/link)
SiMoA	Simoa® Neurology 3-Plex A Kit HD-1 platform (Quanterix)	t-tau Aβ40 Aβ42	CSF plasma	Tau: 0.019 Aβ40: 0.196 Aβ42: 0.045	Quanterix.com. Available online: https://www.quanterix.com/sites/default/files/assays/Simoa_N3PA_Data_Sheet_HD-1_HD-X_Rev04%20%281%29.pdf. Accessed on 29 July 2020
	Simoa® Neurology 4-Plex A Kit HD-1 platform (Quanterix)	t-tau NfL GFAP UCLH-1	CSF plasma	Tau: 0.024 NfL: 0.104 GFAP: 0.221 UCLH-1: 1.74	Quanterix.com. Available online: https://www.quanterix.com/sites/default/files/assays/Simoa_N4PA_Data_Sheet_HD-1_HD-X_DS-0074_rev7.pdf. Accessed on 29 July 2020
	Simoa® 4X-plex neurology Kit (Quanterix) NEW	Aβ40 Aβ42 GFAP NfL	CSF plasma	Aβ40: 0.084 Aβ42: 0.148 GFAP: 1.66 NfL: 1.157	Alzheimer Association International Conference, 2020. Available online: https://alz.confex.com/alz/20amsterdam/meetingapp.cgi/Paper/43506. Accessed on 29 July 2020.
Luminex®xMAP®	The MILLIPLEX® map 4X multiplex immunoassay kit (Millipore, Sigma)	t-tau p-T181 Aβ40 Aβ42	CSF	N.A.	Emdmillipore.com. Available online: https://www.emdmillipore.com/US/en/product/MILLIPLEX-MAP-Human-Amyloid-Beta-and-Tau-Magnetic-Bead-Panel-Multiplex-Assay,MM_NF-HNABTMAG-68K. Accessed on 29 July 2020.
NeuroToolKit	Roche's Elecsys electroluminescence immunoassay platform	t-tau, p-T181 Aβ40, Aβ42 α-synuclein S100b YKL-40 GFAP sTREM2 IL-6 NfL Neurogranin	CSF	N.A.	32573951

Listed are some of the assays available for the simultaneous detection of multiple biomarkers in CSF or plasma. Type of assays and platforms: SiMoA: Single-Molecule enzyme-linked immunosorbent assay; Luminex XMAP: bead-based multiplex immunoassay in a microplate format; NeuroToolKit: based on electroluminescence immunoassay platform. Targets and Fluid samples are specified. Limit of detection (LOD) of the assay is provided when available. References are listed as PMID or hyperlink.

The NeuroToolKit, in development with Roche's Elecsys electroluminescence immunoassay platform [300], includes (1) α-synuclein as a marker of synaptic dysfunction, (2) S100b, YKL-40, and glial fibrillary acidic protein (GFAP) as markers of astrocyte activation, (3) sTREM2 and IL-6 as markers of microglial activation and inflammation, and (4) NfL and neurogranin as markers of axonal injury and synaptic dysfunction.

Simultaneous measurement of Aβ42, t-tau and p-T181 in CSF has been previously developed by the xMAP technology [321]. The MILLIPLEX® map multiplex immunoassay kit is a 4Xplex panel enables the simultaneous measurement of Aβ1-40, Aβ1-42, t-tau and p-T181 in human CSF.

The NEUROLOGY 3-PLEX A (SiMoA, Quanterix) detects t-tau, Aβ1-40 and Aβ1-42 in both CSF and blood.

The NEUROLOGY 4-PLEX A (SiMoA, Quanterix) detects t-tau, NfL, GFAP and ubiquitin carboxyl-terminal hydrolase L1 (UCH-L1) both in CSF and blood.

A new 4-PLEX assay has been recently developed (SiMoA, Quanterix) with the ability to target Aβ1-40, Aβ1-4, GFAP and NfL in both CSF and blood (Alzheimer Association International Conference, 2020. Available online: https://alz.confex.com/alz/20amsterdam/meetingapp.cgi/Paper/43506. Accessed on 29 July 2020), and was validated against the parent assays. We await studies on larger number of patients, with diagnostic and prognostic implications.

Using a single platform with the ability to test multiple targets, such as in this case, would be invaluable in clinical practice, given how precious CSF and even blood samples are. Ideal kits should include markers specific of disease (e.g., Aβ42/40 ratio, p-T217 tau) and biomarkers of severity of disease, as NfL, sTREM2 etc.

8. Immunoassays, Ultrasensitive Platforms and Their Potential Limitations

One main concern in the development of an immunological assay is to exclude any factor that could potentially (1) interfere with the detection of the analyte and (2) alter the antibody binding. The first category includes pre-analytical factors (sample storage, anti-coagulants), anti-analyte antibodies, and hormone binding proteins that can change the measurable concentration of the analyte in the sample; the second group consists instead of antibodies such as heterophile antibodies, human anti-animal antibodies (HAAA), and human anti-mouse antibodies (HAMA) which are found in the biological fluids and are able to interfere with the antibody binding in the assay [322]. Unlike plasma (~7 g protein/100 mL) the CSF has only ~0.025 g protein/100 mL—mainly albumin [323]. Given the different composition of CSF and blood, it is relatively easy to anticipate the different susceptibility to assay interference of these two different biological fluids. While the CSF is a relatively "clean" fluid with respect to protein concentration, plasma contains heterophilic antibodies and other molecules that might interfere with the measurements of a biomarker of interest [245]. The presence of HAMA in human plasma has been described in 30% of the population, and consequent interference by human anti-globulin antibodies in immunoassay has been reported in several studies [324–328]. For these reasons, detecting biomarkers for CNS disease in blood not only calls for highly sensitive and specific assays, but require to efficiently remove all the potential confounders. Different methods for the reduction of heterophile antibody and anti-animal interferences in immunoassays have been previously described and include ways to remove or block the interfering antibody [322,329,330]. In this respect, our group has previously developed a protocol combining NaOAc (sodium acetate) and heat-treatment to 'purify' tau from the blood of transgenic animals undergone tau immunotherapy [328]. This protocol was validated using mouse and human serum. While the NaOAc/heat-treatment did not affect tau reactivity on CSF samples, human plasma samples displayed an impressive reduction of the apparent tau signals after undergoing the heat extraction protocol. The use of the ultrasensitive assays described here has overcome some of these technical issues. In addition, the use of blockers against heterophilic antibodies in the sample diluent is also helpful to achieve reliable quantification [245]. We still believe that the previous considerations need to be considered, especially when analyzing human samples derived from patients undergone immunotherapy, where the risk of assay interference could compromise the interpretations of the disease course and therapy.

Ageing is per se associated with a reduction of the integrity of the BBB, due to a multitude of causes, e.g., prior infections, general inflammatory state, trauma, tumors and more [315,316]. MCI, AD and cognitive changes in ageing have been associated with non-specific BBB permeability in certain brain regions [317]. The resulting permeability may result in falsification of CSF data for reasons analogous to the blood.

9. Novel Approaches to Unbiased Biomarker Discovery: The Case for Metabolomics

A successful preclinical diagnosis of AD may benefit from an unbiased metabolomic analysis of biological fluids. Given that CSF metabolites reflect brain changes better than blood, CSF biomarkers are widely used in research and clinical practice [331]. The strength of metabolomics is in its ability to measure a plethora of metabolites in an unbiased manner, providing a snapshot of an individual's biological status [331,332]. The ideal system would include a CSF metabolomic profile covering the whole lifespan of individuals belonging to both FAD and SAD cohorts, followed by plasma validation. While this analysis would require decades in human AD, or the longitudinal analysis of autosomal dominant families, running such studies on faithful animal models would make for an optimal surrogate, taking advantage of novel knock-in models, as opposed to transgenic ones, which reproduce the exact genetic defect found in humans [333–338].

Metabolomic studies have been performed in CSF, blood and post-mortem tissue from AD and MCI patients [331,339,340]. For example, elevated CSF glutamate and glutamine levels have been described in AD before [332,341,342], and other studies have shown blood and CSF metabolites changes in AD [343–345], some correlating with progression and risk of MCI to progress to AD [346]. Most identified pathways relate to energy metabolism, Krebs cycle, mitochondrial function, neurotransmitter and amino acids metabolism, and lipid biosynthesis. Longitudinal studies in FAD cases would be welcome in the near future to understand both the pathological relevance of the said pathways and their power to predict AD.

10. Discussion and Conclusions

Several studies have by now assessed the use of isolated biomarkers vs. their combinations to predict diagnosis of AD, or progression of MCI to AD. No single biomarker, in CSF, blood, imaging or cognitive alone is capable to predict onset and course reliably. Rather, the combination of multimodal biomarkers is required to reach reliable predictions [100,300,342,347,348]. CSF Aβ1-42 reduction (best proxied by the Aβ42/40 ratio) starts very early before symptoms onset, peaks a few years later when amyloid PET is at the zenith; CSF tau elevation follows Aβ, and represent clinical disease severity very well. NfL increase starts early, before tau, and is a very good indicator of neuronal damage early in the disease, though it is not specific for AD; still, its reliability in blood as well in CSF, makes it an excellent marker to track disease progression and possible response to therapies. Similarly, sTREM2 and YKL-40 are excellent markers of inflammation, and although their best use is in CSF, they could be extremely useful to monitor possible adverse events of therapeutic intervention. Aprioristic analysis of CSF and blood by metabolomic, proteomic, lipidomic and other large-scale approaches could be the key, if done early enough in the pathogenic course, to generate hypothesis on the primordial triggers of the disease, besides to identify AD patients and predict their trajectory. In this respect, autosomal dominant families and patients with Down's syndrome [134,349,350] may be the ideal subjects for dedicated longitudinal studies.

Given this premise, the biomarker field has to drive every resources toward the development of blood-based assays able to provide high specificity and sensitivity to excel in both diagnosis (Aβ, and tau) and prognosis (i.e., NfL) of AD. Implementing AD biomarkers in clinical practice will require blood-based assays (1) easy-to-use in terms of human specimen collection (few mL of blood) and methodology, (2) with high sensitivity (under the pg/mL threshold) and specificity, (3) free of interference produced by several confounders associated with the ageing process. The focus on pre-symptomatic Aβ+ populations is paramount (e.g., autosomal-dominant cohorts) if we really want to diagnose the disease in a phase where significant intervention is still possible.

Author Contributions: Conceptualization, L.D., L.G., C.d.; methodology, C.d., L.G.; writing—original draft preparation, C.d., L.G.; writing—review and editing, L.D., L.G.; visualization, C.d.; supervision, L.D. All authors have read and agreed to the published version of the manuscript.

Acknowledgments: We would like to thank Peter Davies for his continued support and insight.

References

1. Apostolova, L.G. Alzheimer disease. *Continuum Minneap. Minn.* **2016**, *22*, 419–434. [CrossRef] [PubMed]
2. Hebert, L.E.; Weuve, J.; Scherr, P.A.; Evans, D.A. Alzheimer disease in the United States (2010–2050) estimated using the 2010 census. *Neurology* **2013**, *80*, 1778–1783. [CrossRef] [PubMed]
3. Hebert, L.E.; Bienias, J.L.; Aggarwal, N.T.; Wilson, R.S.; Bennett, D.A.; Shah, R.C.; Evans, D.A. Change in risk of Alzheimer disease over time. *Neurology* **2010**, *75*, 786–791. [CrossRef] [PubMed]
4. Fan, C.C.; Banks, S.J.; Thompson, W.K.; Chen, C.H.; McEvoy, L.K.; Tan, C.H.; Kukull, W.; Bennett, D.A.; Farrer, L.A.; Mayeux, R.; et al. Sex-dependent autosomal effects on clinical progression of alzheimer's disease. *Brain* **2020**, *143*, 2272–2280. [CrossRef]
5. Plassman, B.L.; Langa, K.M.; Fisher, G.G.; Heeringa, S.G.; Weir, D.R.; Ofstedal, M.B.; Burke, J.R.; Hurd, M.D.; Potter, G.G.; Rodgers, W.L.; et al. Prevalence of dementia in the united states: The aging, demographics, and memory study. *Neuroepidemiology* **2007**, *29*, 125–132. [CrossRef]
6. Seshadri, S.; Wolf, P.A.; Beiser, A.; Au, R.; McNulty, K.; White, R.; D'Agostino, R.B. Lifetime risk of dementia and alzheimer's disease. The impact of mortality on risk estimates in the framingham study. *Neurology* **1997**, *49*, 1498–1504. [CrossRef]
7. Hebert, L.E.; Scherr, P.A.; McCann, J.J.; Beckett, L.A.; Evans, D.A. Is the risk of developing alzheimer's disease greater for women than for men? *Am. J. Epidemiol.* **2001**, *153*, 132–136. [CrossRef]
8. Chêne, G.; Beiser, A.; Au, R.; Preis, S.R.; Wolf, P.A.; Dufouil, C.; Seshadri, S. Gender and incidence of dementia in the framingham heart study from mid-adult life. *Alzheimer's Dement.* **2015**, *11*, 310–320. [CrossRef]
9. Carter, C.L.; Resnick, E.M.; Mallampalli, M.; Kalbarczyk, A. Sex and gender differences in alzheimer's disease: Recommendations for future research. *J. Womens Health* **2012**, *21*, 1018–1023. [CrossRef]
10. Altmann, A.; Tian, L.; Henderson, V.W.; Greicius, M.D.; Investigators, A.s.D.N.I. Sex modifies the apoe-related risk of developing alzheimer disease. *Ann. Neurol.* **2014**, *75*, 563–573. [CrossRef]
11. Ungar, L.; Altmann, A.; Greicius, M.D. Apolipoprotein E, gender, and alzheimer's disease: An overlooked, but potent and promising interaction. *Brain Imaging Behav.* **2014**, *8*, 262–273. [CrossRef] [PubMed]
12. Yaffe, K.; Haan, M.; Byers, A.; Tangen, C.; Kuller, L. Estrogen use, apoe, and cognitive decline: Evidence of gene-environment interaction. *Neurology* **2000**, *54*, 1949–1954. [CrossRef] [PubMed]
13. Kang, J.H.; Grodstein, F. Postmenopausal hormone therapy, timing of initiation, apoe and cognitive decline. *Neurobiol. Aging* **2012**, *33*, 1129–1137. [CrossRef] [PubMed]
14. Barrett-Connor, E.; Laughlin, G.A. Endogenous and exogenous estrogen, cognitive function, and dementia in postmenopausal women: Evidence from epidemiologic studies and clinical trials. *Semin. Reprod. Med.* **2009**, *27*, 275–282. [CrossRef]
15. O'Brien, J.; Jackson, J.W.; Grodstein, F.; Blacker, D.; Weuve, J. Postmenopausal hormone therapy is not associated with risk of all-cause dementia and alzheimer's disease. *Epidemiol. Rev.* **2014**, *36*, 83–103. [CrossRef]
16. Xu, J.; Murphy, S.L.; Kochanek, K.D.; Bastian, B.A. Deaths: Final data for 2013. *Natl. Vital Stat. Rep.* **2016**, *64*, 1–119.
17. Murray, C.J.; Atkinson, C.; Bhalla, K.; Birbeck, G.; Burstein, R.; Chou, D.; Dellavalle, R.; Danaei, G.; Ezzati, M.; Fahimi, A.; et al. The state of us health, 1990–2010: Burden of diseases, injuries, and risk factors. *JAMA* **2013**, *310*, 591–608. [CrossRef]
18. Gaugler, J.E.; Kane, R.L.; Kane, R.A. Family care for older adults with disabilities: Toward more targeted and interpretable research. *Int. J. Aging Hum. Dev.* **2002**, *54*, 205–231. [CrossRef]
19. Schulz, R.; Czaja, S.J.; Lustig, A.; Zdaniuk, B.; Martire, L.M.; Perdomo, D. Improving the quality of life of caregivers of persons with spinal cord injury: A randomized controlled trial. *Rehabil. Psychol.* **2009**, *54*, 1. [CrossRef]
20. Kasper, J.D.; Freedman, V.A.; Spillman, B.C.; Wolff, J.L. The disproportionate impact of dementia on family and unpaid caregiving to older adults. *Health Aff. Millwood* **2015**, *34*, 1642–1649. [CrossRef]
21. Freedman, V.A.; Spillman, B.C. Disability and care needs among older americans. *Milbank Q.* **2014**, *92*, 509–541. [CrossRef] [PubMed]

22. Anderson, L.A.; Edwards, V.J.; Pearson, W.S.; Talley, R.C.; McGuire, L.C.; Andresen, E.M. Adult caregivers in the united states: Characteristics and differences in well-being, by caregiver age and caregiving status. *Prev. Chronic Dis.* **2013**, *10*, E135. [CrossRef] [PubMed]
23. Hurd, M.D.; Martorell, P.; Delavande, A.; Mullen, K.J.; Langa, K.M. Monetary costs of dementia in the united states. *N. Engl. J. Med.* **2013**, *368*, 1326–1334. [CrossRef] [PubMed]
24. Consensus recommendations for the postmortem diagnosis of alzheimer's disease. The national institute on aging, and reagan institute working group on diagnostic criteria for the neuropathological assessment of alzheimer's disease. *Neurobiol. Aging* **1997**, *18*, S1–S2.
25. Braak, H.; Braak, E. Neuropathological stageing of alzheimer-related changes. *Acta Neuropathol.* **1991**, *82*, 239–259. [CrossRef] [PubMed]
26. Hyman, B.T.; Phelps, C.H.; Beach, T.G.; Bigio, E.H.; Cairns, N.J.; Carrillo, M.C.; Dickson, D.W.; Duyckaerts, C.; Frosch, M.P.; Masliah, E.; et al. National institute on aging-alzheimer's association guidelines for the neuropathologic assessment of alzheimer's disease. *Alzheimer's Dement.* **2012**, *8*, 1–13. [CrossRef] [PubMed]
27. Montine, T.J.; Phelps, C.H.; Beach, T.G.; Bigio, E.H.; Cairns, N.J.; Dickson, D.W.; Duyckaerts, C.; Frosch, M.P.; Masliah, E.; Mirra, S.S.; et al. National institute on aging-alzheimer's association guidelines for the neuropathologic assessment of alzheimer's disease: A practical approach. *Acta Neuropathol.* **2012**, *123*, 1–13. [CrossRef]
28. Holtzman, D.M.; Mandelkow, E.; Selkoe, D.J. Alzheimer disease in 2020. *Cold Spring Harb. Perspect. Med.* **2012**, *2*, a011585. [CrossRef]
29. Braak, H.; Braak, E. Evolution of the neuropathology of alzheimer's disease. *Acta Neurol. Scand.* **1996**, *165*, 3–12. [CrossRef]
30. Sengupta, U.; Nilson, A.N.; Kayed, R. The role of amyloid-β oligomers in toxicity, propagation, and immunotherapy. *EBioMedicine* **2016**, *6*, 42–49. [CrossRef]
31. Goedert, M.; Spillantini, M.G. Ordered assembly of tau protein and neurodegeneration. *Adv. Exp. Med. Biol.* **2019**, *1184*, 3–21. [PubMed]
32. Walsh, D.M.; Klyubin, I.; Fadeeva, J.V.; Rowan, M.J.; Selkoe, D.J. Amyloid-beta oligomers: Their production, toxicity and therapeutic inhibition. *Biochem. Soc. Trans.* **2002**, *30*, 552–557. [CrossRef] [PubMed]
33. Goedert, M.; Eisenberg, D.S.; Crowther, R.A. Propagation of tau aggregates and neurodegeneration. *Annu. Rev. Neurosci.* **2017**, *40*, 189–210. [CrossRef] [PubMed]
34. Ittner, A.; Ittner, L.M. Dendritic tau in alzheimer's disease. *Neuron* **2018**, *99*, 13–27. [CrossRef] [PubMed]
35. Stancu, I.C.; Vasconcelos, B.; Terwel, D.; Dewachter, I. Models of β-amyloid induced tau-pathology: The long and "folded" road to understand the mechanism. *Mol. Neurodegener.* **2014**, *9*, 51. [CrossRef]
36. van der Kant, R.; Goldstein, L.S.B.; Ossenkoppele, R. Amyloid-β-independent regulators of tau pathology in alzheimer disease. *Nat. Rev. Neurosci.* **2020**, *21*, 21–35. [CrossRef]
37. La Joie, R.; Visani, A.V.; Baker, S.L.; Brown, J.A.; Bourakova, V.; Cha, J.; Chaudhary, K.; Edwards, L.; Iaccarino, L.; Janabi, M.; et al. Prospective longitudinal atrophy in alzheimer's disease correlates with the intensity and topography of baseline tau-pet. *Sci. Transl. Med.* **2020**, *12*, 5732–5745. [CrossRef]
38. Franzmeier, N.; Neitzel, J.; Rubinski, A.; Smith, R.; Strandberg, O.; Ossenkoppele, R.; Hansson, O.; Ewers, M.; (ADNI), A.s.D.N.I. Functional brain architecture is associated with the rate of tau accumulation in alzheimer's disease. *Nat. Commun.* **2020**, *11*, 347. [CrossRef]
39. DeTure, M.A.; Dickson, D.W. The neuropathological diagnosis of alzheimer's disease. *Mol. Neurodegener.* **2019**, *14*, 32. [CrossRef]
40. Serrano-Pozo, A.; Mielke, M.L.; Gómez-Isla, T.; Betensky, R.A.; Growdon, J.H.; Frosch, M.P.; Hyman, B.T. Reactive glia not only associates with plaques but also parallels tangles in alzheimer's disease. *Am. J. Pathol.* **2011**, *179*, 1373–1384. [CrossRef]
41. Wake, H.; Moorhouse, A.J.; Jinno, S.; Kohsaka, S.; Nabekura, J. Resting microglia directly monitor the functional state of synapses in vivo and determine the fate of ischemic terminals. *J. Neurosci.* **2009**, *29*, 3974–3980. [CrossRef] [PubMed]
42. Vehmas, A.K.; Kawas, C.H.; Stewart, W.F.; Troncoso, J.C. Immune reactive cells in senile plaques and cognitive decline in alzheimer's disease. *Neurobiol. Aging* **2003**, *24*, 321–331. [CrossRef]
43. Serrano-Pozo, A.; Frosch, M.P.; Masliah, E.; Hyman, B.T. Neuropathological alterations in alzheimer disease. *Cold Spring Harb. Perspect. Med.* **2011**, *1*, a006189. [CrossRef] [PubMed]
44. Perl, D.P. Neuropathology of alzheimer's disease. *Mt. Sinai J. Med.* **2010**, *77*, 32–42. [CrossRef] [PubMed]

45. Thal, D.R.; Schultz, C.; Botez, G.; Del Tredici, K.; Mrak, R.E.; Griffin, W.S.; Wiestler, O.D.; Braak, H.; Ghebremedhin, E. The impact of argyrophilic grain disease on the development of dementia and its relationship to concurrent alzheimer's disease-related pathology. *Neuropathol. Appl. Neurobiol.* **2005**, *31*, 270–279. [CrossRef] [PubMed]
46. Hansen, L.; Salmon, D.; Galasko, D.; Masliah, E.; Katzman, R.; DeTeresa, R.; Thal, L.; Pay, M.M.; Hofstetter, R.; Klauber, M. The lewy body variant of alzheimer's disease: A clinical and pathologic entity. *Neurology* **1990**, *40*, 1. [CrossRef]
47. Nelson, P.T.; Gal, Z.; Wang, W.X.; Niedowicz, D.M.; Artiushin, S.C.; Wycoff, S.; Wei, A.; Jicha, G.A.; Fardo, D.W. Tdp-43 proteinopathy in aging: Associations with risk-associated gene variants and with brain parenchymal thyroid hormone levels. *Neurobiol. Dis.* **2019**, *125*, 67–76. [CrossRef]
48. Josephs, K.A.; Murray, M.E.; Whitwell, J.L.; Parisi, J.E.; Petrucelli, L.; Jack, C.R.; Petersen, R.C.; Dickson, D.W. Staging tdp-43 pathology in alzheimer's disease. *Acta Neuropathol.* **2014**, *127*, 441–450. [CrossRef]
49. Prasad, A.; Bharathi, V.; Sivalingam, V.; Girdhar, A.; Patel, B.K. Molecular mechanisms of tdp-43 misfolding and pathology in amyotrophic lateral sclerosis. *Front. Mol. Neurosci.* **2019**, *12*, 25. [CrossRef]
50. Gómez-Isla, T.; Hollister, R.; West, H.; Mui, S.; Growdon, J.H.; Petersen, R.C.; Parisi, J.E.; Hyman, B.T. Neuronal loss correlates with but exceeds neurofibrillary tangles in alzheimer's disease. *Ann. Neurol.* **1997**, *41*, 17–24. [CrossRef]
51. Forner, S.; Baglietto-Vargas, D.; Martini, A.C.; Trujillo-Estrada, L.; LaFerla, F.M. Synaptic impairment in alzheimer's disease: A dysregulated symphony. *Trends Neurosci.* **2017**, *40*, 347–357. [CrossRef] [PubMed]
52. Overk, C.R.; Masliah, E. Pathogenesis of synaptic degeneration in alzheimer's disease and lewy body disease. *Biochem. Pharmacol.* **2014**, *88*, 508–516. [CrossRef] [PubMed]
53. Sabbagh, M.N.; Lue, L.F.; Fayard, D.; Shi, J. Increasing precision of clinical diagnosis of alzheimer's disease using a combined algorithm incorporating clinical and novel biomarker data. *Neurol. Ther.* **2017**, *6*, 83–95. [CrossRef]
54. Dubois, B.; Feldman, H.H.; Jacova, C.; Hampel, H.; Molinuevo, J.L.; Blennow, K.; DeKosky, S.T.; Gauthier, S.; Selkoe, D.; Bateman, R.; et al. Advancing research diagnostic criteria for alzheimer's disease: The iwg-2 criteria. *Lancet Neurol.* **2014**, *13*, 614–629. [CrossRef]
55. Boise, L.; Camicioli, R.; Morgan, D.L.; Rose, J.H.; Congleton, L. Diagnosing dementia: Perspectives of primary care physicians. *Gerontologist* **1999**, *39*, 457–464. [CrossRef] [PubMed]
56. Beach, T.G.; Monsell, S.E.; Phillips, L.E.; Kukull, W. Accuracy of the clinical diagnosis of alzheimer disease at national institute on aging alzheimer disease centers, 2005–2010. *J. Neuropathol. Exp. Neurol.* **2012**, *71*, 266–273. [CrossRef]
57. Cacace, R.; Sleegers, K.; Van Broeckhoven, C. Molecular genetics of early-onset alzheimer's disease revisited. *Alzheimer's Dement.* **2016**, *12*, 733–748. [CrossRef]
58. Kimberly, W.T.; LaVoie, M.J.; Ostaszewski, B.L.; Ye, W.; Wolfe, M.S.; Selkoe, D.J. Gamma-secretase is a membrane protein complex comprised of presenilin, nicastrin, aph-1, and pen-2. *Proc. Natl. Acad. Sci. USA* **2003**, *100*, 6382–6387. [CrossRef]
59. Van Broeckhoven, C. Presenilins and alzheimer disease. *Nat. Genet.* **1995**, *11*, 230–232. [CrossRef]
60. Rademakers, R.; Cruts, M.; Van Broeckhoven, C. Genetics of early-onset alzheimer dementia. *Sci. World J.* **2003**, *3*, 497–519. [CrossRef]
61. Sherrington, R.; Rogaev, E.I.; Liang, Y.; Rogaeva, E.A.; Levesque, G.; Ikeda, M.; Chi, H.; Lin, C.; Li, G.; Holman, K.; et al. Cloning of a gene bearing missense mutations in early-onset familial alzheimer's disease. *Nature* **1995**, *375*, 754–760. [CrossRef]
62. Levy-Lahad, E.; Wasco, W.; Poorkaj, P.; Romano, D.M.; Oshima, J.; Pettingell, W.H.; Yu, C.E.; Jondro, P.D.; Schmidt, S.D.; Wang, K. Candidate gene for the chromosome 1 familial alzheimer's disease locus. *Science* **1995**, *269*, 973–977. [CrossRef] [PubMed]
63. Welzel, A.T.; Maggio, J.E.; Shankar, G.M.; Walker, D.E.; Ostaszewski, B.L.; Li, S.; Klyubin, I.; Rowan, M.J.; Seubert, P.; Walsh, D.M.; et al. Secreted amyloid β-proteins in a cell culture model include n-terminally extended peptides that impair synaptic plasticity. *Biochemistry* **2014**, *53*, 3908–3921. [CrossRef] [PubMed]
64. Riedel, B.C.; Thompson, P.M.; Brinton, R.D. Age, apoe and sex: Triad of risk of alzheimer's disease. *J. Steroid Biochem. Mol. Biol.* **2016**, *160*, 134–147. [CrossRef] [PubMed]
65. Yamazaki, Y.; Zhao, N.; Caulfield, T.R.; Liu, C.C.; Bu, G. Apolipoprotein e and alzheimer disease: Pathobiology and targeting strategies. *Nat. Rev. Neurol.* **2019**, *15*, 501–518. [CrossRef] [PubMed]

66. Gratuze, M.; Leyns, C.E.G.; Holtzman, D.M. New insights into the role of trem2 in alzheimer's disease. *Mol. Neurodegener.* **2018**, *13*, 66. [CrossRef] [PubMed]
67. Cai, Q.; Tammineni, P. Alterations in mitochondrial quality control in alzheimer's disease. *Front. Cell. Neurosci.* **2016**, *10*, 24. [CrossRef]
68. Devi, L.; Prabhu, B.M.; Galati, D.F.; Avadhani, N.G.; Anandatheerthavarada, H.K. Accumulation of amyloid precursor protein in the mitochondrial import channels of human alzheimer's disease brain is associated with mitochondrial dysfunction. *J. Neurosci.* **2006**, *26*, 9057–9068. [CrossRef]
69. Lamprecht, R.; LeDoux, J. Structural plasticity and memory. *Nat. Rev. Neurosci.* **2004**, *5*, 45–54. [CrossRef]
70. Kashyap, G.; Bapat, D.; Das, D.; Gowaikar, R.; Amritkar, R.E.; Rangarajan, G.; Ravindranath, V.; Ambika, G. Synapse loss and progress of alzheimer's disease—A network model. *Sci. Rep.* **2019**, *9*, 6555. [CrossRef]
71. Fabiani, C.; Antollini, S.S. Alzheimer's disease as a membrane disorder: Spatial cross-talk among beta-amyloid peptides, nicotinic acetylcholine receptors and lipid rafts. *Front. Cell. Neurosci.* **2019**, *13*, 309. [CrossRef] [PubMed]
72. Di Scala, C.; Yahi, N.; Boutemeur, S.; Flores, A.; Rodriguez, L.; Chahinian, H.; Fantini, J. Common molecular mechanism of amyloid pore formation by alzheimer's β-amyloid peptide and α-synuclein. *Sci. Rep.* **2016**, *6*, 28781. [CrossRef] [PubMed]
73. Lasagna-Reeves, C.A.; Sengupta, U.; Castillo-Carranza, D.; Gerson, J.E.; Guerrero-Munoz, M.; Troncoso, J.C.; Jackson, G.R.; Kayed, R. The formation of tau pore-like structures is prevalent and cell specific: Possible implications for the disease phenotypes. *Acta Neuropathol. Commun.* **2014**, *2*, 56. [CrossRef] [PubMed]
74. Tseng, B.P.; Green, K.N.; Chan, J.L.; Blurton-Jones, M.; LaFerla, F.M. Abeta inhibits the proteasome and enhances amyloid and tau accumulation. *Neurobiol. Aging* **2008**, *29*, 1607–1618. [CrossRef] [PubMed]
75. Myeku, N.; Clelland, C.L.; Emrani, S.; Kukushkin, N.V.; Yu, W.H.; Goldberg, A.L.; Duff, K.E. Tau-driven 26s proteasome impairment and cognitive dysfunction can be prevented early in disease by activating camp-pka signaling. *Nat. Med.* **2016**, *22*, 46–53. [CrossRef]
76. Yamazaki, Y.; Kanekiyo, T. Blood-brain barrier dysfunction and the pathogenesis of alzheimer's disease. *Int. J. Mol. Sci.* **2017**, *18*, 1965. [CrossRef]
77. Venegas, C.; Kumar, S.; Franklin, B.S.; Dierkes, T.; Brinkschulte, R.; Tejera, D.; Vieira-Saecker, A.; Schwartz, S.; Santarelli, F.; Kummer, M.P.; et al. Microglia-derived asc specks cross-seed amyloid-β in alzheimer's disease. *Nature* **2017**, *552*, 355–361. [CrossRef]
78. Perea, J.R.; Llorens-Martín, M.; Ávila, J.; Bolós, M. The role of microglia in the spread of tau: Relevance for tauopathies. *Front. Cell. Neurosci.* **2018**, *12*, 172. [CrossRef]
79. Heneka, M.T.; Carson, M.J.; El Khoury, J.; Landreth, G.E.; Brosseron, F.; Feinstein, D.L.; Jacobs, A.H.; Wyss-Coray, T.; Vitorica, J.; Ransohoff, R.M.; et al. Neuroinflammation in alzheimer's disease. *Lancet Neurol.* **2015**, *14*, 388–405. [CrossRef]
80. Jack, C.R.; Bennett, D.A.; Blennow, K.; Carrillo, M.C.; Feldman, H.H.; Frisoni, G.B.; Hampel, H.; Jagust, W.J.; Johnson, K.A.; Knopman, D.S.; et al. A/t/n: An unbiased descriptive classification scheme for alzheimer disease biomarkers. *Neurology* **2016**, *87*, 539–547. [CrossRef]
81. Ekman, U.; Ferreira, D.; Westman, E. The a/t/n biomarker scheme and patterns of brain atrophy assessed in mild cognitive impairment. *Sci. Rep.* **2018**, *8*, 8431. [CrossRef] [PubMed]
82. Ross, D.E.; Ochs, A.L.; Seabaugh, J.; Henshaw, T. Neuroquant®revealed hippocampal atrophy in a patient with traumatic brain injury. *J. Neuropsychiatry Clin. Neurosci.* **2012**, *24*, E33. [CrossRef] [PubMed]
83. Brewer, J.B.; Magda, S.; Airriess, C.; Smith, M.E. Fully-automated quantification of regional brain volumes for improved detection of focal atrophy in alzheimer disease. *AJNR Am. J. Neuroradiol.* **2009**, *30*, 578–580. [CrossRef] [PubMed]
84. Piccini, A.; Russo, C.; Gliozzi, A.; Relini, A.; Vitali, A.; Borghi, R.; Giliberto, L.; Armirotti, A.; D'Arrigo, C.; Bachi, A.; et al. Beta-amyloid is different in normal aging and in alzheimer disease. *J. Biol. Chem.* **2005**, *280*, 34186–34192. [CrossRef]
85. Panza, F.; Lozupone, M.; Logroscino, G.; Imbimbo, B.P. A critical appraisal of amyloid-β-targeting therapies for alzheimer disease. *Nat. Rev. Neurol.* **2019**, *15*, 73–88. [CrossRef]
86. Selkoe, D.J. Resolving controversies on the path to alzheimer's therapeutics. *Nat. Med.* **2011**, *17*, 1060–1065. [CrossRef]
87. Hane, F.T.; Robinson, M.; Lee, B.Y.; Bai, O.; Leonenko, Z.; Albert, M.S. Recent progress in alzheimer's disease research, part 3: Diagnosis and treatment. *J. Alzheimer's Dis.* **2017**, *57*, 645–665. [CrossRef]

88. Orgogozo, J.M.; Gilman, S.; Dartigues, J.F.; Laurent, B.; Puel, M.; Kirby, L.C.; Jouanny, P.; Dubois, B.; Eisner, L.; Flitman, S.; et al. Subacute meningoencephalitis in a subset of patients with ad after abeta42 immunization. *Neurology* **2003**, *61*, 46–54. [CrossRef]
89. Vellas, B.; Black, R.; Thal, L.J.; Fox, N.C.; Daniels, M.; McLennan, G.; Tompkins, C.; Leibman, C.; Pomfret, M.; Grundman, M.; et al. Long-term follow-up of patients immunized with an1792: Reduced functional decline in antibody responders. *Curr. Alzheimer Res.* **2009**, *6*, 144–151. [CrossRef]
90. Lemere, C.A.; Masliah, E. Can alzheimer disease be prevented by amyloid-beta immunotherapy? *Nat. Rev. Neurol.* **2010**, *6*, 108–119. [CrossRef]
91. Wiessner, C.; Wiederhold, K.H.; Tissot, A.C.; Frey, P.; Danner, S.; Jacobson, L.H.; Jennings, G.T.; Lüönd, R.; Ortmann, R.; Reichwald, J.; et al. The second-generation active aβ immunotherapy cad106 reduces amyloid accumulation in app transgenic mice while minimizing potential side effects. *J. Neurosci.* **2011**, *31*, 9323–9331. [CrossRef] [PubMed]
92. Doody, R.S.; Thomas, R.G.; Farlow, M.; Iwatsubo, T.; Vellas, B.; Joffe, S.; Kieburtz, K.; Raman, R.; Sun, X.; Aisen, P.S.; et al. Phase 3 trials of solanezumab for mild-to-moderate alzheimer's disease. *N. Engl. J. Med.* **2014**, *370*, 311–321. [CrossRef] [PubMed]
93. Liu-Seifert, H.; Siemers, E.; Holdridge, K.C.; Andersen, S.W.; Lipkovich, I.; Carlson, C.; Sethuraman, G.; Hoog, S.; Hayduk, R.; Doody, R.; et al. Delayed-start analysis: Mild alzheimer's disease patients in solanezumab trials, 3.5 years. *Alzheimer's Dement. N. Y.* **2015**, *1*, 111–121. [CrossRef] [PubMed]
94. Siemers, E.R.; Sundell, K.L.; Carlson, C.; Case, M.; Sethuraman, G.; Liu-Seifert, H.; Dowsett, S.A.; Pontecorvo, M.J.; Dean, R.A.; Demattos, R. Phase 3 solanezumab trials: Secondary outcomes in mild alzheimer's disease patients. *Alzheimer's Dement.* **2016**, *12*, 110–120. [CrossRef]
95. Sevigny, J.; Chiao, P.; Bussière, T.; Weinreb, P.H.; Williams, L.; Maier, M.; Dunstan, R.; Salloway, S.; Chen, T.; Ling, Y.; et al. The antibody aducanumab reduces aβ plaques in alzheimer's disease. *Nature* **2016**, *537*, 50–56. [CrossRef]
96. Novak, P.; Zilka, N.; Zilkova, M.; Kovacech, B.; Skrabana, R.; Ondrus, M.; Fialova, L.; Kontsekova, E.; Otto, M.; Novak, M. Aadvac1, an active immunotherapy for alzheimer's disease and non alzheimer tauopathies: An overview of preclinical and clinical development. *J. Prev. Alzheimer's Dis.* **2019**, *6*, 63–69.
97. Theunis, C.; Crespo-Biel, N.; Gafner, V.; Pihlgren, M.; López-Deber, M.P.; Reis, P.; Hickman, D.T.; Adolfsson, O.; Chuard, N.; Ndao, D.M.; et al. Efficacy and safety of a liposome-based vaccine against protein tau, assessed in tau.P301l mice that model tauopathy. *PLoS ONE* **2013**, *8*, e72301. [CrossRef]
98. Davies, P.; Maloney, A.J. Selective loss of central cholinergic neurons in alzheimer's disease. *Lancet* **1976**, *2*, 1403. [CrossRef]
99. Jack, C.R.; Bennett, D.A.; Blennow, K.; Carrillo, M.C.; Dunn, B.; Haeberlein, S.B.; Holtzman, D.M.; Jagust, W.; Jessen, F.; Karlawish, J.; et al. Nia-aa research framework: Toward a biological definition of alzheimer's disease. *Alzheimer's Dement.* **2018**, *14*, 535–562. [CrossRef]
100. Pedrero-Prieto, C.M.; García-Carpintero, S.; Frontiñán-Rubio, J.; Llanos-González, E.; Aguilera García, C.; Alcaín, F.J.; Lindberg, I.; Durán-Prado, M.; Peinado, J.R.; Rabanal-Ruiz, Y. A comprehensive systematic review of csf proteins and peptides that define alzheimer's disease. *Clin. Proteom.* **2020**, *17*, 21. [CrossRef]
101. Villemagne, V.L.; Doré, V.; Burnham, S.C.; Masters, C.L.; Rowe, C.C. Imaging tau and amyloid-β proteinopathies in alzheimer disease and other conditions. *Nat. Rev. Neurol.* **2018**, *14*, 225–236. [CrossRef] [PubMed]
102. Mattsson-Carlgren, N.; Andersson, E.; Janelidze, S.; Ossenkoppele, R.; Insel, P.; Strandberg, O.; Zetterberg, H.; Rosen, H.J.; Rabinovici, G.; Chai, X.; et al. Aβ deposition is associated with increases in soluble and phosphorylated tau that precede a positive tau pet in alzheimer's disease. *Sci. Adv.* **2020**, *6*, eaaz2387. [CrossRef] [PubMed]
103. Lombardi, G.; Crescioli, G.; Cavedo, E.; Lucenteforte, E.; Casazza, G.; Bellatorre, A.G.; Lista, C.; Costantino, G.; Frisoni, G.; Virgili, G.; et al. Structural magnetic resonance imaging for the early diagnosis of dementia due to alzheimer's disease in people with mild cognitive impairment. *Cochrane Database Syst. Rev.* **2020**, *3*, CD009628. [CrossRef] [PubMed]
104. Khosravi, M.; Peter, J.; Wintering, N.A.; Serruya, M.; Shamchi, S.P.; Werner, T.J.; Alavi, A.; Newberg, A.B. 18f-fdg is a superior indicator of cognitive performance compared to 18f-florbetapir in alzheimer's disease and mild cognitive impairment evaluation: A global quantitative analysis. *J. Alzheimer's Dis.* **2019**, *70*, 1197–1207. [CrossRef]

105. Zetterberg, H.; Skillbäck, T.; Mattsson, N.; Trojanowski, J.Q.; Portelius, E.; Shaw, L.M.; Weiner, M.W.; Blennow, K.; Initiative, A.s.D.N. Association of cerebrospinal fluid neurofilament light concentration with alzheimer disease progression. *JAMA Neurol.* **2016**, *73*, 60–67. [CrossRef]
106. Janelidze, S.; Hertze, J.; Zetterberg, H.; Landqvist Waldö, M.; Santillo, A.; Blennow, K.; Hansson, O. Cerebrospinal fluid neurogranin and ykl-40 as biomarkers of alzheimer's disease. *Ann. Clin. Transl. Neurol.* **2016**, *3*, 12–20. [CrossRef]
107. Jack, C.R.; Albert, M.S.; Knopman, D.S.; McKhann, G.M.; Sperling, R.A.; Carrillo, M.C.; Thies, B.; Phelps, C.H. Introduction to the recommendations from the national institute on aging-alzheimer's association workgroups on diagnostic guidelines for alzheimer's disease. *Alzheimer's Dement.* **2011**, *7*, 257–262. [CrossRef]
108. McKhann, G.M.; Knopman, D.S.; Chertkow, H.; Hyman, B.T.; Jack, C.R.; Kawas, C.H.; Klunk, W.E.; Koroshetz, W.J.; Manly, J.J.; Mayeux, R.; et al. The diagnosis of dementia due to alzheimer's disease: Recommendations from the national institute on aging-alzheimer's association workgroups on diagnostic guidelines for alzheimer's disease. *Alzheimer's Dement.* **2011**, *7*, 263–269. [CrossRef]
109. Albert, M.S.; DeKosky, S.T.; Dickson, D.; Dubois, B.; Feldman, H.H.; Fox, N.C.; Gamst, A.; Holtzman, D.M.; Jagust, W.J.; Petersen, R.C.; et al. The diagnosis of mild cognitive impairment due to alzheimer's disease: Recommendations from the national institute on aging-alzheimer's association workgroups on diagnostic guidelines for alzheimer's disease. *Alzheimer's Dement.* **2011**, *7*, 270–279. [CrossRef]
110. Sperling, R.A.; Aisen, P.S.; Beckett, L.A.; Bennett, D.A.; Craft, S.; Fagan, A.M.; Iwatsubo, T.; Jack, C.R.; Kaye, J.; Montine, T.J.; et al. Toward defining the preclinical stages of alzheimer's disease: Recommendations from the national institute on aging-alzheimer's association workgroups on diagnostic guidelines for alzheimer's disease. *Alzheimer's Dement.* **2011**, *7*, 280–292. [CrossRef]
111. Dubois, B.; Feldman, H.H.; Jacova, C.; Dekosky, S.T.; Barberger-Gateau, P.; Cummings, J.; Delacourte, A.; Galasko, D.; Gauthier, S.; Jicha, G.; et al. Research criteria for the diagnosis of alzheimer's disease: Revising the nincds-adrda criteria. *Lancet Neurol.* **2007**, *6*, 734–746. [CrossRef]
112. Dubois, B.; Hampel, H.; Feldman, H.H.; Scheltens, P.; Aisen, P.; Andrieu, S.; Bakardjian, H.; Benali, H.; Bertram, L.; Blennow, K.; et al. Preclinical alzheimer's disease: Definition, natural history, and diagnostic criteria. *Alzheimer's Dement.* **2016**, *12*, 292–323. [CrossRef] [PubMed]
113. Hampel, H.; O'Bryant, S.E.; Molinuevo, J.L.; Zetterberg, H.; Masters, C.L.; Lista, S.; Kiddle, S.J.; Batrla, R.; Blennow, K. Blood-based biomarkers for alzheimer disease: Mapping the road to the clinic. *Nat. Rev. Neurol.* **2018**, *14*, 639–652. [CrossRef] [PubMed]
114. Twohig, D.; Rodriguez-Vieitez, E.; Sando, S.B.; Berge, G.; Lauridsen, C.; Møller, I.; Grøntvedt, G.R.; Bråthen, G.; Patra, K.; Bu, G.; et al. The relevance of cerebrospinal fluid α-synuclein levels to sporadic and familial alzheimer's disease. *Acta Neuropathol. Commun.* **2018**, *6*, 130. [CrossRef] [PubMed]
115. Olsson, B.; Lautner, R.; Andreasson, U.; Öhrfelt, A.; Portelius, E.; Bjerke, M.; Hölttä, M.; Rosén, C.; Olsson, C.; Strobel, G.; et al. Csf and blood biomarkers for the diagnosis of alzheimer's disease: A systematic review and meta-analysis. *Lancet Neurol.* **2016**, *15*, 673–684. [CrossRef]
116. Li, Q.X.; Villemagne, V.L.; Doecke, J.D.; Rembach, A.; Sarros, S.; Varghese, S.; McGlade, A.; Laughton, K.M.; Pertile, K.K.; Fowler, C.J.; et al. Alzheimer's disease normative cerebrospinal fluid biomarkers validated in pet amyloid-β characterized subjects from the australian imaging, biomarkers and lifestyle (aibl) study. *J. Alzheimer's Dis.* **2015**, *48*, 175–187. [CrossRef]
117. Mattsson, N.; Palmqvist, S.; Stomrud, E.; Vogel, J.; Hansson, O. Staging β-amyloid pathology with amyloid positron emission tomography. *JAMA Neurol.* **2019**, *76*, 1319–1329. [CrossRef]
118. Fagan, A.M.; Xiong, C.; Jasielec, M.S.; Bateman, R.J.; Goate, A.M.; Benzinger, T.L.; Ghetti, B.; Martins, R.N.; Masters, C.L.; Mayeux, R.; et al. Longitudinal change in csf biomarkers in autosomal-dominant alzheimer's disease. *Sci. Transl. Med.* **2014**, *6*, 226ra230. [CrossRef]
119. Lewczuk, P.; Matzen, A.; Blennow, K.; Parnetti, L.; Molinuevo, J.L.; Eusebi, P.; Kornhuber, J.; Morris, J.C.; Fagan, A.M. Cerebrospinal fluid aβ42/40 corresponds better than aβ42 to amyloid pet in alzheimer's disease. *J. Alzheimer's Dis.* **2017**, *55*, 813–822. [CrossRef]
120. Doecke, J.D.; Rembach, A.; Villemagne, V.L.; Varghese, S.; Rainey-Smith, S.; Sarros, S.; Evered, L.A.; Fowler, C.J.; Pertile, K.K.; Rumble, R.L.; et al. Concordance between cerebrospinal fluid biomarkers with alzheimer's disease pathology between three independent assay platforms. *J. Alzheimer's Dis.* **2018**, *61*, 169–183. [CrossRef]

121. Xia, D.; Watanabe, H.; Wu, B.; Lee, S.H.; Li, Y.; Tsvetkov, E.; Bolshakov, V.Y.; Shen, J.; Kelleher, R.J. Presenilin-1 knockin mice reveal loss-of-function mechanism for familial alzheimer's disease. *Neuron* **2015**, *85*, 967–981. [CrossRef] [PubMed]
122. Selkoe, D.J.; Hardy, J. The amyloid hypothesis of alzheimer's disease at 25 years. *EMBO Mol. Med.* **2016**, *8*, 595–608. [CrossRef] [PubMed]
123. Saido, T.C.; Iwatsubo, T.; Mann, D.M.; Shimada, H.; Ihara, Y.; Kawashima, S. Dominant and differential deposition of distinct beta-amyloid peptide species, a beta n3(pe), in senile plaques. *Neuron* **1995**, *14*, 457–466. [CrossRef]
124. Portelius, E.; Bogdanovic, N.; Gustavsson, M.K.; Volkmann, I.; Brinkmalm, G.; Zetterberg, H.; Winblad, B.; Blennow, K. Mass spectrometric characterization of brain amyloid beta isoform signatures in familial and sporadic alzheimer's disease. *Acta Neuropathol.* **2010**, *120*, 185–193. [CrossRef]
125. Nussbaum, J.M.; Schilling, S.; Cynis, H.; Silva, A.; Swanson, E.; Wangsanut, T.; Tayler, K.; Wiltgen, B.; Hatami, A.; Rönicke, R.; et al. Prion-like behaviour and tau-dependent cytotoxicity of pyroglutamylated amyloid-β. *Nature* **2012**, *485*, 651–655. [CrossRef]
126. Plant, L.D.; Boyle, J.P.; Smith, I.F.; Peers, C.; Pearson, H.A. The production of amyloid beta peptide is a critical requirement for the viability of central neurons. *J. Neurosci.* **2003**, *23*, 5531–5535. [CrossRef]
127. Sjögren, M.; Gisslén, M.; Vanmechelen, E.; Blennow, K. Low cerebrospinal fluid beta-amyloid 42 in patients with acute bacterial meningitis and normalization after treatment. *Neurosci. Lett.* **2001**, *314*, 33–36. [CrossRef]
128. Emmerling, M.R.; Morganti-Kossmann, M.C.; Kossmann, T.; Stahel, P.F.; Watson, M.D.; Evans, L.M.; Mehta, P.D.; Spiegel, K.; Kuo, Y.M.; Roher, A.E.; et al. Traumatic brain injury elevates the alzheimer's amyloid peptide a beta 42 in human csf. A possible role for nerve cell injury. *Ann. N. Y. Acad. Sci.* **2000**, *903*, 118–122. [CrossRef]
129. Mondello, S.; Buki, A.; Barzo, P.; Randall, J.; Provuncher, G.; Hanlon, D.; Wilson, D.; Kobeissy, F.; Jeromin, A. Csf and plasma amyloid-beta temporal profiles and relationships with neurological status and mortality after severe traumatic brain injury. *Sci. Rep.* **2014**, *4*, 6446. [CrossRef]
130. Olsson, A.; Csajbok, L.; Ost, M.; Höglund, K.; Nylén, K.; Rosengren, L.; Nellgård, B.; Blennow, K. Marked increase of beta-amyloid(1-42) and amyloid precursor protein in ventricular cerebrospinal fluid after severe traumatic brain injury. *J. Neurol.* **2004**, *251*, 870–876. [CrossRef]
131. Hortobágyi, T.; Wise, S.; Hunt, N.; Cary, N.; Djurovic, V.; Fegan-Earl, A.; Shorrock, K.; Rouse, D.; Al-Sarraj, S. Traumatic axonal damage in the brain can be detected using beta-app immunohistochemistry within 35 min after head injury to human adults. *Neuropathol. Appl. Neurobiol.* **2007**, *33*, 226–237. [CrossRef] [PubMed]
132. Tsitsopoulos, P.P.; Marklund, N. Amyloid-beta peptides and tau protein as biomarkers in cerebrospinal and interstitial fluid following traumatic brain injury: A review of experimental and clinical studies. *Front. Neurol.* **2013**, *4*, 79. [CrossRef] [PubMed]
133. Schindler, S.E.; Li, Y.; Todd, K.W.; Herries, E.M.; Henson, R.L.; Gray, J.D.; Wang, G.; Graham, D.L.; Shaw, L.M.; Trojanowski, J.Q.; et al. Emerging cerebrospinal fluid biomarkers in autosomal dominant alzheimer's disease. *Alzheimer's Dement.* **2019**, *15*, 655–665. [CrossRef] [PubMed]
134. Henson, R.L.; Doran, E.; Christian, B.T.; Handen, B.L.; Klunk, W.E.; Lai, F.; Lee, J.H.; Rosas, H.D.; Schupf, N.; Zaman, S.H.; et al. Cerebrospinal fluid biomarkers of alzheimer's disease in a cohort of adults with down syndrome. *Alzheimer's Dement.* **2020**, *12*, e12057. [CrossRef] [PubMed]
135. Mo, J.A.; Lim, J.H.; Sul, A.R.; Lee, M.; Youn, Y.C.; Kim, H.J. Cerebrospinal fluid β-amyloid1-42 levels in the differential diagnosis of alzheimer's disease–systematic review and meta-analysis. *PLoS ONE* **2015**, *10*, e0116802. [CrossRef]
136. Englund, H.; Annerén, G.; Gustafsson, J.; Wester, U.; Wiltfang, J.; Lannfelt, L.; Blennow, K.; Höglund, K. Increase in beta-amyloid levels in cerebrospinal fluid of children with down syndrome. *Dement. Geriatr. Cogn. Disord.* **2007**, *24*, 369–374. [CrossRef] [PubMed]
137. Peskind, E.R.; Riekse, R.; Quinn, J.F.; Kaye, J.; Clark, C.M.; Farlow, M.R.; Decarli, C.; Chabal, C.; Vavrek, D.; Raskind, M.A.; et al. Safety and acceptability of the research lumbar puncture. *Alzheimer Dis. Assoc. Disord.* **2005**, *19*, 220–225. [CrossRef]
138. Palmert, M.R.; Podlisny, M.B.; Witker, D.S.; Oltersdorf, T.; Younkin, L.H.; Selkoe, D.J.; Younkin, S.G. The beta-amyloid protein precursor of alzheimer disease has soluble derivatives found in human brain and cerebrospinal fluid. *Proc. Natl. Acad. Sci. USA* **1989**, *86*, 6338–6342. [CrossRef]

139. Ghiso, J.; Tagliavini, F.; Timmers, W.F.; Frangione, B. Alzheimer's disease amyloid precursor protein is present in senile plaques and cerebrospinal fluid: Immunohistochemical and biochemical characterization. *Biochem. Biophys. Res. Commun.* **1989**, *163*, 430–437. [CrossRef]
140. Palmert, M.R.; Siedlak, S.L.; Podlisny, M.B.; Greenberg, B.; Shelton, E.R.; Chan, H.W.; Usiak, M.; Selkoe, D.J.; Perry, G.; Younkin, S.G. Soluble derivatives of the beta amyloid protein precursor of alzheimer's disease are labeled by antisera to the beta amyloid protein. *Biochem. Biophys. Res. Commun.* **1989**, *165*, 182–188. [CrossRef]
141. Chong, J.K.; Miller, B.E.; Ghanbari, H.A. Detection of amyloid beta protein precursor immunoreactivity in normal and alzheimer's disease cerebrospinal fluid. *Life Sci.* **1990**, *47*, 1163–1171. [CrossRef]
142. Van Nostrand, W.E.; Wagner, S.L.; Shankle, W.R.; Farrow, J.S.; Dick, M.; Rozemuller, J.M.; Kuiper, M.A.; Wolters, E.C.; Zimmerman, J.; Cotman, C.W. Decreased levels of soluble amyloid beta-protein precursor in cerebrospinal fluid of live alzheimer disease patients. *Proc. Natl. Acad. Sci. USA* **1992**, *89*, 2551–2555. [CrossRef] [PubMed]
143. Urakami, K.; Takahashi, K.; Okada, A.; Oshima, T.; Adachi, Y.; Nakamura, S.; Kitaguchi, N.; Tokushima, Y.; Yamamoto, S.; Tanaka, S. Clinical course and csf amyloid beta protein precursor having the site of application of the protease inhibitor (appi) levels in patients with dementia of the alzheimer type. *Dementia* **1993**, *4*, 59–60.
144. Vigo-Pelfrey, C.; Lee, D.; Keim, P.; Lieberburg, I.; Schenk, D.B. Characterization of beta-amyloid peptide from human cerebrospinal fluid. *J. Neurochem.* **1993**, *61*, 1965–1968. [CrossRef]
145. van Gool, W.A.; Schenk, D.B.; Bolhuis, P.A. Concentrations of amyloid-beta protein in cerebrospinal fluid increase with age in patients free from neurodegenerative disease. *Neurosci. Lett.* **1994**, *172*, 122–124. [CrossRef]
146. Tabaton, M.; Nunzi, M.G.; Xue, R.; Usiak, M.; Autilio-Gambetti, L.; Gambetti, P. Soluble amyloid beta-protein is a marker of alzheimer amyloid in brain but not in cerebrospinal fluid. *Biochem. Biophys. Res. Commun.* **1994**, *200*, 1598–1603. [CrossRef]
147. Jensen, M.; Schröder, J.; Blomberg, M.; Engvall, B.; Pantel, J.; Ida, N.; Basun, H.; Wahlund, L.O.; Werle, E.; Jauss, M.; et al. Cerebrospinal fluid a beta42 is increased early in sporadic alzheimer's disease and declines with disease progression. *Ann. Neurol.* **1999**, *45*, 504–511. [CrossRef]
148. Fagan, A.M.; Roe, C.M.; Xiong, C.; Mintun, M.A.; Morris, J.C.; Holtzman, D.M. Cerebrospinal fluid tau/beta-amyloid(42) ratio as a prediction of cognitive decline in nondemented older adults. *Arch. Neurol.* **2007**, *64*, 343–349. [CrossRef]
149. Fagan, A.M.; Perrin, R.J. Upcoming candidate cerebrospinal fluid biomarkers of alzheimer's disease. *Biomark. Med.* **2012**, *6*, 455–476. [CrossRef]
150. Hansson, O.; Lehmann, S.; Otto, M.; Zetterberg, H.; Lewczuk, P. Advantages and disadvantages of the use of the csf amyloid β (aβ) 42/40 ratio in the diagnosis of alzheimer's disease. *Alzheimer's Res. Ther.* **2019**, *11*, 34. [CrossRef]
151. Holtzman, D.M. Csf biomarkers for alzheimer's disease: Current utility and potential future use. *Neurobiol. Aging* **2011**, *32* (Suppl. 1), S4–S9. [CrossRef]
152. Dumurgier, J.; Gabelle, A.; Vercruysse, O.; Bombois, S.; Laplanche, J.L.; Peoc'h, K.; Schraen, S.; Sablonnière, B.; Pasquier, F.; Touchon, J.; et al. Exacerbated csf abnormalities in younger patients with alzheimer's disease. *Neurobiol. Dis.* **2013**, *54*, 486–491. [CrossRef] [PubMed]
153. Reijn, T.S.; Rikkert, M.O.; van Geel, W.J.; de Jong, D.; Verbeek, M.M. Diagnostic accuracy of elisa and xmap technology for analysis of amyloid beta(42) and tau proteins. *Clin. Chem.* **2007**, *53*, 859–865. [CrossRef] [PubMed]
154. Mattsson, N.; Zetterberg, H.; Hansson, O.; Andreasen, N.; Parnetti, L.; Jonsson, M.; Herukka, S.K.; van der Flier, W.M.; Blankenstein, M.A.; Ewers, M.; et al. Csf biomarkers and incipient alzheimer disease in patients with mild cognitive impairment. *JAMA* **2009**, *302*, 385–393. [CrossRef] [PubMed]
155. Kapaki, E.N.; Paraskevas, G.P.; Tzerakis, N.G.; Sfagos, C.; Seretis, A.; Kararizou, E.; Vassilopoulos, D. Cerebrospinal fluid tau, phospho-tau181 and beta-amyloid1-42 in idiopathic normal pressure hydrocephalus: A discrimination from alzheimer's disease. *Eur. J. Neurol.* **2007**, *14*, 168–173. [CrossRef] [PubMed]
156. Kapaki, E.; Liappas, I.; Paraskevas, G.P.; Theotoka, I.; Rabavilas, A. The diagnostic value of tau protein, beta-amyloid (1-42) and their ratio for the discrimination of alcohol-related cognitive disorders from alzheimer's disease in the early stages. *Int. J. Geriatr. Psychiatry* **2005**, *20*, 722–729. [CrossRef]

157. Ewers, M.; Mattsson, N.; Minthon, L.; Molinuevo, J.L.; Antonell, A.; Popp, J.; Jessen, F.; Herukka, S.K.; Soininen, H.; Maetzler, W.; et al. Csf biomarkers for the differential diagnosis of alzheimer's disease: A large-scale international multicenter study. *Alzheimer's Dement.* **2015**, *11*, 1306–1315. [CrossRef]
158. Selnes, P.; Blennow, K.; Zetterberg, H.; Grambaite, R.; Rosengren, L.; Johnsen, L.; Stenset, V.; Fladby, T. Effects of cerebrovascular disease on amyloid precursor protein metabolites in cerebrospinal fluid. *Cerebrospinal Fluid Res.* **2010**, *7*, 10. [CrossRef]
159. Vos, S.J.; van Rossum, I.A.; Verhey, F.; Knol, D.L.; Soininen, H.; Wahlund, L.O.; Hampel, H.; Tsolaki, M.; Minthon, L.; Frisoni, G.B.; et al. Prediction of alzheimer disease in subjects with amnestic and nonamnestic mci. *Neurology* **2013**, *80*, 1124–1132. [CrossRef]
160. Hampel, H.; Teipel, S.J.; Fuchsberger, T.; Andreasen, N.; Wiltfang, J.; Otto, M.; Shen, Y.; Dodel, R.; Du, Y.; Farlow, M.; et al. Value of csf beta-amyloid1-42 and tau as predictors of alzheimer's disease in patients with mild cognitive impairment. *Mol. Psychiatry* **2004**, *9*, 705–710. [CrossRef]
161. Perneczky, R.; Tsolakidou, A.; Arnold, A.; Diehl-Schmid, J.; Grimmer, T.; Förstl, H.; Kurz, A.; Alexopoulos, P. Csf soluble amyloid precursor proteins in the diagnosis of incipient alzheimer disease. *Neurology* **2011**, *77*, 35–38. [CrossRef] [PubMed]
162. Lewczuk, P.; Kornhuber, J.; Vanderstichele, H.; Vanmechelen, E.; Esselmann, H.; Bibl, M.; Wolf, S.; Otto, M.; Reulbach, U.; Kölsch, H.; et al. Multiplexed quantification of dementia biomarkers in the csf of patients with early dementias and mci: A multicenter study. *Neurobiol. Aging* **2008**, *29*, 812–818. [CrossRef] [PubMed]
163. Bibl, M.; Gallus, M.; Welge, V.; Esselmann, H.; Wolf, S.; Rüther, E.; Wiltfang, J. Cerebrospinal fluid amyloid-β 2-42 is decreased in alzheimer's, but not in frontotemporal dementia. *J. Neural Transm.* **2012**, *119*, 805–813. [CrossRef] [PubMed]
164. Lewczuk, P.; Lelental, N.; Spitzer, P.; Maler, J.M.; Kornhuber, J. Amyloid-β 42/40 cerebrospinal fluid concentration ratio in the diagnostics of alzheimer's disease: Validation of two novel assays. *J. Alzheimer's Dis.* **2015**, *43*, 183–191. [CrossRef]
165. Struyfs, H.; Van Broeck, B.; Timmers, M.; Fransen, E.; Sleegers, K.; Van Broeckhoven, C.; De Deyn, P.P.; Streffer, J.R.; Mercken, M.; Engelborghs, S. Diagnostic accuracy of cerebrospinal fluid amyloid-β isoforms for early and differential dementia diagnosis. *J. Alzheimer's Dis.* **2015**, *45*, 813–822. [CrossRef]
166. Hansson, O.; Zetterberg, H.; Buchhave, P.; Andreasson, U.; Londos, E.; Minthon, L.; Blennow, K. Prediction of alzheimer's disease using the csf abeta42/abeta40 ratio in patients with mild cognitive impairment. *Dement. Geriatr. Cogn. Disord.* **2007**, *23*, 316–320. [CrossRef]
167. Janelidze, S.; Zetterberg, H.; Mattsson, N.; Palmqvist, S.; Vanderstichele, H.; Lindberg, O.; van Westen, D.; Stomrud, E.; Minthon, L.; Blennow, K.; et al. Csf aβ42/aβ40 and aβ42/aβ38 ratios: Better diagnostic markers of alzheimer disease. *Ann. Clin. Transl. Neurol.* **2016**, *3*, 154–165. [CrossRef]
168. Fukumoto, H.; Tennis, M.; Locascio, J.J.; Hyman, B.T.; Growdon, J.H.; Irizarry, M.C. Age but not diagnosis is the main predictor of plasma amyloid beta-protein levels. *Arch. Neurol.* **2003**, *60*, 958–964. [CrossRef]
169. Rissin, D.M.; Kan, C.W.; Campbell, T.G.; Howes, S.C.; Fournier, D.R.; Song, L.; Piech, T.; Patel, P.P.; Chang, L.; Rivnak, A.J.; et al. Single-molecule enzyme-linked immunosorbent assay detects serum proteins at subfemtomolar concentrations. *Nat. Biotechnol.* **2010**, *28*, 595–599. [CrossRef]
170. Janelidze, S.; Stomrud, E.; Palmqvist, S.; Zetterberg, H.; van Westen, D.; Jeromin, A.; Song, L.; Hanlon, D.; Tan Hehir, C.A.; Baker, D.; et al. Plasma β-amyloid in alzheimer's disease and vascular disease. *Sci. Rep.* **2016**, *6*, 26801. [CrossRef]
171. Zetterberg, H.; Mörtberg, E.; Song, L.; Chang, L.; Provuncher, G.K.; Patel, P.P.; Ferrell, E.; Fournier, D.R.; Kan, C.W.; Campbell, T.G.; et al. Hypoxia due to cardiac arrest induces a time-dependent increase in serum amyloid β levels in humans. *PLoS ONE* **2011**, *6*, e28263. [CrossRef] [PubMed]
172. Yang, S.Y.; Chiu, M.J.; Chen, T.F.; Horng, H.E. Detection of plasma biomarkers using immunomagnetic reduction: A promising method for the early diagnosis of alzheimer's disease. *Neurol. Ther.* **2017**, *6*, 37–56. [CrossRef] [PubMed]
173. Wang, L.S.; Leung, Y.Y.; Chang, S.K.; Leight, S.; Knapik-Czajka, M.; Baek, Y.; Shaw, L.M.; Lee, V.M.; Trojanowski, J.Q.; Clark, C.M. Comparison of xmap and elisa assays for detecting cerebrospinal fluid biomarkers of alzheimer's disease. *J. Alzheimer's Dis.* **2012**, *31*, 439–445. [CrossRef] [PubMed]
174. Pan, C.; Korff, A.; Galasko, D.; Ginghina, C.; Peskind, E.; Li, G.; Quinn, J.; Montine, T.J.; Cain, K.; Shi, M.; et al. Diagnostic values of cerebrospinal fluid t-tau and aβ_{42} using meso scale discovery assays for alzheimer's disease. *J. Alzheimer's Dis.* **2015**, *45*, 709–719. [CrossRef]

175. Nakamura, A.; Kaneko, N.; Villemagne, V.L.; Kato, T.; Doecke, J.; Doré, V.; Fowler, C.; Li, Q.X.; Martins, R.; Rowe, C.; et al. High performance plasma amyloid-β biomarkers for alzheimer's disease. *Nature* **2018**, *554*, 249–254. [CrossRef]
176. Schindler, S.E.; Bollinger, J.G.; Ovod, V.; Mawuenyega, K.G.; Li, Y.; Gordon, B.A.; Holtzman, D.M.; Morris, J.C.; Benzinger, T.L.S.; Xiong, C.; et al. High-precision plasma β-amyloid 42/40 predicts current and future brain amyloidosis. *Neurology* **2019**, *93*, e1647–e1659. [CrossRef]
177. Verberk, I.M.W.; Slot, R.E.; Verfaillie, S.C.J.; Heijst, H.; Prins, N.D.; van Berckel, B.N.M.; Scheltens, P.; Teunissen, C.E.; van der Flier, W.M. Plasma amyloid as prescreener for the earliest alzheimer pathological changes. *Ann. Neurol.* **2018**, *84*, 648–658. [CrossRef]
178. Kaneko, N.; Nakamura, A.; Washimi, Y.; Kato, T.; Sakurai, T.; Arahata, Y.; Bundo, M.; Takeda, A.; Niida, S.; Ito, K.; et al. Novel plasma biomarker surrogating cerebral amyloid deposition. *Proc. Jpn. Acad. Ser. B Phys. Biol. Sci.* **2014**, *90*, 353–364. [CrossRef]
179. Ovod, V.; Ramsey, K.N.; Mawuenyega, K.G.; Bollinger, J.G.; Hicks, T.; Schneider, T.; Sullivan, M.; Paumier, K.; Holtzman, D.M.; Morris, J.C.; et al. Amyloid β concentrations and stable isotope labeling kinetics of human plasma specific to central nervous system amyloidosis. *Alzheimer's Dement.* **2017**, *13*, 841–849. [CrossRef]
180. Pannee, J.; Törnqvist, U.; Westerlund, A.; Ingelsson, M.; Lannfelt, L.; Brinkmalm, G.; Persson, R.; Gobom, J.; Svensson, J.; Johansson, P.; et al. The amyloid-β degradation pattern in plasma–a possible tool for clinical trials in alzheimer's disease. *Neurosci. Lett.* **2014**, *573*, 7–12. [CrossRef]
181. Li, Q.X.; Berndt, M.C.; Bush, A.I.; Rumble, B.; Mackenzie, I.; Friedhuber, A.; Beyreuther, K.; Masters, C.L. Membrane-associated forms of the beta a4 amyloid protein precursor of alzheimer's disease in human platelet and brain: Surface expression on the activated human platelet. *Blood* **1994**, *84*, 133–142. [CrossRef] [PubMed]
182. Palmqvist, S.; Insel, P.S.; Stomrud, E.; Janelidze, S.; Zetterberg, H.; Brix, B.; Eichenlaub, U.; Dage, J.L.; Chai, X.; Blennow, K.; et al. Cerebrospinal fluid and plasma biomarker trajectories with increasing amyloid deposition in alzheimer's disease. *EMBO Mol. Med.* **2019**, *11*, e11170. [CrossRef]
183. Augustinack, J.C.; Schneider, A.; Mandelkow, E.M.; Hyman, B.T. Specific tau phosphorylation sites correlate with severity of neuronal cytopathology in alzheimer's disease. *Acta Neuropathol.* **2002**, *103*, 26–35. [CrossRef] [PubMed]
184. Haroutunian, V.; Davies, P.; Vianna, C.; Buxbaum, J.D.; Purohit, D.P. Tau protein abnormalities associated with the progression of alzheimer disease type dementia. *Neurobiol. Aging* **2007**, *28*, 1–7. [CrossRef] [PubMed]
185. Zetterberg, H.; Bendlin, B.B. Biomarkers for alzheimer's disease-preparing for a new era of disease-modifying therapies. *Mol. Psychiatry* **2020**, 1–13. [CrossRef] [PubMed]
186. Fossati, S.; Ramos Cejudo, J.; Debure, L.; Pirraglia, E.; Sone, J.Y.; Li, Y.; Chen, J.; Butler, T.; Zetterberg, H.; Blennow, K.; et al. Plasma tau complements csf tau and p-tau in the diagnosis of alzheimer's disease. *Alzheimer's Dement.* **2019**, *11*, 483–492. [CrossRef] [PubMed]
187. Vandermeeren, M.; Mercken, M.; Vanmechelen, E.; Six, J.; van de Voorde, A.; Martin, J.J.; Cras, P. Detection of tau proteins in normal and alzheimer's disease cerebrospinal fluid with a sensitive sandwich enzyme-linked immunosorbent assay. *J. Neurochem.* **1993**, *61*, 1828–1834. [CrossRef]
188. Kandimalla, R.J.; Prabhakar, S.; Bk, B.; Wani, W.Y.; Sharma, D.R.; Grover, V.K.; Bhardwaj, N.; Jain, K.; Gill, K.D. Cerebrospinal fluid profile of amyloid β42 (aβ42), htau and ubiquitin in north indian alzheimer's disease patients. *Neurosci. Lett.* **2011**, *487*, 134–138. [CrossRef]
189. Kandimalla, R.J.; Prabhakar, S.; Binukumar, B.K.; Wani, W.Y.; Gupta, N.; Sharma, D.R.; Sunkaria, A.; Grover, V.K.; Bhardwaj, N.; Jain, K.; et al. Apo-eε4 allele in conjunction with aβ42 and tau in csf: Biomarker for alzheimer's disease. *Curr. Alzheimer Res.* **2011**, *8*, 187–196. [CrossRef]
190. Tapiola, T.; Alafuzoff, I.; Herukka, S.K.; Parkkinen, L.; Hartikainen, P.; Soininen, H.; Pirttilä, T. Cerebrospinal fluid {beta}-amyloid 42 and tau proteins as biomarkers of alzheimer-type pathologic changes in the brain. *Arch Neurol.* **2009**, *66*, 382–389. [CrossRef]
191. Haense, C.; Buerger, K.; Kalbe, E.; Drzezga, A.; Teipel, S.J.; Markiewicz, P.; Herholz, K.; Heiss, W.D.; Hampel, H. Csf total and phosphorylated tau protein, regional glucose metabolism and dementia severity in alzheimer's disease. *Eur. J. Neurol.* **2008**, *15*, 1155–1162. [CrossRef] [PubMed]
192. Hampel, H.; Goernitz, A.; Buerger, K. Advances in the development of biomarkers for alzheimer's disease: From csf total tau and abeta(1-42) proteins to phosphorylated tau protein. *Brain Res. Bull.* **2003**, *61*, 243–253. [CrossRef]

193. Gordon, B.A.; Blazey, T.M.; Christensen, J.; Dincer, A.; Flores, S.; Keefe, S.; Chen, C.; Su, Y.; McDade, E.M.; Wang, G.; et al. Tau pet in autosomal dominant alzheimer's disease: Relationship with cognition, dementia and other biomarkers. *Brain* **2019**, *142*, 1063–1076. [CrossRef]
194. Quiroz, Y.T.; Sperling, R.A.; Norton, D.J.; Baena, A.; Arboleda-Velasquez, J.F.; Cosio, D.; Schultz, A.; Lapoint, M.; Guzman-Velez, E.; Miller, J.B.; et al. Association between amyloid and tau accumulation in young adults with autosomal dominant alzheimer disease. *JAMA Neurol.* **2018**, *75*, 548–556. [CrossRef] [PubMed]
195. Fleisher, A.S.; Chen, K.; Quiroz, Y.T.; Jakimovich, L.J.; Gutierrez Gomez, M.; Langois, C.M.; Langbaum, J.B.; Roontiva, A.; Thiyyagura, P.; Lee, W.; et al. Associations between biomarkers and age in the presenilin 1 e280a autosomal dominant alzheimer disease kindred: A cross-sectional study. *JAMA Neurol.* **2015**, *72*, 316–324. [CrossRef] [PubMed]
196. Toledo, J.B.; Xie, S.X.; Trojanowski, J.Q.; Shaw, L.M. Longitudinal change in csf tau and aβ biomarkers for up to 48 months in adni. *Acta Neuropathol.* **2013**, *126*, 659–670. [CrossRef]
197. McDade, E.; Wang, G.; Gordon, B.A.; Hassenstab, J.; Benzinger, T.L.S.; Buckles, V.; Fagan, A.M.; Holtzman, D.M.; Cairns, N.J.; Goate, A.M.; et al. Longitudinal cognitive and biomarker changes in dominantly inherited alzheimer disease. *Neurology* **2018**, *91*, e1295–e1306. [CrossRef]
198. Fitzpatrick, A.W.P.; Falcon, B.; He, S.; Murzin, A.G.; Murshudov, G.; Garringer, H.J.; Crowther, R.A.; Ghetti, B.; Goedert, M.; Scheres, S.H.W. Cryo-em structures of tau filaments from alzheimer's disease. *Nature* **2017**, *547*, 185–190. [CrossRef]
199. Falcon, B.; Zhang, W.; Schweighauser, M.; Murzin, A.G.; Vidal, R.; Garringer, H.J.; Ghetti, B.; Scheres, S.H.W.; Goedert, M. Tau filaments from multiple cases of sporadic and inherited alzheimer's disease adopt a common fold. *Acta Neuropathol.* **2018**, *136*, 699–708. [CrossRef]
200. Zhang, W.; Falcon, B.; Murzin, A.G.; Fan, J.; Crowther, R.A.; Goedert, M.; Scheres, S.H. Heparin-induced tau filaments are polymorphic and differ from those in alzheimer's and pick's diseases. *Elife* **2019**, *8*, e43584. [CrossRef]
201. Arakhamia, T.; Lee, C.E.; Carlomagno, Y.; Duong, D.M.; Kundinger, S.R.; Wang, K.; Williams, D.; DeTure, M.; Dickson, D.W.; Cook, C.N.; et al. Posttranslational modifications mediate the structural diversity of tauopathy strains. *Cell* **2020**, *180*, 633–644. [CrossRef] [PubMed]
202. Jicha, G.A.; Bowser, R.; Kazam, I.G.; Davies, P. Alz-50 and mc-1, a new monoclonal antibody raised to paired helical filaments, recognize conformational epitopes on recombinant tau. *J. Neurosci. Res.* **1997**, *48*, 128–132. [CrossRef]
203. Jicha, G.A.; Lane, E.; Vincent, I.; Otvos, L.; Hoffmann, R.; Davies, P. A conformation- and phosphorylation-dependent antibody recognizing the paired helical filaments of alzheimer's disease. *J. Neurochem.* **1997**, *69*, 2087–2095. [CrossRef] [PubMed]
204. Weaver, C.L.; Espinoza, M.; Kress, Y.; Davies, P. Conformational change as one of the earliest alterations of tau in alzheimer's disease. *Neurobiol. Aging* **2000**, *21*, 719–727. [CrossRef]
205. Cicognola, C.; Brinkmalm, G.; Wahlgren, J.; Portelius, E.; Gobom, J.; Cullen, N.C.; Hansson, O.; Parnetti, L.; Constantinescu, R.; Wildsmith, K.; et al. Novel tau fragments in cerebrospinal fluid: Relation to tangle pathology and cognitive decline in alzheimer's disease. *Acta Neuropathol.* **2019**, *137*, 279–296. [CrossRef]
206. Amadoro, G.; Corsetti, V.; Sancesario, G.M.; Lubrano, A.; Melchiorri, G.; Bernardini, S.; Calissano, P.; Sancesario, G. Cerebrospinal fluid levels of a 20-22 kda nh2 fragment of human tau provide a novel neuronal injury biomarker in alzheimer's disease and other dementias. *J. Alzheimer's Dis.* **2014**, *42*, 211–226. [CrossRef]
207. Blennow, K.; Chen, C.; Cicognola, C.; Wildsmith, K.R.; Manser, P.T.; Bohorquez, S.M.S.; Zhang, Z.; Xie, B.; Peng, J.; Hansson, O.; et al. Cerebrospinal fluid tau fragment correlates with tau pet: A candidate biomarker for tangle pathology. *Brain* **2020**, *143*, 650–660. [CrossRef]
208. Quinn, J.P.; Corbett, N.J.; Kellett, K.A.B.; Hooper, N.M. Tau proteolysis in the pathogenesis of tauopathies: Neurotoxic fragments and novel biomarkers. *J. Alzheimer's Dis.* **2018**, *63*, 13–33. [CrossRef]
209. Maia, L.F.; Kaeser, S.A.; Reichwald, J.; Hruscha, M.; Martus, P.; Staufenbiel, M.; Jucker, M. Changes in amyloid-β and tau in the cerebrospinal fluid of transgenic mice overexpressing amyloid precursor protein. *Sci. Transl. Med.* **2013**, *5*, 194re192. [CrossRef]
210. Sato, C.; Barthélemy, N.R.; Mawuenyega, K.G.; Patterson, B.W.; Gordon, B.A.; Jockel-Balsarotti, J.; Sullivan, M.; Crisp, M.J.; Kasten, T.; Kirmess, K.M.; et al. Tau kinetics in neurons and the human central nervous system. *Neuron* **2018**, *97*, 1284–1298. [CrossRef]

211. Buerger, K.; Ewers, M.; Pirttilä, T.; Zinkowski, R.; Alafuzoff, I.; Teipel, S.J.; DeBernardis, J.; Kerkman, D.; McCulloch, C.; Soininen, H.; et al. Csf phosphorylated tau protein correlates with neocortical neurofibrillary pathology in alzheimer's disease. *Brain* **2006**, *129*, 3035–3041. [CrossRef] [PubMed]
212. Molinuevo, J.L.; Ayton, S.; Batrla, R.; Bednar, M.M.; Bittner, T.; Cummings, J.; Fagan, A.M.; Hampel, H.; Mielke, M.M.; Mikulskis, A.; et al. Current state of alzheimer's fluid biomarkers. *Acta Neuropathol.* **2018**, *136*, 821–853. [CrossRef] [PubMed]
213. Blennow, K.; Hampel, H.; Weiner, M.; Zetterberg, H. Cerebrospinal fluid and plasma biomarkers in alzheimer disease. *Nat. Rev. Neurol.* **2010**, *6*, 131–144. [CrossRef] [PubMed]
214. Lleó, A.; Irwin, D.J.; Illán-Gala, I.; McMillan, C.T.; Wolk, D.A.; Lee, E.B.; Van Deerlin, V.M.; Shaw, L.M.; Trojanowski, J.Q.; Grossman, M. A 2-step cerebrospinal algorithm for the selection of frontotemporal lobar degeneration subtypes. *JAMA Neurol.* **2018**, *75*, 738–745. [CrossRef]
215. Schoonenboom, N.S.; Reesink, F.E.; Verwey, N.A.; Kester, M.I.; Teunissen, C.E.; van de Ven, P.M.; Pijnenburg, Y.A.; Blankenstein, M.A.; Rozemuller, A.J.; Scheltens, P.; et al. Cerebrospinal fluid markers for differential dementia diagnosis in a large memory clinic cohort. *Neurology* **2012**, *78*, 47–54. [CrossRef]
216. Buchhave, P.; Minthon, L.; Zetterberg, H.; Wallin, A.K.; Blennow, K.; Hansson, O. Cerebrospinal fluid levels of β-amyloid 1-42, but not of tau, are fully changed already 5 to 10 years before the onset of alzheimer dementia. *Arch. Gen. Psychiatry* **2012**, *69*, 98–106. [CrossRef]
217. Vos, S.J.; Xiong, C.; Visser, P.J.; Jasielec, M.S.; Hassenstab, J.; Grant, E.A.; Cairns, N.J.; Morris, J.C.; Holtzman, D.M.; Fagan, A.M. Preclinical alzheimer's disease and its outcome: A longitudinal cohort study. *Lancet Neurol.* **2013**, *12*, 957–965. [CrossRef]
218. Hansson, O.; Mikulskis, A.; Fagan, A.M.; Teunissen, C.; Zetterberg, H.; Vanderstichele, H.; Molinuevo, J.L.; Shaw, L.M.; Vandijck, M.; Verbeek, M.M.; et al. The impact of preanalytical variables on measuring cerebrospinal fluid biomarkers for alzheimer's disease diagnosis: A review. *Alzheimer's Dement.* **2018**, *14*, 1313–1333. [CrossRef]
219. Shaw, L.M.; Arias, J.; Blennow, K.; Galasko, D.; Molinuevo, J.L.; Salloway, S.; Schindler, S.; Carrillo, M.C.; Hendrix, J.A.; Ross, A.; et al. Appropriate use criteria for lumbar puncture and cerebrospinal fluid testing in the diagnosis of alzheimer's disease. *Alzheimer's Dement.* **2018**, *14*, 1505–1521. [CrossRef]
220. Janelidze, S.; Stomrud, E.; Smith, R.; Palmqvist, S.; Mattsson, N.; Airey, D.C.; Proctor, N.K.; Chai, X.; Shcherbinin, S.; Sims, J.R.; et al. Cerebrospinal fluid p-tau217 performs better than p-tau181 as a biomarker of alzheimer's disease. *Nat. Commun.* **2020**, *11*, 1683. [CrossRef]
221. Hampel, H.; Buerger, K.; Zinkowski, R.; Teipel, S.J.; Goernitz, A.; Andreasen, N.; Sjoegren, M.; DeBernardis, J.; Kerkman, D.; Ishiguro, K.; et al. Measurement of phosphorylated tau epitopes in the differential diagnosis of alzheimer disease: A comparative cerebrospinal fluid study. *Arch. Gen. Psychiatry* **2004**, *61*, 95–102. [CrossRef]
222. Spiegel, J.; Pirraglia, E.; Osorio, R.S.; Glodzik, L.; Li, Y.; Tsui, W.; Saint Louis, L.A.; Randall, C.; Butler, T.; Xu, J.; et al. Greater specificity for cerebrospinal fluid p-tau231 over p-tau181 in the differentiation of healthy controls from alzheimer's disease. *J. Alzheimer's Dis.* **2016**, *49*, 93–100. [CrossRef]
223. Buerger, K.; Alafuzoff, I.; Ewers, M.; Pirttilä, T.; Zinkowski, R.; Hampel, H. No correlation between csf tau protein phosphorylated at threonine 181 with neocortical neurofibrillary pathology in alzheimer's disease. *Brain* **2007**, *130*, e82. [CrossRef] [PubMed]
224. Braak, H.; Braak, E. On areas of transition between entorhinal allocortex and temporal isocortex in the human brain. Normal morphology and lamina-specific pathology in alzheimer's disease. *Acta Neuropathol.* **1985**, *68*, 325–332. [CrossRef] [PubMed]
225. Barthélemy, N.R.; Bateman, R.J.; Hirtz, C.; Marin, P.; Becher, F.; Sato, C.; Gabelle, A.; Lehmann, S. Cerebrospinal fluid phospho-tau t217 outperforms t181 as a biomarker for the differential diagnosis of alzheimer's disease and pet amyloid-positive patient identification. *Alzheimer's Res. Ther.* **2020**, *12*, 26. [CrossRef] [PubMed]
226. Barthélemy, N.R.; Li, Y.; Joseph-Mathurin, N.; Gordon, B.A.; Hassenstab, J.; Benzinger, T.L.S.; Buckles, V.; Fagan, A.M.; Perrin, R.J.; Goate, A.M.; et al. A soluble phosphorylated tau signature links tau, amyloid and the evolution of stages of dominantly inherited alzheimer's disease. *Nat. Med.* **2020**, *26*, 398–407. [CrossRef]
227. Chen, Z.; Mengel, D.; Keshavan, A.; Rissman, R.A.; Billinton, A.; Perkinton, M.; Percival-Alwyn, J.; Schultz, A.; Properzi, M.; Johnson, K.; et al. Learnings about the complexity of extracellular tau aid development of a blood-based screen for alzheimer's disease. *Alzheimer's Dement.* **2019**, *15*, 487–496. [CrossRef] [PubMed]

228. Ramos-Cejudo, J.; Wisniewski, T.; Marmar, C.; Zetterberg, H.; Blennow, K.; de Leon, M.J.; Fossati, S. Traumatic brain injury and alzheimer's disease: The cerebrovascular link. *EBioMedicine* **2018**, *28*, 21–30. [CrossRef] [PubMed]
229. Mendez, M.F. What is the relationship of traumatic brain injury to dementia? *J. Alzheimer's Dis.* **2017**, *57*, 667–681. [CrossRef]
230. Blennow, K.; Brody, D.L.; Kochanek, P.M.; Levin, H.; McKee, A.; Ribbers, G.M.; Yaffe, K.; Zetterberg, H. Traumatic brain injuries. *Nat. Rev. Dis. Primers* **2016**, *2*, 16084. [CrossRef]
231. Clinton, J.; Ambler, M.W.; Roberts, G.W. Post-traumatic alzheimer's disease: Preponderance of a single plaque type. *Neuropathol. Appl. Neurobiol.* **1991**, *17*, 69–74. [CrossRef] [PubMed]
232. Mortimer, J.A.; van Duijn, C.M.; Chandra, V.; Fratiglioni, L.; Graves, A.B.; Heyman, A.; Jorm, A.F.; Kokmen, E.; Kondo, K.; Rocca, W.A. Head trauma as a risk factor for alzheimer's disease: A collaborative re-analysis of case-control studies. Eurodem risk factors research group. *Int. J. Epidemiol.* **1991**, *20* (Suppl. 2), S28–S35. [CrossRef]
233. Shahim, P.; Blennow, K.; Zetterberg, H. Tau, s-100 calcium-binding protein b, and neuron-specific enolase as biomarkers of concussion-reply. *JAMA Neurol.* **2014**, *71*, 926–927. [CrossRef] [PubMed]
234. Shahim, P.; Tegner, Y.; Wilson, D.H.; Randall, J.; Skillback, T.; Pazooki, D.; Kallberg, B.; Blennow, K.; Zetterberg, H. Blood biomarkers for brain injury in concussed professional ice hockey players. *JAMA Neurol.* **2014**, *71*, 684–692. [CrossRef] [PubMed]
235. Rubenstein, R.; Chang, B.; Davies, P.; Wagner, A.K.; Robertson, C.S.; Wang, K.K. A novel, ultrasensitive assay for tau: Potential for assessing traumatic brain injury in tissues and biofluids. *J. Neurotrauma* **2015**, *32*, 342–352. [CrossRef]
236. Hu, W.T.; Watts, K.; Grossman, M.; Glass, J.; Lah, J.J.; Hales, C.; Shelnutt, M.; Van Deerlin, V.; Trojanowski, J.Q.; Levey, A.I. Reduced csf p-tau181 to tau ratio is a biomarker for ftld-tdp. *Neurology* **2013**, *81*, 1945–1952. [CrossRef]
237. Vanmechelen, E.; Vanderstichele, H.; Davidsson, P.; Van Kerschaver, E.; Van Der Perre, B.; Sjögren, M.; Andreasen, N.; Blennow, K. Quantification of tau phosphorylated at threonine 181 in human cerebrospinal fluid: A sandwich elisa with a synthetic phosphopeptide for standardization. *Neurosci. Lett.* **2000**, *285*, 49–52. [CrossRef]
238. Wagshal, D.; Sankaranarayanan, S.; Guss, V.; Hall, T.; Berisha, F.; Lobach, I.; Karydas, A.; Voltarelli, L.; Scherling, C.; Heuer, H.; et al. Divergent csf τ alterations in two common tauopathies: Alzheimer's disease and progressive supranuclear palsy. *J. Neurol. Neurosurg. Psychiatry* **2015**, *86*, 244–250. [CrossRef]
239. O'Brien, J.T.; Herholz, K. Amyloid imaging for dementia in clinical practice. *BMC Med.* **2015**, *13*, 163. [CrossRef]
240. Henriksen, K.; O'Bryant, S.E.; Hampel, H.; Trojanowski, J.Q.; Montine, T.J.; Jeromin, A.; Blennow, K.; Lonneborg, A.; Wyss-Coray, T.; Soares, H.; et al. The future of blood-based biomarkers for alzheimer's disease. *Alzheimer's Dement. J. Assoc.* **2014**, *10*, 115–131. [CrossRef]
241. de Almeida, S.M.; Shumaker, S.D.; LeBlanc, S.K.; Delaney, P.; Marquie-Beck, J.; Ueland, S.; Alexander, T.; Ellis, R.J. Incidence of post-dural puncture headache in research volunteers. *Headache* **2011**, *51*, 1503–1510. [CrossRef] [PubMed]
242. Mukaetova-Ladinska, E.B.; Abdell-All, Z.; Andrade, J.; da Silva, J.A.; Boksha, I.; Burbaeva, G.; Kalaria, R.N.; TO'Brien, J. Platelet tau protein as a potential peripheral biomarker in alzheimer's disease: An explorative study. *Curr. Alzheimer Res.* **2018**, *15*, 800–808. [CrossRef] [PubMed]
243. Slachevsky, A.; Guzmán-Martínez, L.; Delgado, C.; Reyes, P.; Farías, G.A.; Muñoz-Neira, C.; Bravo, E.; Farías, M.; Flores, P.; Garrido, C.; et al. Tau platelets correlate with regional brain atrophy in patients with alzheimer's disease. *J. Alzheimer's Dis.* **2017**, *55*, 1595–1603. [CrossRef] [PubMed]
244. Tzen, K.Y.; Yang, S.Y.; Chen, T.F.; Cheng, T.W.; Horng, H.E.; Wen, H.P.; Huang, Y.Y.; Shiue, C.Y.; Chiu, M.J. Plasma aβ but not tau is related to brain pib retention in early alzheimer's disease. *ACS Chem. Neurosci.* **2014**, *5*, 830–836. [CrossRef]
245. Zetterberg, H.; Blennow, K. Blood biomarkers: Democratizing alzheimer's diagnostics. *Neuron* **2020**, *106*, 881–883. [CrossRef]
246. Mattsson, N.; Zetterberg, H.; Janelidze, S.; Insel, P.S.; Andreasson, U.; Stomrud, E.; Palmqvist, S.; Baker, D.; Tan Hehir, C.A.; Jeromin, A.; et al. Plasma tau in alzheimer disease. *Neurology* **2016**, *87*, 1827–1835. [CrossRef]

247. Mielke, M.M.; Hagen, C.E.; Wennberg, A.M.V.; Airey, D.C.; Savica, R.; Knopman, D.S.; Machulda, M.M.; Roberts, R.O.; Jack, C.R.; Petersen, R.C.; et al. Association of plasma total tau level with cognitive decline and risk of mild cognitive impairment or dementia in the mayo clinic study on aging. *JAMA Neurol.* **2017**, *74*, 1073–1080. [CrossRef]
248. Dage, J.L.; Wennberg, A.M.V.; Airey, D.C.; Hagen, C.E.; Knopman, D.S.; Machulda, M.M.; Roberts, R.O.; Jack, C.R.; Petersen, R.C.; Mielke, M.M. Levels of tau protein in plasma are associated with neurodegeneration and cognitive function in a population-based elderly cohort. *Alzheimer's Dement.* **2016**, *12*, 1226–1234. [CrossRef]
249. Pereira, J.B.; Westman, E.; Hansson, O.; Initiative, A.s.D.N. Association between cerebrospinal fluid and plasma neurodegeneration biomarkers with brain atrophy in alzheimer's disease. *Neurobiol. Aging* **2017**, *58*, 14–29. [CrossRef]
250. Mielke, M.M.; Hagen, C.E.; Xu, J.; Chai, X.; Vemuri, P.; Lowe, V.J.; Airey, D.C.; Knopman, D.S.; Roberts, R.O.; Machulda, M.M.; et al. Plasma phospho-tau181 increases with alzheimer's disease clinical severity and is associated with tau- and amyloid-positron emission tomography. *Alzheimer's Dement.* **2018**, *14*, 989–997. [CrossRef]
251. Tatebe, H.; Kasai, T.; Ohmichi, T.; Kishi, Y.; Kakeya, T.; Waragai, M.; Kondo, M.; Allsop, D.; Tokuda, T. Quantification of plasma phosphorylated tau to use as a biomarker for brain alzheimer pathology: Pilot case-control studies including patients with alzheimer's disease and down syndrome. *Mol. Neurodegener.* **2017**, *12*, 63. [CrossRef] [PubMed]
252. Yang, C.C.; Chiu, M.J.; Chen, T.F.; Chang, H.L.; Liu, B.H.; Yang, S.Y. Assay of plasma phosphorylated tau protein (threonine 181) and total tau protein in early-stage alzheimer's disease. *J. Alzheimer's Dis.* **2018**, *61*, 1323–1332. [CrossRef] [PubMed]
253. Karikari, T.K.; Pascoal, T.A.; Ashton, N.J.; Janelidze, S.; Benedet, A.L.; Rodriguez, J.L.; Chamoun, M.; Savard, M.; Kang, M.S.; Therriault, J.; et al. Blood phosphorylated tau 181 as a biomarker for alzheimer's disease: A diagnostic performance and prediction modelling study using data from four prospective cohorts. *Lancet Neurol.* **2020**, *19*, 422–433. [CrossRef]
254. Thijssen, E.H.; La Joie, R.; Wolf, A.; Strom, A.; Wang, P.; Iaccarino, L.; Bourakova, V.; Cobigo, Y.; Heuer, H.; Spina, S.; et al. Diagnostic value of plasma phosphorylated tau181 in alzheimer's disease and frontotemporal lobar degeneration. *Nat. Med.* **2020**, *26*, 387–397. [CrossRef] [PubMed]
255. Janelidze, S.; Mattsson, N.; Palmqvist, S.; Smith, R.; Beach, T.G.; Serrano, G.E.; Chai, X.; Proctor, N.K.; Eichenlaub, U.; Zetterberg, H.; et al. Plasma p-tau181 in alzheimer's disease: Relationship to other biomarkers, differential diagnosis, neuropathology and longitudinal progression to Alzheimer's Dementia. *Nat. Med.* **2020**, *26*, 379–386. [CrossRef] [PubMed]
256. Barthélemy, N.R.; Horie, K.; Sato, C.; Bateman, R.J. Blood plasma phosphorylated-tau isoforms track cns change in alzheimer's disease. *J. Exp. Med.* **2020**, *217*, e20200861. [CrossRef]
257. Lifke, V.; Kollmorgen, G.; Manuilova, E.; Oelschlaegel, T.; Hillringhaus, L.; Widmann, M.; von Arnim, C.A.F.; Otto, M.; Christenson, R.H.; Powers, J.L.; et al. Elecsys. *Clin. Biochem.* **2019**, *72*, 30–38. [CrossRef]
258. Chiasserini, D.; Biscetti, L.; Farotti, L.; Eusebi, P.; Salvadori, N.; Lisetti, V.; Baschieri, F.; Chipi, E.; Frattini, G.; Stoops, E.; et al. Performance evaluation of an automated elisa system for alzheimer's disease detection in clinical routine. *J. Alzheimer's Dis.* **2016**, *54*, 55–67. [CrossRef]
259. Rissin, D.M.; Fournier, D.R.; Piech, T.; Kan, C.W.; Campbell, T.G.; Song, L.; Chang, L.; Rivnak, A.J.; Patel, P.P.; Provuncher, G.K.; et al. Simultaneous detection of single molecules and singulated ensembles of molecules enables immunoassays with broad dynamic range. *Anal Chem.* **2011**, *83*, 2279–2285. [CrossRef]
260. Barthélemy, N.R.; Fenaille, F.; Hirtz, C.; Sergeant, N.; Schraen-Maschke, S.; Vialaret, J.; Buée, L.; Gabelle, A.; Junot, C.; Lehmann, S.; et al. Tau protein quantification in human cerebrospinal fluid by targeted mass spectrometry at high sequence coverage provides insights into its primary structure heterogeneity. *J. Proteome Res.* **2016**, *15*, 667–676. [CrossRef]
261. Barthélemy, N.R.; Mallipeddi, N.; Moiseyev, P.; Sato, C.; Bateman, R.J. Tau phosphorylation rates measured by mass spectrometry differ in the intracellular brain vs. Extracellular cerebrospinal fluid compartments and are differentially affected by alzheimer's disease. *Front. Aging Neurosci.* **2019**, *11*, 121. [CrossRef] [PubMed]
262. Khalil, M.; Teunissen, C.E.; Otto, M.; Piehl, F.; Sormani, M.P.; Gattringer, T.; Barro, C.; Kappos, L.; Comabella, M.; Fazekas, F.; et al. Neurofilaments as biomarkers in neurological disorders. *Nat. Rev. Neurol.* **2018**, *14*, 577–589. [CrossRef] [PubMed]

263. Gaetani, L.; Blennow, K.; Calabresi, P.; Di Filippo, M.; Parnetti, L.; Zetterberg, H. Neurofilament light chain as a biomarker in neurological disorders. *J. Neurol. Neurosurg. Psychiatry* **2019**, *90*, 870–881. [CrossRef] [PubMed]
264. Bridel, C.; van Wieringen, W.N.; Zetterberg, H.; Tijms, B.M.; Teunissen, C.E.; Alvarez-Cermeño, J.C.; Andreasson, U.; Axelsson, M.; Bäckström, D.C.; Bartos, A.; et al. Diagnostic value of cerebrospinal fluid neurofilament light protein in neurology: A systematic review and meta-analysis. *JAMA Neurol.* **2019**, *76*, 1035–1048. [CrossRef] [PubMed]
265. Weston, P.S.J.; Poole, T.; O'Connor, A.; Heslegrave, A.; Ryan, N.S.; Liang, Y.; Druyeh, R.; Mead, S.; Blennow, K.; Schott, J.M.; et al. Longitudinal measurement of serum neurofilament light in presymptomatic familial alzheimer's disease. *Alzheimer's Res. Ther.* **2019**, *11*, 19. [CrossRef] [PubMed]
266. Schultz, S.A.; Strain, J.F.; Adedokun, A.; Wang, Q.; Preische, O.; Kuhle, J.; Flores, S.; Keefe, S.; Dincer, A.; Ances, B.M.; et al. Serum neurofilament light chain levels are associated with white matter integrity in autosomal dominant alzheimer's disease. *Neurobiol. Dis.* **2020**, *142*, 104960. [CrossRef]
267. Kuhle, J.; Barro, C.; Andreasson, U.; Derfuss, T.; Lindberg, R.; Sandelius, Å.; Liman, V.; Norgren, N.; Blennow, K.; Zetterberg, H. Comparison of three analytical platforms for quantification of the neurofilament light chain in blood samples: Elisa, electrochemiluminescence immunoassay and simoa. *Clin. Chem. Lab Med.* **2016**, *54*, 1655–1661. [CrossRef]
268. Kvartsberg, H.; Duits, F.H.; Ingelsson, M.; Andreasen, N.; Öhrfelt, A.; Andersson, K.; Brinkmalm, G.; Lannfelt, L.; Minthon, L.; Hansson, O.; et al. Cerebrospinal fluid levels of the synaptic protein neurogranin correlates with cognitive decline in prodromal alzheimer's disease. *Alzheimer's Dement.* **2015**, *11*, 1180–1190. [CrossRef]
269. De Vos, A.; Jacobs, D.; Struyfs, H.; Fransen, E.; Andersson, K.; Portelius, E.; Andreasson, U.; De Surgeloose, D.; Hernalsteen, D.; Sleegers, K.; et al. C-terminal neurogranin is increased in cerebrospinal fluid but unchanged in plasma in alzheimer's disease. *Alzheimer's Dement.* **2015**, *11*, 1461–1469. [CrossRef]
270. Ashton, N.J.; Nevado-Holgado, A.J.; Barber, I.S.; Lynham, S.; Gupta, V.; Chatterjee, P.; Goozee, K.; Hone, E.; Pedrini, S.; Blennow, K.; et al. A plasma protein classifier for predicting amyloid burden for preclinical alzheimer's disease. *Sci. Adv.* **2019**, *5*, eaau7220. [CrossRef]
271. Bouchon, A.; Dietrich, J.; Colonna, M. Cutting edge: Inflammatory responses can be triggered by trem-1, a novel receptor expressed on neutrophils and monocytes. *J. Immunol.* **2000**, *164*, 4991–4995. [CrossRef] [PubMed]
272. Ulland, T.K.; Song, W.M.; Huang, S.C.; Ulrich, J.D.; Sergushichev, A.; Beatty, W.L.; Loboda, A.A.; Zhou, Y.; Cairns, N.J.; Kambal, A.; et al. Trem2 maintains microglial metabolic fitness in alzheimer's disease. *Cell* **2017**, *170*, 649–663. [CrossRef] [PubMed]
273. Schlepckow, K.; Kleinberger, G.; Fukumori, A.; Feederle, R.; Lichtenthaler, S.F.; Steiner, H.; Haass, C. An alzheimer-associated trem2 variant occurs at the adam cleavage site and affects shedding and phagocytic function. *EMBO Mol. Med.* **2017**, *9*, 1356–1365. [CrossRef]
274. Yeh, F.L.; Wang, Y.; Tom, I.; Gonzalez, L.C.; Sheng, M. Trem2 binds to apolipoproteins, including apoe and clu/apoj, and thereby facilitates uptake of amyloid-beta by microglia. *Neuron* **2016**, *91*, 328–340. [CrossRef] [PubMed]
275. Filipello, F.; Morini, R.; Corradini, I.; Zerbi, V.; Canzi, A.; Michalski, B.; Erreni, M.; Markicevic, M.; Starvaggi-Cucuzza, C.; Otero, K.; et al. The microglial innate immune receptor trem2 is required for synapse elimination and normal brain connectivity. *Immunity* **2018**, *48*, 979–991. [CrossRef] [PubMed]
276. Kleinberger, G.; Yamanishi, Y.; Suárez-Calvet, M.; Czirr, E.; Lohmann, E.; Cuyvers, E.; Struyfs, H.; Pettkus, N.; Wenninger-Weinzierl, A.; Mazaheri, F.; et al. Trem2 mutations implicated in neurodegeneration impair cell surface transport and phagocytosis. *Sci. Transl. Med.* **2014**, *6*, 243ra286. [CrossRef]
277. Guerreiro, R.; Wojtas, A.; Bras, J.; Carrasquillo, M.; Rogaeva, E.; Majounie, E.; Cruchaga, C.; Sassi, C.; Kauwe, J.S.; Younkin, S.; et al. Trem2 variants in alzheimer's disease. *N. Engl. J. Med.* **2013**, *368*, 117–127. [CrossRef]
278. Yaghmoor, F.; Noorsaeed, A.; Alsaggaf, S.; Aljohani, W.; Scholtzova, H.; Boutajangout, A.; Wisniewski, T. The role of trem2 in alzheimer's disease and other neurological disorders. *J. Alzheimer's Dis. Parkinsonism* **2014**, *4*, 160. [CrossRef]

279. Jonsson, T.; Stefansson, H.; Steinberg, S.; Jonsdottir, I.; Jonsson, P.V.; Snaedal, J.; Bjornsson, S.; Huttenlocher, J.; Levey, A.I.; Lah, J.J.; et al. Variant of trem2 associated with the risk of alzheimer's disease. *N. Engl. J. Med.* **2013**, *368*, 107–116. [CrossRef]
280. Lill, C.M.; Rengmark, A.; Pihlstrøm, L.; Fogh, I.; Shatunov, A.; Sleiman, P.M.; Wang, L.S.; Liu, T.; Lassen, C.F.; Meissner, E.; et al. The role of trem2 r47h as a risk factor for alzheimer's disease, frontotemporal lobar degeneration, amyotrophic lateral sclerosis, and parkinson's disease. *Alzheimer's Dement.* **2015**, *11*, 1407–1416. [CrossRef]
281. Bekris, L.M.; Khrestian, M.; Dyne, E.; Shao, Y.; Pillai, J.A.; Rao, S.M.; Bemiller, S.M.; Lamb, B.; Fernandez, H.H.; Leverenz, J.B. Soluble trem2 and biomarkers of central and peripheral inflammation in neurodegenerative disease. *J. Neuroimmunol.* **2018**, *319*, 19–27. [CrossRef] [PubMed]
282. Ashton, N.J.; Suárez-Calvet, M.; Heslegrave, A.; Hye, A.; Razquin, C.; Pastor, P.; Sanchez-Valle, R.; Molinuevo, J.L.; Visser, P.J.; Blennow, K.; et al. Plasma levels of soluble trem2 and neurofilament light chain in trem2 rare variant carriers. *Alzheimer's Res. Ther.* **2019**, *11*, 94. [CrossRef] [PubMed]
283. Piccio, L.; Deming, Y.; Del-Águila, J.L.; Ghezzi, L.; Holtzman, D.M.; Fagan, A.M.; Fenoglio, C.; Galimberti, D.; Borroni, B.; Cruchaga, C. Cerebrospinal fluid soluble trem2 is higher in alzheimer disease and associated with mutation status. *Acta Neuropathol.* **2016**, *131*, 925–933. [CrossRef] [PubMed]
284. Suárez-Calvet, M.; Kleinberger, G.; Araque Caballero, M.; Brendel, M.; Rominger, A.; Alcolea, D.; Fortea, J.; Lleó, A.; Blesa, R.; Gispert, J.D.; et al. Strem2 cerebrospinal fluid levels are a potential biomarker for microglia activity in early-stage alzheimer's disease and associate with neuronal injury markers. *EMBO Mol. Med.* **2016**, *8*, 466–476. [CrossRef]
285. Hakala, B.E.; White, C.; Recklies, A.D. Human cartilage gp-39, a major secretory product of articular chondrocytes and synovial cells, is a mammalian member of a chitinase protein family. *J. Biol. Chem.* **1993**, *268*, 25803–25810.
286. Colton, C.A.; Mott, R.T.; Sharpe, H.; Xu, Q.; Van Nostrand, W.E.; Vitek, M.P. Expression profiles for macrophage alternative activation genes in ad and in mouse models of ad. *J. Neuroinflam.* **2006**, *3*, 27. [CrossRef]
287. Johansen, J.S. Studies on serum ykl-40 as a biomarker in diseases with inflammation, tissue remodelling, fibroses and cancer. *Dan Med. Bull.* **2006**, *53*, 172–209.
288. Johansen, J.S.; Schultz, N.A.; Jensen, B.V. Plasma ykl-40: A potential new cancer biomarker? *Future Oncol.* **2009**, *5*, 1065–1082. [CrossRef]
289. Craig-Schapiro, R.; Perrin, R.J.; Roe, C.M.; Xiong, C.; Carter, D.; Cairns, N.J.; Mintun, M.A.; Peskind, E.R.; Li, G.; Galasko, D.R.; et al. Ykl-40: A novel prognostic fluid biomarker for preclinical alzheimer's disease. *Biol. Psychiatry* **2010**, *68*, 903–912. [CrossRef]
290. Mattsson, N.; Tabatabaei, S.; Johansson, P.; Hansson, O.; Andreasson, U.; Månsson, J.E.; Johansson, J.O.; Olsson, B.; Wallin, A.; Svensson, J.; et al. Cerebrospinal fluid microglial markers in alzheimer's disease: Elevated chitotriosidase activity but lack of diagnostic utility. *Neuromol. Med.* **2011**, *13*, 151–159. [CrossRef]
291. Teunissen, C.E.; Elias, N.; Koel-Simmelink, M.J.; Durieux-Lu, S.; Malekzadeh, A.; Pham, T.V.; Piersma, S.R.; Beccari, T.; Meeter, L.H.; Dopper, E.G.; et al. Novel diagnostic cerebrospinal fluid biomarkers for pathologic subtypes of frontotemporal dementia identified by proteomics. *Alzheimer's Dement.* **2016**, *2*, 86–94. [CrossRef] [PubMed]
292. Choi, J.; Lee, H.W.; Suk, K. Plasma level of chitinase 3-like 1 protein increases in patients with early alzheimer's disease. *J. Neurol.* **2011**, *258*, 2181–2185. [CrossRef] [PubMed]
293. Shen, X.N.; Niu, L.D.; Wang, Y.J.; Cao, X.P.; Liu, Q.; Tan, L.; Zhang, C.; Yu, J.T. Inflammatory markers in alzheimer's disease and mild cognitive impairment: A meta-analysis and systematic review of 170 studies. *J. Neurol. Neurosurg. Psychiatry* **2019**, *90*, 590–598. [CrossRef] [PubMed]
294. Park, J.C.; Han, S.H.; Mook-Jung, I. Peripheral inflammatory biomarkers in alzheimer's disease: A brief review. *BMB Rep.* **2020**, *53*, 10–19. [CrossRef] [PubMed]
295. Zuena, A.R.; Casolini, P.; Lattanzi, R.; Maftei, D. Chemokines in alzheimer's disease: New insights into prokineticins, chemokine-like proteins. *Front. Pharmacol.* **2019**, *10*, 622. [CrossRef]
296. Colangelo, A.M.; Alberghina, L.; Papa, M. Astrogliosis as a therapeutic target for neurodegenerative diseases. *Neurosci. Lett.* **2014**, *565*, 59–64. [CrossRef]
297. Liddelow, S.; Barres, B. Snapshot: Astrocytes in health and disease. *Cell* **2015**, *162*, 1170. [CrossRef]

298. Liddelow, S.A.; Guttenplan, K.A.; Clarke, L.E.; Bennett, F.C.; Bohlen, C.J.; Schirmer, L.; Bennett, M.L.; Münch, A.E.; Chung, W.S.; Peterson, T.C.; et al. Neurotoxic reactive astrocytes are induced by activated microglia. *Nature* **2017**, *541*, 481–487. [CrossRef]
299. Liddelow, S.A. Modern approaches to investigating non-neuronal aspects of alzheimer's disease. *FASEB J.* **2019**, *33*, 1528–1535. [CrossRef]
300. Milà-Alomà, M.; Salvadó, G.; Gispert, J.D.; Vilor-Tejedor, N.; Grau-Rivera, O.; Sala-Vila, A.; Sánchez-Benavides, G.; Arenaza-Urquijo, E.M.; Crous-Bou, M.; González-de-Echávarri, J.M.; et al. Amyloid beta, tau, synaptic, neurodegeneration, and glial biomarkers in the preclinical stage of the alzheimer's continuum. *Alzheimer's Dement.* **2020**. [CrossRef]
301. Elahi, F.M.; Casaletto, K.B.; La Joie, R.; Walters, S.M.; Harvey, D.; Wolf, A.; Edwards, L.; Rivera-Contreras, W.; Karydas, A.; Cobigo, Y.; et al. Plasma biomarkers of astrocytic and neuronal dysfunction in early- and late-onset alzheimer's disease. *Alzheimer's Dement.* **2020**, *16*, 681–695. [CrossRef] [PubMed]
302. James, B.D.; Wilson, R.S.; Boyle, P.A.; Trojanowski, J.Q.; Bennett, D.A.; Schneider, J.A. Tdp-43 stage, mixed pathologies, and clinical alzheimer's-type dementia. *Brain* **2016**, *139*, 2983–2993. [CrossRef] [PubMed]
303. Majumder, V.; Gregory, J.M.; Barria, M.A.; Green, A.; Pal, S. Tdp-43 as a potential biomarker for amyotrophic lateral sclerosis: A systematic review and meta-analysis. *BMC Neurol.* **2018**, *18*, 90. [CrossRef] [PubMed]
304. Feneberg, E.; Gray, E.; Ansorge, O.; Talbot, K.; Turner, M.R. Towards a tdp-43-based biomarker for als and ftld. *Mol. Neurobiol.* **2018**, *55*, 7789–7801. [CrossRef] [PubMed]
305. Huang, W.; Zhou, Y.; Tu, L.; Ba, Z.; Huang, J.; Huang, N.; Luo, Y. Tdp-43: From alzheimer's disease to limbic-predominant age-related tdp-43 encephalopathy. *Front. Mol. Neurosci.* **2020**, *13*, 26. [CrossRef] [PubMed]
306. Meade, R.M.; Fairlie, D.P.; Mason, J.M. Alpha-synuclein structure and parkinson's disease—Lessons and emerging principles. *Mol. Neurodegener.* **2019**, *14*, 29. [CrossRef] [PubMed]
307. Paciotti, S.; Bellomo, G.; Gatticchi, L.; Parnetti, L. Are we ready for detecting α-synuclein prone to aggregation in patients? The case of "protein-misfolding cyclic amplification" and "real-time quaking-induced conversion" as diagnostic tools. *Front. Neurol.* **2018**, *9*, 415. [CrossRef]
308. Groveman, B.R.; Orrù, C.D.; Hughson, A.G.; Raymond, L.D.; Zanusso, G.; Ghetti, B.; Campbell, K.J.; Safar, J.; Galasko, D.; Caughey, B. Rapid and ultra-sensitive quantitation of disease-associated α-synuclein seeds in brain and cerebrospinal fluid by αsyn rt-quic. *Acta Neuropathol. Commun.* **2018**, *6*, 7. [CrossRef]
309. Schweighauser, M.; Shi, Y.; Tarutani, A.; Kametani, F.; Murzin, A.G.; Ghetti, B.; Matsubara, T.; Tomita, T.; Ando, T.; Hasegawa, K.; et al. Structures of α-synuclein filaments from multiple system atrophy. *Nature* **2020**, 1–6. [CrossRef]
310. Montagne, A.; Zhao, Z.; Zlokovic, B.V. Alzheimer's disease: A matter of blood-brain barrier dysfunction? *J. Exp. Med.* **2017**, *214*, 3151–3169. [CrossRef]
311. Bennett, R.E.; Robbins, A.B.; Hu, M.; Cao, X.; Betensky, R.A.; Clark, T.; Das, S.; Hyman, B.T. Tau induces blood vessel abnormalities and angiogenesis-related gene expression in p301l transgenic mice and human alzheimer's disease. *Proc. Natl. Acad. Sci. USA* **2018**, *115*, E1289–E1298. [CrossRef]
312. Snyder, H.M.; Corriveau, R.A.; Craft, S.; Faber, J.E.; Greenberg, S.M.; Knopman, D.; Lamb, B.T.; Montine, T.J.; Nedergaard, M.; Schaffer, C.B.; et al. Vascular contributions to cognitive impairment and dementia including alzheimer's disease. *Alzheimer's Dement.* **2015**, *11*, 710–717. [CrossRef] [PubMed]
313. Gottesman, R.F.; Schneider, A.L.; Zhou, Y.; Coresh, J.; Green, E.; Gupta, N.; Knopman, D.S.; Mintz, A.; Rahmim, A.; Sharrett, A.R.; et al. Association between midlife vascular risk factors and estimated brain amyloid deposition. *JAMA* **2017**, *317*, 1443–1450. [CrossRef] [PubMed]
314. Sweeney, M.D.; Sagare, A.P.; Zlokovic, B.V. Blood-brain barrier breakdown in alzheimer disease and other neurodegenerative disorders. *Nat. Rev. Neurol.* **2018**, *14*, 133–150. [CrossRef] [PubMed]
315. Montagne, A.; Barnes, S.R.; Sweeney, M.D.; Halliday, M.R.; Sagare, A.P.; Zhao, Z.; Toga, A.W.; Jacobs, R.E.; Liu, C.Y.; Amezcua, L.; et al. Blood-brain barrier breakdown in the aging human hippocampus. *Neuron* **2015**, *85*, 296–302. [CrossRef] [PubMed]
316. Verheggen, I.C.M.; de Jong, J.J.A.; van Boxtel, M.P.J.; Gronenschild, E.H.B.M.; Palm, W.M.; Postma, A.A.; Jansen, J.F.A.; Verhey, F.R.J.; Backes, W.H. Increase in blood-brain barrier leakage in healthy, older adults. *Geroscience* **2020**, *42*, 1183–1193. [CrossRef] [PubMed]

317. Nation, D.A.; Sweeney, M.D.; Montagne, A.; Sagare, A.P.; D'Orazio, L.M.; Pachicano, M.; Sepehrband, F.; Nelson, A.R.; Buennagel, D.P.; Harrington, M.G.; et al. Blood-brain barrier breakdown is an early biomarker of human cognitive dysfunction. *Nat. Med.* **2019**, *25*, 270–276. [CrossRef]
318. Wang, H.; Golob, E.J.; Su, M.Y. Vascular volume and blood-brain barrier permeability measured by dynamic contrast enhanced mri in hippocampus and cerebellum of patients with mci and normal controls. *J. Magn. Reson. Imaging* **2006**, *24*, 695–700. [CrossRef]
319. Starr, J.M.; Farrall, A.J.; Armitage, P.; McGurn, B.; Wardlaw, J. Blood-brain barrier permeability in alzheimer's disease: A case-control mri study. *Psychiatry Res.* **2009**, *171*, 232–241. [CrossRef]
320. Sagare, A.P.; Sweeney, M.D.; Makshanoff, J.; Zlokovic, B.V. Shedding of soluble platelet-derived growth factor receptor-β from human brain pericytes. *Neurosci. Lett.* **2015**, *607*, 97–101. [CrossRef]
321. Olsson, A.; Vanderstichele, H.; Andreasen, N.; De Meyer, G.; Wallin, A.; Holmberg, B.; Rosengren, L.; Vanmechelen, E.; Blennow, K. Simultaneous measurement of beta-amyloid(1-42), total tau, and phosphorylated tau (thr181) in cerebrospinal fluid by the xmap technology. *Clin. Chem.* **2005**, *51*, 336–345. [CrossRef] [PubMed]
322. Tate, J.; Ward, G. Interferences in immunoassay. *Clin. Biochem. Rev.* **2004**, *25*, 105–120. [PubMed]
323. Spector, R.; Robert Snodgrass, S.; Johanson, C.E. A balanced view of the cerebrospinal fluid composition and functions: Focus on adult humans. *Exp. Neurol.* **2015**, *273*, 57–68. [CrossRef] [PubMed]
324. Maiolini, R.; Bagrel, A.; Chavance, C.; Krebs, B.; Herbeth, B.; Masseyeff, R. Study of an enzyme immunoassay kit for carcinoembryonic antigen. *Clin. Chem.* **1980**, *26*, 1718–1722. [CrossRef]
325. Pimm, M.V.; Perkins, A.C.; Armitage, N.C.; Baldwin, R.W. The characteristics of blood-borne radiolabels and the effect of anti-mouse igg antibodies on localization of radiolabeled monoclonal antibody in cancer patients. *J. Nucl. Med. Off. Publ. Soc. Nucl. Med.* **1985**, *26*, 1011–1023.
326. Primus, F.J.; Kelley, E.A.; Hansen, H.J.; Goldenberg, D.M. "Sandwich"-type immunoassay of carcinoembryonic antigen in patients receiving murine monoclonal antibodies for diagnosis and therapy. *Clin. Chem.* **1988**, *34*, 261–264. [CrossRef]
327. Thompson, R.J.; Jackson, A.P.; Langlois, N. Circulating antibodies to mouse monoclonal immunoglobulins in normal subjects–incidence, species specificity, and effects on a two-site assay for creatine kinase-mb isoenzyme. *Clin. Chem.* **1986**, *32*, 476–481. [CrossRef]
328. d'Abramo, C.; Acker, C.M.; Schachter, J.B.; Terracina, G.; Wang, X.; Forest, S.K.; Davies, P. Detecting tau in serum of transgenic animal models after tau immunotherapy treatment. *Neurobiol. Aging* **2016**, *37*, 58–65. [CrossRef]
329. Kricka, L.J. Human anti-animal antibody interferences in immunological assays. *Clin. Chem.* **1999**, *45*, 942–956. [CrossRef]
330. Selby, C. Interference in immunoassay. *Ann Clin Biochem* **1999**, *36 Pt 6*, 704–721. [CrossRef]
331. Wilkins, J.M.; Trushina, E. Application of metabolomics in alzheimer's disease. *Front. Neurol.* **2017**, *8*, 719. [CrossRef] [PubMed]
332. Trushina, E.; Mielke, M.M. Recent advances in the application of metabolomics to alzheimer's disease. *Biochim. Biophys. Acta* **2014**, *1842*, 1232–1239. [CrossRef] [PubMed]
333. Tambini, M.D.; Yao, W.; D'Adamio, L. Facilitation of glutamate, but not gaba, release in familial alzheimer's app mutant knock-in rats with increased β-cleavage of app. *Aging Cell* **2019**, *18*, e13033. [CrossRef]
334. Tambini, M.D.; D'Adamio, L. Knock-in rats with homozygous. *J. Biol. Chem.* **2020**, *295*, 7442–7451. [CrossRef] [PubMed]
335. Tambini, M.D.; Norris, K.A.; D'Adamio, L. Opposite changes in app processing and human aβ levels in rats carrying either a protective or a pathogenic app mutation. *Elife* **2020**, *9*, e52612. [CrossRef]
336. Saito, T.; Matsuba, Y.; Mihira, N.; Takano, J.; Nilsson, P.; Itohara, S.; Iwata, N.; Saido, T.C. Single app knock-in mouse models of alzheimer's disease. *Nat. Neurosci.* **2014**, *17*, 661–663. [CrossRef]
337. Saito, T.; Mihira, N.; Matsuba, Y.; Sasaguri, H.; Hashimoto, S.; Narasimhan, S.; Zhang, B.; Murayama, S.; Higuchi, M.; Lee, V.M.Y.; et al. Humanization of the entire murine. *J. Biol. Chem.* **2019**, *294*, 12754–12765. [CrossRef]
338. Tambini, M.D.; D'Adamio, L. Trem2 splicing and expression are preserved in a human aβ-producing, rat knock-in model of trem2-r47h alzheimer's risk variant. *Sci. Rep.* **2020**, *10*, 4122. [CrossRef]
339. Niedzwiecki, M.M.; Walker, D.I.; Howell, J.C.; Watts, K.D.; Jones, D.P.; Miller, G.W.; Hu, W.T. High-resolution metabolomic profiling of alzheimer's disease in plasma. *Ann. Clin. Transl. Neurol.* **2020**, *7*, 36–45. [CrossRef]

340. Ibáñez, C.; Simó, C.; Barupal, D.K.; Fiehn, O.; Kivipelto, M.; Cedazo-Mínguez, A.; Cifuentes, A. A new metabolomic workflow for early detection of alzheimer's disease. *J. Chromatogr. A* **2013**, *1302*, 65–71. [CrossRef]
341. Pomara, N.; Singh, R.; Deptula, D.; Chou, J.C.; Schwartz, M.B.; LeWitt, P.A. Glutamate and other csf amino acids in alzheimer's disease. *Am. J. Psychiatry* **1992**, *149*, 251–254. [PubMed]
342. Madeira, C.; Vargas-Lopes, C.; Brandão, C.O.; Reis, T.; Laks, J.; Panizzutti, R.; Ferreira, S.T. Elevated glutamate and glutamine levels in the cerebrospinal fluid of patients with probable alzheimer's disease and depression. *Front. Psychiatry* **2018**, *9*, 561. [CrossRef] [PubMed]
343. Orešič, M.; Hyötyläinen, T.; Herukka, S.K.; Sysi-Aho, M.; Mattila, I.; Seppänan-Laakso, T.; Julkunen, V.; Gopalacharyulu, P.V.; Hallikainen, M.; Koikkalainen, J.; et al. Metabolome in progression to alzheimer's disease. *Transl. Psychiatry* **2011**, *1*, e57. [CrossRef] [PubMed]
344. Trushina, E.; Dutta, T.; Persson, X.M.; Mielke, M.M.; Petersen, R.C. Identification of altered metabolic pathways in plasma and csf in mild cognitive impairment and alzheimer's disease using metabolomics. *PLoS ONE* **2013**, *8*, e63644. [CrossRef] [PubMed]
345. Kaddurah-Daouk, R.; Rozen, S.; Matson, W.; Han, X.; Hulette, C.M.; Burke, J.R.; Doraiswamy, P.M.; Welsh-Bohmer, K.A. Metabolomic changes in autopsy-confirmed alzheimer's disease. *Alzheimer's Dement.* **2011**, *7*, 309–317. [CrossRef] [PubMed]
346. Mapstone, M.; Cheema, A.K.; Fiandaca, M.S.; Zhong, X.; Mhyre, T.R.; MacArthur, L.H.; Hall, W.J.; Fisher, S.G.; Peterson, D.R.; Haley, J.M.; et al. Plasma phospholipids identify antecedent memory impairment in older adults. *Nat. Med.* **2014**, *20*, 415–418. [CrossRef]
347. Frölich, L.; Peters, O.; Lewczuk, P.; Gruber, O.; Teipel, S.J.; Gertz, H.J.; Jahn, H.; Jessen, F.; Kurz, A.; Luckhaus, C.; et al. Incremental value of biomarker combinations to predict progression of mild cognitive impairment to Alzheimer's Dementia. *Alzheimer's Res. Ther.* **2017**, *9*, 84. [CrossRef]
348. Spies, P.E.; Claassen, J.A.; Peer, P.G.; Blankenstein, M.A.; Teunissen, C.E.; Scheltens, P.; van der Flier, W.M.; Olde Rikkert, M.G.; Verbeek, M.M. A prediction model to calculate probability of alzheimer's disease using cerebrospinal fluid biomarkers. *Alzheimer's Dement.* **2013**, *9*, 262–268. [CrossRef]
349. Antonaros, F.; Ghini, V.; Pulina, F.; Ramacieri, G.; Cicchini, E.; Mannini, E.; Martelli, A.; Feliciello, A.; Lanfranchi, S.; Onnivello, S.; et al. Plasma metabolome and cognitive skills in down syndrome. *Sci. Rep.* **2020**, *10*, 10491. [CrossRef]
350. Orozco, J.S.; Hertz-Picciotto, I.; Abbeduto, L.; Slupsky, C.M. Metabolomics analysis of children with autism, idiopathic-developmental delays, and down syndrome. *Transl. Psychiatry* **2019**, *9*, 243. [CrossRef]

11

Potential Drug Candidates to Treat TRPC6 Channel Deficiencies in the Pathophysiology of Alzheimer's Disease and Brain Ischemia

Veronika Prikhodko [1,2,3], Daria Chernyuk [1], Yurii Sysoev [1,2,3,4], Nikita Zernov [1], Sergey Okovityi [2,3] and Elena Popugaeva [1,*]

1 Laboratory of Molecular Neurodegeneration, Peter the Great St. Petersburg Polytechnic University, 195251 St. Petersburg, Russia; veronika.prihodko@pharminnotech.com (V.P.); dasha0703@mail.ru (D.C.); susoyev92@mail.ru (Y.S.); quakenbush97@gmail.com (N.Z.)

2 Department of Pharmacology and Clinical Pharmacology, Saint Petersburg State Chemical Pharmaceutical University, 197022 St. Petersburg, Russia; okovityy@mail.ru

3 N.P. Bechtereva Institute of the Human Brain of the Russian Academy of Sciences, 197376 St. Petersburg, Russia

4 Institute of Translational Biomedicine, Saint Petersburg State University, 199034 St. Petersburg, Russia

* Correspondence: lena.popugaeva@gmail.com

Abstract: Alzheimer's disease and cerebral ischemia are among the many causative neurodegenerative diseases that lead to disabilities in the middle-aged and elderly population. There are no effective disease-preventing therapies for these pathologies. Recent in vitro and in vivo studies have revealed the TRPC6 channel to be a promising molecular target for the development of neuroprotective agents. TRPC6 channel is a non-selective cation plasma membrane channel that is permeable to Ca^{2+}. Its Ca^{2+}-dependent pharmacological effect is associated with the stabilization and protection of excitatory synapses. Downregulation as well as upregulation of TRPC6 channel functions have been observed in Alzheimer's disease and brain ischemia models. Thus, in order to protect neurons from Alzheimer's disease and cerebral ischemia, proper TRPC6 channels modulators have to be used. TRPC6 channels modulators are an emerging research field. New chemical structures modulating the activity of TRPC6 channels are being currently discovered. The recent publication of the cryo-EM structure of TRPC6 channels should speed up the discovery process even more. This review summarizes the currently available information about potential drug candidates that may be used as basic structures to develop selective, highly potent TRPC6 channel modulators to treat neurodegenerative disorders, such as Alzheimer's disease and cerebral ischemia.

Keywords: TRPC6; Alzheimer's disease; cerebral ischemia; pharmaceutical agents

---

1. Introduction

Due to increased life expectancies, neurodegenerative diseases (NDD), such as Alzheimer's disease (AD), dementia, and cerebrovascular diseases, are considered by WHO the main cause of disability in the coming decades. Currently, there are no effective disease-modifying or preventing therapies for those NDDs.

AD is caused by the progressive loss of neurons in brain structures that are responsible for memory acquisition and preservation, such as the hippocampus and cortical areas. The exact mechanism that causes neurons to die is not known. Among the most studied toxic changes of proteins that cause neuronal degeneration in AD are extracellular amyloid-beta (Aβ) aggregates and intracellular hyperphosphorylated tau (p-tau) that forms neurofibrillary tangles. Recently, disruption of immune system signaling in glial cells has started to receive growing attention due to the appearance of genome-wide association study (GWAS) data for late-onset AD patients [1].

Brain ischemia is a cerebrovascular disease that is caused by a restriction in blood supply, leading to oxygen deprivation and the rapid death of neurons. Several mechanisms, including excitotoxicity, ionic imbalance, oxidative and nitrosative stress, and apoptosis, have been implicated in ischemic neuronal death [2,3]. Acute brain ischemia can be treated successfully in modern healthcare settings, although treatment success depends on how quickly the patient receives medical care as well as the brain volume affected. However, there are currently no effective treatment options for chronic brain ischemia, which is usually caused by cerebral atherosclerosis.

Although the pathophysiological mechanisms causing AD and cerebral ischemia may differ, cerebral ischemia serves as a risk factor for AD development [4], and vice versa [5,6], indicating that a common intracellular mechanism may be disrupted in these two distinct pathologies. Such a common mechanism may be associated with Ca^{2+} dyshomeostasis. The N-methyl-D-aspartate (NMDA) receptor, an important excitatory neurotransmitter receptor, has been reported as the key player in the Ca^{2+} signaling in AD [7] and cerebral ischemia [8]. However, the NMDA receptor blocker memantine only relieves the symptoms temporarily in the early to moderate stage of AD patients [9,10]. Moreover, blocking NMDA receptors to prevent ischemic neuronal damage in clinical trials has caused severe adverse effects [11,12]. Although multiple factors might have contributed to the unsuccessful clinical trials, it is possible that the disruption of neuroprotective pathways, which precedes NMDA receptors hyperactivation, could be responsible for either AD and/or ischemic brain damage.

One of such neuroprotective pathways is the transient receptor potential cation channel, subfamily C, member 6 (TRPC6)-dependent regulation of excitatory synapse formation. TRPC6 overexpression has been shown to increase dendritic spine density [13] and rescue mushroom spine loss in mouse AD models [14], as well as protect neurons from ischemic brain damage [15,16]. TRPC6 upregulates the cAMP-response element-binding protein (CREB) pathway that is important for dendritic growth [17] and promotes synapse and dendritic spine formation, spatial memory, and learning [13]. In addition, TRPC6 also acts as a negative regulator that suppresses NMDA-induced Ca^{2+} influx in hippocampal neurons [15], which may protect neurons from excitotoxicity in the first stages of the disease. TRPC6 overexpression has been observed in breast cancer cells [18]. Overactivation of TRPC6 is toxic to immune cells (reviewed here [19]). Gain-of-function mutations of TRPC6 have been associated with familial forms of focal segmental glomerular sclerosis [20]. The mentioned studies indicate that despite the positive effect of TRPC6 activation in the brain, excessive TRPC6 activation has toxic effects on other cellular systems in the body.

Current prevalent evidence suggests that the TRPC6 channel function is downregulated in AD and cerebral ischemia [14,21–23]. However, there are reports in the literature that observe TRPC6 overactivation in AD [24] and cerebral ischemia models [25,26]. Existing contradictions on TRPC6 channel function in AD and ischemia indicate that these NDDs might be heterogenic, meaning that in one group of patients, the disease leads to hypofunction of the TRPC6 channel; however, there is another group (most likely smaller than the first one) where TRPC6 is hyperactivated. Thus, in order to preserve brain function, TRPC6 activity has to be in its physiological state, and deviations towards hypoactivity as well as hyperactivity are toxic to the cells. In terms of patient treatment, a careful investigation of the dysfunction of the TRPC6-dependent molecular pathway has to be performed in order to develop appropriate pharmacological treatments for said pathologies.

This review is devoted to the description of the role of TRPC6 channels in AD and brain ischemia with a particular focus on the dysfunction of them as Ca^{2+}-dependent channels. Potential drug candidates that have shown their therapeutic effects in different cellular and animal models are discussed. When available, the pros and cons of each particular TRPC6 channel modulator are mentioned. TRPC6 is also involved in certain Ca^{2+}-independent processes, such as amyloid precursor protein (APP) interaction [27]. However, in order to keep the review focused, this Ca^{2+}-independent process observed in AD and brain ischemia pathogenesis is omitted.

2. TRPC Channels and Their Regulation in Cells

Transient receptor potential (TRP) cation channels form a large family of multifunctional cell sensors. There are 29 TRP channels that can be described and divided into six subfamilies based on sequence homology: seven canonical channels (TRPC), six vanilloid channels (TRPV), eight melastatin-related channels (TRPM), three polycystic channels (TRPP), three mucolipins (TPRML), and one ankyrin channel (TRPA) [28].

TRPCs participate in different physiological processes in the development of the nervous system [29]. TRPC subfamily consists of seven members: TRPC1, TRPC2, TRPC3, TRPC4, TRPC5, TRPC6, and TRPC7. TRPC2 is a pseudogene in a number of vertebrates, including humans [30].

Analysis of the expression of different types of TRPC channels in situ using the Allen Brain Atlas and of gene expression in different regions of the mouse brain has demonstrated that TRPC6 is highly expressed in the hippocampus [14]. Western blot analysis of the rat hippocampus has shown that TRPC6 levels are enhanced in postsynaptic structures compared with synaptosomes. Moreover, electron microscopy has shown that TRPC6 is mostly located in the postsynaptic sites [13].

TRPs are cloned and identified, assuming that they are calcium-selective and activated by the emptying of internal Ca^{2+} stores (store-operated channels (SOC)) [31]. After their initial functional characterization, it has turned out that both assumptions do not hold true, especially for TRPCs [31]. These ion channels only show a moderate Ca^{2+} selectivity (PCa/PNa from ~0.5 to 9), and the TRPC3/6/7 subfamily of TRPC channels can be activated by the second messenger diacylglycerol (DAG) produced by receptor-activated phospholipase C (PLC) without any involvement of internal stores (receptor-operated channels (ROC)) [32].

Store-operated Ca^{2+} entry (SOCE) via TRPCs happens when 1,4,5-trisphosphate (IP3) or some other intracellular mechanism empties Ca^{2+} stored in the endoplasmic reticulum (ER). The fall in the ER Ca^{2+} concentration signals to the plasma membrane to open store-operated channels [33]. The major breakthrough in the understanding of SOCE physiology happened when Ca^{2+}-sensing stromal interaction molecule (STIM) ER proteins and plasma membrane (PM) Orai 1-3 channels have been described [34–37]. STIM1 and 2 proteins reside in the ER and monitor ER Ca^{2+} concentration with their EF-hand motif. When the ER Ca^{2+} concentration drops, Ca^{2+} dissociates from EF-hand, thus allowing STIM proteins to oligomerize and move to ER-PM tight junctions where they interact with PM Orai and TRP channels in order to facilitate Ca^{2+} flow.

3. Role of TRPC6 in the Formation of Excitatory Synapses

TRPC6 plays a certain physiological role in the formation of excitatory synapses. Particularly, TRPC6 overexpression increases dendritic spine density [13] and attenuates mushroom spine loss in presenilin 1 knock-in (PS1-KI) and amyloid precursor protein knock in (APP-KI) hippocampal neurons to the level of wild type neurons [14]. At the same time, overexpression of TRPC1, TRPC3-5, and TRPC7 does not affect spine morphology [14]. Meanwhile, the downregulation of TRPC6 expression leads to spine density reduction, lowers the frequency of spontaneous miniature excitatory postsynaptic currents (mEPSCs) [13], decreases the expression of postsynaptic density protein 95 (PSD95), and inhibits phosphorylation of calcium-calmodulin-dependent protein kinase II (pCaMKII) [14].

Activation of TRPC6 can promote spine formation via the STIM2-neuronal SOCE-CaMKII pathway. The expression level of STIM2 is downregulated in hippocampal neurons from PS1-M146V-KI [38] and APP-KI [14] mice as well as in a cellular model of amyloid synaptotoxicity [39]. The STIM2 reduction may be a compensatory response to ER Ca^{2+} overload in these models and may lead to the loss of mushroom spines in PS1-M146V-KI and APP-KI hippocampal neurons. TRPC6 and Orai2 channels are suggested to be the key components of neuronal SOCE in hippocampal cells [14]. It is hypothesized that the downstream molecule for TRPC6-mediated SOCE in hippocampal neurons is CaMKII since upregulation of neuronal SOCE activity recovers phosphorylation of CaMKII, restores the number of mushroom spines in hippocampal neurons in mouse models of AD [38,39], and induces long-term potentiation in PS1-KI, APP-KI, and 5xFAD hippocampal slices [14,21].

Alternative TRPC6-downstream signaling pathways are the Ca^{2+}/calmodulin-dependent kinase IV (CaMKIV) pathway and the cAMP-response element-binding protein (CREB) pathway, which is important for dendritic growth in hippocampal neurons [17]; another study has shown that the CaMKIV-CREB pathway is important in promoting synapse and dendritic spine formation, spatial memory, and learning [13]. TRPC6 also acts as a negative regulator that suppresses NMDA-induced Ca^{2+} influx in hippocampal neurons [15]. In addition, NMDAR has been shown to regulate transcription and degradation of TRPC6 in neurons in a bidirectional manner through NMDAR subunit 2A (NR2A) or NR2B activation [40].

4. Hypo- and Hyperactivation of TRPC6 Channels in Different Pathogenetic Forms of AD

There is evidence that different genetically inherited familial forms of AD (fAD) can cause TRPC6 dysfunction [14,21,24]. Both hypo- [14,21,22] and hyperactivation [24] of TRPC6 channels have been reported for different fAD-associated mutations in *APP* and *PS* genes.

fAD-associated PS2-N141I, M239V mutations cause downregulation of TRPC6-mediated Ca^{2+} entry in transiently transfected HEK cells. Lessard et al. suggested that TRPC6 downregulation by PS2-N141I, M239V does not depend on ER Ca^{2+} content but rather involves the interaction of PS2 with an intermediate protein of unknown origin [22]. Later on, contradictory results were obtained on ER Ca^{2+} content in PS2-N141I expressing cells [41,42]. In double knockout fibroblasts, PS2-N141I increases ER Ca^{2+} content [41] but lowers it in Hela cells [42]. According to the classical understanding of the SOCE physiology, overloaded ER Ca^{2+} stores downregulate SOCE [33]; thus, the data provided by Tu et al. [41] seem to be more relevant.

PS1-M146V is an fAD-associated mutation that has been reported to downregulate TRPC6-dependent Ca^{2+} entry in hippocampal neurons in store-operated mode [14]. PS1-M146V has been shown to increase ER Ca^{2+} content in mouse embryonic fibroblasts (MEFs) [41] and in neurons [43]. It has been demonstrated in previous studies [38,44] that ER Ca^{2+} stores are overloaded in neurons from AD mouse models. Furthermore, it has been discovered that overloaded ER Ca^{2+} stores cause compensatory downregulation of TRPC6 channels in PS1-M146V neurons [14]. A similar impact on TRPC6 function has been reported for fAD-associated mutations in APP (KM670/671NL and I716F) [14] as well as for Aβ toxicity in a cell culture model of AD [21]. There are fAD mutations in PSEN1 (PSEN1M146L, PSEN1S170F, PSEN1I213F, PSEN1E318G, PSEN1P117R, PSEN1L226F, PSENA246E) [45,46] and PSEN2 (PSEN2M239I, PSEN2T122R) [42], which have been reported to downregulate SOCE, although their role in the regulation of TRPC6 function has not been investigated yet. TRPC6 activators have been shown to recover the percentage of mushroom spines in cell culture models of fAD and induce long-term potentiation in hippocampal brain slices taken from AD mouse models [14,21]. Based on these results, it is suggested that activators of TRPC6 may have a therapeutic value for the treatment of fAD with TRPC6 hypofunction [14,47–49].

PS1-ΔE9 mutation has been reported to empty ER Ca^{2+} stores [41] and enhance SOCE [24,50]. There are other fAD mutations in PSEN1 (PSEN1D257A, PSEN1D385A), which have been reported to enhance SOCE [51]; however, their role in the regulation of TRPC6 function has not been investigated yet. Today, there is only one fAD-associated PS1-ΔE9 mutation that has been shown to upregulate the TRPC6 function in store-operated mode [24]. A TRPC6 inhibitor has been shown to recover mushroom spine percentage in a cell culture model of fAD [24]. Inhibitors of TRPC6 have been proposed to have therapeutic effects in fAD with TRPC6 hyperfunction [24,49].

To conclude the section, in order to normalize TRPC6 function in neurons and preserve the stability of excitatory synaptic contacts, suitable pharmacological agents have to be used for distinct genetic forms of AD.

5. Cerebral Ischemia as a Risk Factor for AD Development

Recent experimental and clinical findings have demonstrated a high degree of correlation between cerebral ischemia and AD [4,52,53]. While some studies have indicated that ischemic stroke significantly increases the risk of AD [4], others, in turn, have associated AD with a higher risk of stroke [5,6]. Previous studies have suggested that almost 30% of AD subjects bear evidence of cerebral infarction at autopsy [54,55]. A meta-analysis that comprises seven cohort studies and two nested case-control studies has found that a history of stroke is associated with the development of AD [4]. Notably, several lines of evidence suggest that AD patients have a high risk of cerebral ischemia [5,6]. For example, among AD patients with no history of previous stroke, vascular dementia, or other cerebral degenerative diseases, the incidence of ischemic stroke amounts to 37.8 per 1000 persons (versus 23.2 in non-AD controls) [5]. In another register-based matched cohort study [6], patients with Alzheimer's dementia have a higher risk of hemorrhagic stroke, while there is no difference in ischemic stroke incidence. When the results are analyzed within different age groups, the risk of ischemic stroke is found to be increased among AD patients younger than 80 years [6].

6. Role of TRPC6 in the Development of Ischemia

Ca^{2+} overload is one of the main molecular mechanisms involved in ischemic cell damage and death [56]. TRPC6, along with a few other prominent members of the family, has recently gained considerable attention as a promising target for the prevention of Ca^{2+} overload [23]. Dysregulation of TRPC6 activity has been implicated in ischemic stroke [23,57], as well as retinal ischemia [58], and renal hypoxia following cerebral ischemia [59].

On the one hand, upregulation and maintenance of TRPC6 activity prevent NMDAR hyperactivation and the subsequent Ca^{2+} influx, development of excitotoxicity, and neuronal death. In supporting this notion, both direct activation by 1-oleoyl-2-acetyl-sn-glycerol (a synthetic analog of diacylglycerol, the main endogenous TRPC6 agonist) and overexpression of TRPC6 inhibit NMDA-induced currents in cultured hippocampal neurons [15], and TRPC overexpression attenuates excitotoxic damage in hippocampal and cortical neurons [16]. *Trpc6*-transgenic mice with an elevated basal level of TRPC6 expression are less susceptible to cerebral ischemia than their wild-type littermates and have lower mortality rates, reduced infarct volumes, and better neurological outcomes after middle cerebral artery occlusion (MCAO) [16]. Recent studies have shown that TRPC6-mediated signaling promotes neuronal survival [60], the brain-derived neurotrophic factor-mediated axonal growth cone guidance [61], dendritic outgrowth and branching [17], and excitatory synapse formation [13]. In addition, positive modulation of TRPC6 activity allows for the sustained activation of the CREB/CaMK-IV and Ras/MEK/ERK pathways, which is vital for neuronal development, survival, and proper functioning [23]. Blocking CREB signaling hinders post-stroke recovery [62], and CaMK-IV inhibition impairs blood–brain barrier integrity and exacerbates ischemic injury [63]. In turn, elevated CREB and CaMK-IV activity is associated with improved post-stroke outcomes in a number of animal studies [62–66].

On the other hand, some experimental data suggest that the upregulation of TRPC6 activity increases intracellular Ca^{2+} concentrations concomitantly with NMDAR activation, further exacerbating excitotoxic damage to neurons [16]. Oxygen-glucose deprivation in cultured cortical neurons and MCAO in wild-type mice are associated with elevated TRPC6 expression and activity, while TRPC6 deletion attenuates glutamate- and NMDA-induced cytotoxicity and reduced infarct volumes [25]. Knockdown of TRPC3, 6, and 7 prevents apoptosis in cultured astrocytes and ameliorates ischemic brain injury in mice [26]. Moreover, prevention of TRPC6 hyperactivation results in increased neuronal viability, reduced infarct volumes and brain edema, and improved functional recovery following acute ischemic stroke in rats [67–69] and crab-eating macaques [67]. Other TRPC6 inhibitors have also been reported to exert beneficial effects in experimental models to some extent relevant to ischemic brain injury (e.g., acute renal ischemia/reperfusion injury) [70–74].

Existing controversies regarding the TRPC6 function in the development of brain ischemia might be due to different experimental settings (i.e., rodent model, sex, age, the method used to model ischemia). However, similarly to AD, brain ischemia seems to be heterogenic, meaning that one group of patients has TRPC6 hypofunction, and another one has TRPC6 hyperfunction. This indicates the need to develop pathology-dependent strategies to treat different NDD patients.

7. Available Drug Candidates to Modulate TRPC6 Activity

To date, two strategies have been proposed for the pharmacological modulation of TRPC6 activity for the treatment of Alzheimer's disease and cerebral ischemia: (1) TRPC6 activation to allow Ca^{2+} influx via neuronal SOCE and sustain the stability of postsynaptic contacts (for AD) and to attenuate NMDAR activity and prevent calcium-dependent excitotoxicity [15,16] (for ischemia); (2) inhibition of TRPC6 in order to prevent calcium overload and the subsequent cell damage [23,64] (for AD and ischemia). Although apparently mutually exclusive, both of these strategies are aimed to keep the intracellular Ca^{2+} concentration within the normal range, which requires limiting its entry via transmembrane channels and/or release from intracellular stores [75]. Given the pivotal role of NMDAR in excitotoxic neuronal damage, NMDAR blockers have been proposed as potential neuroprotective agents, although most of them have failed to show substantial effectiveness in human patients so far [76]. Due to that fact, TRPC6 has emerged as an alternative therapeutic target for AD and ischemic stroke [23].

7.1. TRPC6 Activators

TRPC6 activation can be induced by several endogenous diacylglycerols (DAGs) [32], lysophosphatidylcholines [75], and 20-hydroxyeicosatetraenoic acid, which is a metabolite of arachidonic acid [77]. A number of DAG analogs, including 1,2-dioctanoyl-*sn*-glycerol, DAG-containing arachidonic and docosahexaenoic acids [78,79], and the docosanoid neuroprotectin D1 [80], have also been reported as TRPC6 agonists. This channel can also be activated by agents of synthetic or natural origin that are structurally different from DAG. Direct TRPC6 agonists acting in receptor-operated mode include synthetic compounds, such as flufenamic acid [81] and several pyrazolopyrimidine [82] and piperazine [83] derivatives. The benzimidazole-based small molecule agonist GSK1702934A, its azobenzene derivative OptoBI-1 [84], and the chromone-containing compound C20 [85] are also thought to be direct (ROC) stimulators of TRPC6 activity. In contrast, certain naturally occurring chemicals are known to potentiate TRPC6 effects in an indirect manner. These include the stilbenoid resveratrol [66], the isoflavone calycosin [86], and (−)-epigallocatechin-3-gallate, a catechin-type polyphenol [87]. Recently, a novel potent ethanolamine derivative, bis-{2-[(2E)-4-hydroxy-4-oxobut-2-enoyloxy]-N,N-diethylethanaminium} butandioate (FDES), has been demonstrated to exert neuroprotective effects due to selective TRPC6 channel activation in store-operated mode [88,89]. The aminoquinazoline derivative, NSN21778, was demonstrated by Zhang et al. to have a store-dependent mechanism of action where DAG is required as a co-factor for TRPC6 activation [14]. The piperazine derivative, 51164, has been shown to activate TRPC6 in store-operated mode requiring DAG as a co-factor [21].

7.1.1. Endogenous Ligands and Analogs

DAG

A compound containing both DAG and arachidonic acid fragments, 1-stearoyl-2-arachidonyl-sn-glycerol (SAG), elicits a rapid Ca^{2+} flux into HEK293 cells, while 1-stearoyl-2-docosahexaenoyl-sn-glycerol (SDG), which does not contain an arachidonic acid moiety, has significantly lower potency [78]. 1-oleoyl-2-acetyl-*sn*-glycerol (OAG), a diacylglycerol analog and a TRPC3/6/7 channel modulator, is found to cross the plasma membrane and intracellularly activate the channels [32,90].

OAG has been shown to activate Ca^{2+}-permeable channels, displaying TRPC6-like properties in cultured cortical neurons [91]. In addition, OAG has been demonstrated to increase field excitatory postsynaptic potential (fEPSP) levels in a TRPC-dependent manner in hippocampal slices from wild-type mice [92], indicating that it might have neuroprotective effects. However, as far as we are aware, those compounds have not yet been evaluated in in vivo models of AD and cerebral ischemia.

Lysophosphatidylcholine

Lysophosphatidylcholine (LPC) is produced from phosphatidylcholines via partial hydrolysis generally catalyzed by phospholipase A2. Increased LPC production has been observed in various disorders of the central nervous system, including stroke and AD [93], and is associated with acute and chronic brain ischemia [94,95]. Results of a cohort study have suggested that LPC levels could be used as a tool for ischemic stroke risk stratification in patients who have suffered a transitory ischemic attack before [96]. LPC is shown to activate TRPC6 channels and promote Ca^{2+} flux into endothelial cells, hampering their migration and preventing endothelial healing, thus contributing to atherogenesis [97,98].

20-Hydroxy-5Z,8Z,11Z,14Z-Eicosatetraenoic Acid

20-hydroxy-5Z,8Z,11Z,14Z-eicosatetraenoic acid (20-HETE) is the main eicosanoid metabolite of arachidonic acid and a potent inflammatory vasoconstrictor. In HEK293 cells, 20-HETE (half maximal effective concentration, EC_{50} of 0.8 μM) elicits a three-fold increase in TRPC6 activity (as indicated by an increased inward, the non-selective current observed in whole-cell patch-clamp recordings) but does not affect intracellular Ca^{2+} concentrations [77]. In isolated guinea pig airway smooth muscle cells, it induces a dose-dependent inotropic effect via TRPC6 activation and the subsequent promotion of Ca^{2+} entry [99]. Nevertheless, 20-HETE has been shown to have detrimental effects in ischemic and traumatic brain injury, which might be explained by its vasoconstrictor properties, and has even been proposed as a predictor of poor prognosis in stroke patients [100]. To our knowledge, 20-HETE has not yet been tested in AD models, but it has been shown to activate TRPV1 channels in dorsal root ganglia cultures [101].

10*R*,17*R*-Dihydroxydocosa-4*Z*,7*Z*,11*E*,13*E*,15*Z*,19*Z*-Hexaenoic Acid

10*R*,17*R*-dihydroxydocosa-4*Z*,7*Z*,11*E*,13*E*,15*Z*,19*Z*-hexaenoic acid (Neuroprotectin D1, NPD1, Table 1) is a docosahexaenoic acid ((4Z,7Z,10Z,13Z,16Z,19Z)-docosa-4,7,10,13,16,19-hexaenoic acid, DHA)-derived endogenous anti-inflammatory mediator commonly found in fish oil [102]. NPD1, among other neuroprotectins, is synthesized in ischemic brain tissue as a result of DHA enzymatic lipoxygenation. In a rat model of ischemic stroke, NPD1 administration is associated with a significantly elevated TRPC6 and CREB activity, while the inhibition of the MEK/ERK pathway results in a decrease in NPD1 neuroprotective activity. Continuous intracerebroventricular administration of NPD1 over 10 min at 2 h after reperfusion sustains TRPC6/CREB activity, reduces infarct volumes, and promotes functional recovery [80]. The role of NPD1 in TRPC6-mediated neuroprotection in AD has not been described yet.

Table 1. Pharmacological modulators of TRPC6 in cerebral ischemia and AD models.

No.	Compound Name and Structural Formula	Experimental Model	Mode of Administration	Effect(s)	Reference(s)
		TRPC6 Activators			
		Endogenous ligands			
1	Neuroprotectin D1 10*R*,17*R*-Dihydroxydocosa-4*Z*,7*Z*,11*E*,13*E*,15*Z*,19*Z*-hexaenoic acid 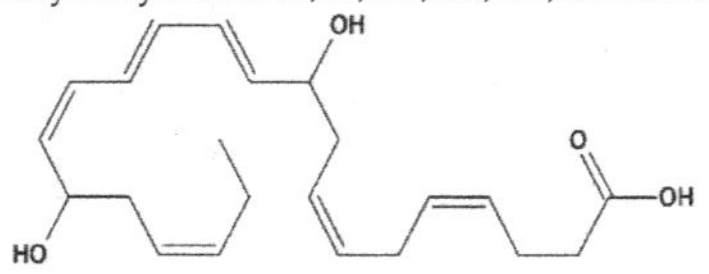	Rat transient MCAO	Icv injection at 2 h after reperfusion	reduced infarct volume reduced sensory and motor deficits	[80]
		Phytochemicals			
2	Hyperforin (1*R*,5*S*,6*R*,7*S*)-4-Hydroxy-6-methyl-1,3,7-tris(3-methylbut-2-en-1-yl)-6-(4-methylpent-3-en-1-yl)-5-(2-methylpropanoyl) bicyclo[3.3.1]non-3-ene-2,9-dione 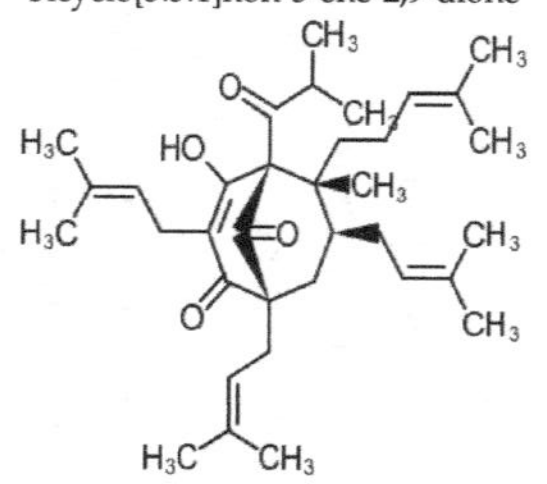	Lipopolysaccharide stimulation in 28 d post-MCAO isolated mouse astrocytes	Co-incubation for 16 h	increased viability	[103]
		Lipopolysaccharide stimulation in 28 d post-MCAO isolated mouse cortical neurons		increased viability	[103]
		NMDA toxicity in rat hippocampal slices	Co-incubation for 30 min	reduced edema	[104]
		Male Sprague-Dawley rats injected with fibrillary Aβ	Intrahippocampal co-injection of Aβ with the drug for 14 days	amyloid deposits disaggregation reduced spatial memory deficit	[105]
		Rat hippocampal slice cultures	Co-incubation for 24 h	increased proportion of mature stubby spines	[106]
		Hippocampal cultures from PS1-M146VKI and APPKI transgenic mice	Incubation for 16 h	increased percentage of mushroom spines in TRPC6-dependent manner increased neuronal SOCE in postsynaptic spines	[14]
		Hippocampal cultures treated with synthetic Aβ42 peptides	Co-incubation for 16 h	increased percentage of mushroom spines increased neuronal SOCE in postsynaptic spines	[21]
		Mouse transient MCAO	Intranasal administration q.d. for 7 d starting at day 7 post-MCAO	increased hippocampal neurogenesis improved post-stroke depression and anxiety reduced memory deficit	[107]
			Icv injections at 1, 24, and 48 h after MCAO	reduced microglial activation reduced infarct volume reduced neurological deficit	[108]
			Icv injections q.d. for 14 d starting at day 14 post-MCAO	increased angiogenesis reduced motor deficit	[109]
				increased angiogenesis increased subventricular neurogenesis reduced motor deficit	[103]
		Mouse permanent MCAO	Ip injection before ischemia onset	no effect on infarct volume or brain edema	[104]
		Mouse water intoxication			
		Rat transient MCAO	Icv injection at 6, 12, or 24 h after reperfusion	prevented neuronal apoptosis reduced infarct volume reduced neurological deficit	[110]

Table 1. *Cont.*

No.	Compound Name and Structural Formula	Experimental Model	Mode of Administration	Effect(s)	Reference(s)
3	Tetrahydrohyperforin (1S,5S,7S,8R)-4,9-dihydroxy-1-(1-hydroxy-2-methylpropyl)-8-methyl-3,5,7-tris(3-methylbut-2-enyl)-8-(4-methylpent-3-enyl)bicyclo[3.3.1]non-3-en-2-one 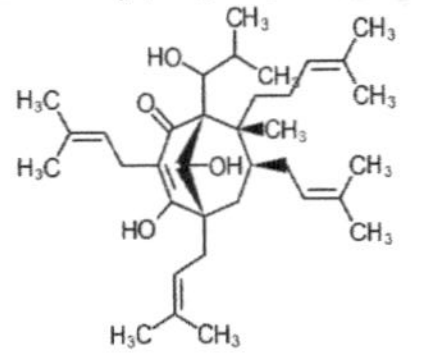	APPSEN1ΔE9 mice	Ip injections for 4 weeks	reduced memory deficit reduced amyloid deposition attenuated neuroinflammation and oxidative stress	[111]
4	Resveratrol 5-[(*E*)-2-(4-Hydroxyphenyl)ethenyl] benzene-1,3-diol 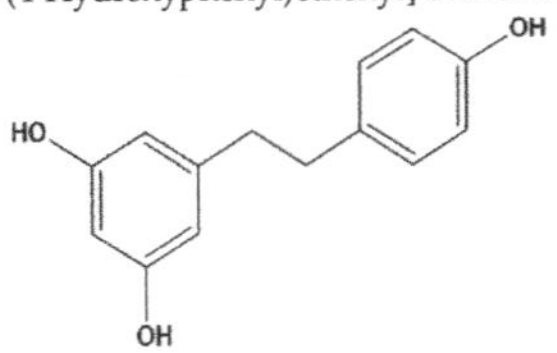	Oxygen/glucose deprivation in isolated rat brain endothelial cells	Preincubation for 3 d	increased viability	[112]
		Mouse transient MCAO	Ip injection at 48 h before MCAO	reduced infarct volume no effect on cerebral blood flow	[113]
			Oral gavage q.d. for 7 d starting from 24 h after MCAO, or for 5 d starting from 72 h after MCAO	increased vascular density in the basal ganglia region and cortex reduced infarct volume reduced neurological deficit	[114]
		Rat transient MCAO	Ip injections q.d. for 7 d before MCAO	reduced infarct volume reduced neurological deficit	[66]
		Rat recurrent transient MCAO	Oral gavage q.d. for 3 d between strokes	reduced infarct volume following an initial and recurrent stroke reduced blood–brain barrier disruption following a recurrent stroke reduced brain edema following a recurrent stroke reduced astrogliosis following a recurrent stroke no effect on cerebral blood flow during or after recurrent stroke	[112]
		Rat asphyxial cardiac arrest	Ip injection at 48 h before cardiac arrest	enhanced ATP synthesis efficiency in hippocampal mitochondria prevented hippocampal neuronal apoptosis	[115]
		Gerbil transient bilateral common carotid artery occlusion	Ip injections during occlusion or at reperfusion + at 24 h after reperfusion	reduced hippocampal microglial activation prevented hippocampal-delayed neuronal death	[116]
		Clinical trials in patients	diverse	affected neuroinflammation, Aβ deposition, and adaptive immunity in patients with mild to moderate Alzheimer's disease	for a review, see [117]

Table 1. *Cont.*

No.	Compound Name and Structural Formula	Experimental Model	Mode of Administration	Effect(s)	Reference(s)
		Synthetic compounds			
5	Flufenamic acid 2-[[3-(Trifluoromethyl)phenyl]amino]benzoic acid 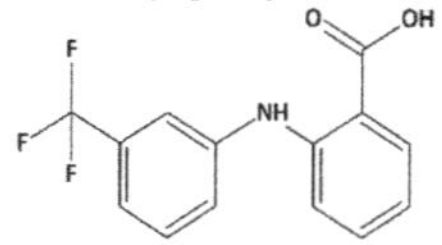	Oxygen/glucose deprivation in isolated mouse embryonic cortical neurons	Incubation from 15 min before oxygen/glucose deprivation until 24 h of reoxygenation	increased viability of male neurons no effect on female neurons	[118]
		Glutamate toxicity in isolated rat embryonic hippocampal neurons	Co-incubation for 10 min	increased viability	[119]
6	PPZ1 [4-(5-Chloro-2-methylphenyl)piperazin-1-yl]-3-fluorophenylmethanone 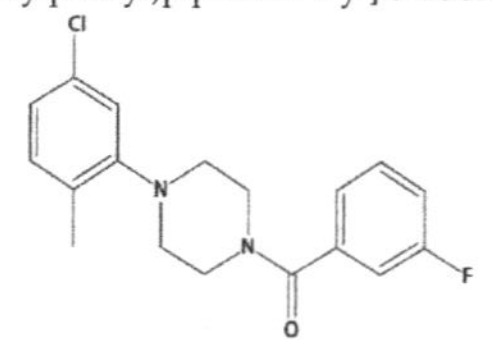	Serum deprivation in isolated rat cerebellar granule neurons	Incubation for 24 h before and 24 h after serum deprivation	increased neurite outgrowth increased cell viability	[83]
7	PPZ2 2-[4-(2,3-Dimethylphenyl)piperazin-1-yl]-N-(2-ethoxyphenyl)acetamide 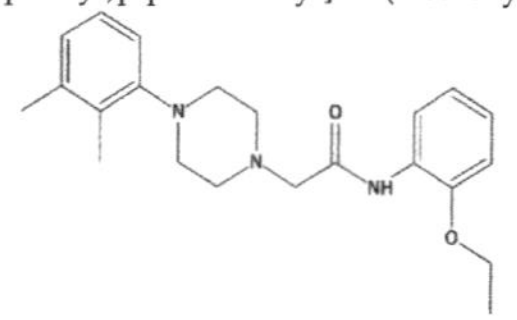				
8	51164 N-(2-chlorophenyl)-2-(4-phenylpiperazin-1-yl)acetamide 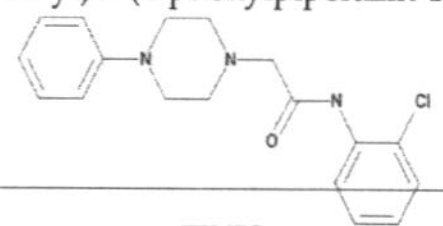	Aβ42-induced toxicity in primary hippocampal neurons	Co-incubation for 16 h	restored mushroom spines percentage induced neuronal SOCE in postsynaptic spines	[21]
		6 month-old 5xFAD mouse hippocampal slices	30 min incubation	restored LTP induction	
9	FDES Bis-{2-[(2E)-4-hydroxy-4-oxobut-2-enoyloxy]-N,N-diethylethanaminium} butandioate 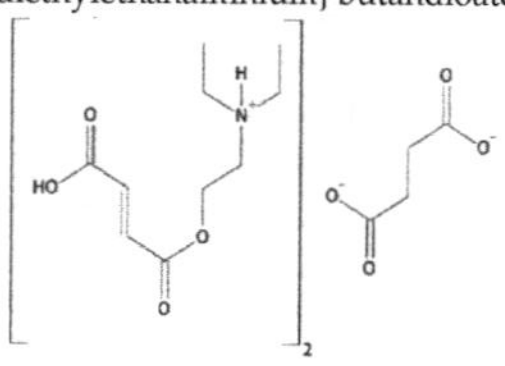	Aβ42-induced toxicity in primary hippocampal neurons	Incubation for 16 h	restored mushroom spines percentage induced neuronal SOCE in postsynaptic spines	[89]
		Rat transient MCAO	Ip injections at 1 h after reperfusion + q.d. for 7 d after reperfusion	improved spatial memory retention no effect on mortality	
		Rat permanent bilateral common carotid artery ligation	Oral gavage at 30 min before MCAO + q.d. for 21 d after reperfusion	reduced mortality reduced motor deficit reduced aggressiveness reduced emotional lability increased exploratory behavior	[120]

Table 1. *Cont.*

No.	Compound Name and Structural Formula	Experimental Model	Mode of Administration	Effect(s)	Reference(s)
10	NSN21778 N-[4-[2-[(6-aminoquinazolin-4-yl)amino]ethyl]phenyl]acetamide 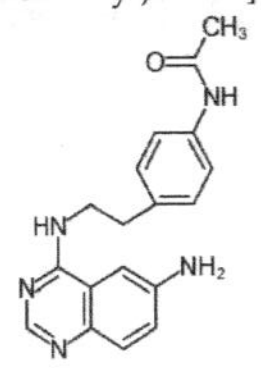	Primary hippocampal cell culture models from PS1-M146V and APPKI mice	Incubation for 16 h	increased percentage of mushroom spines in TRPC6-dependent manner increased neuronal SOCE in postsynaptic spines	[14]
		Hippocampal brain slices from PS1-M146V and APPKI mice	Pretreatment for 30 min	recovered LTP induction	
		TRPC6 inhibitors			
11	HET0016 N-Hydroxy-N′-(4-n-butyl-2-methylphenyl)formamidine 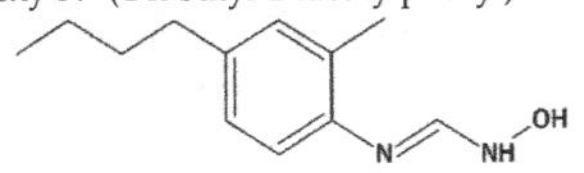	Rat pediatric asphyxial cardiac arrest	Iv injection at reperfusion	increased cortical CBF reduced brain edema	[69]
			Iv injection at reperfusion + ip injections every 6 h for 24 h after reperfusion	reduced neurological deficit reduced neurodegeneration	
		Rat transient MCAO	Iv injection immediately before reperfusion	reduced infarct volume	[68]
			Ip injections q.d. for 3 d before and 3 d after MCAO	increased CBF reduced infarct volume	[121]
		Piglet neonatal hypoxia/ ischemia	5 min-infusion at 5 min after reperfusion + hypothermia at 3 h after reperfusion	increased neuronal viability in the putamen, cortex, and thalamus prevention of seizures	[122]
			Iv injection at 5 min after reperfusion	increased neuronal viability in the putamen reduced neurological deficit no effect on cerebral blood flow (CBF)	[123]
12	TS-011 N-(3-Chloro-4-morpholin-4-yl)phenyl-N′-hydroxyimidoformamide 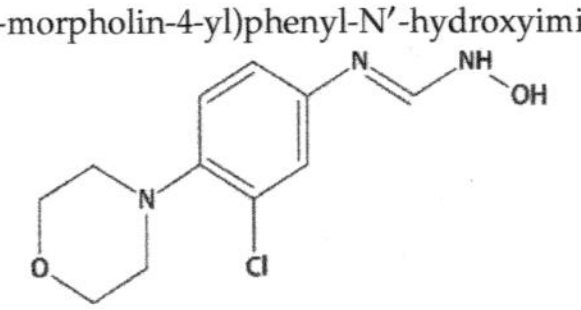	Rat transient MCAO	Iv injection at 30 min before MCAO + 1 or 2 h-infusion during MCAO	reduced cortical, subcortical, and total infarct volumes reduced the delayed drop in CBF no effect on volume at risk	[68]
			Iv injection at 20 min after MCAO + 2 h-infusion at reperfusion	reduced cortical and total infarct volumes no effect on volume at risk no effect on CBF	
			1 h-infusion at reperfusion, 1, 2, or 4 h after reperfusion	reduced infarct volumes	[67]
			1 h-infusion at reperfusion + iv injections q.d. for 7 d	reduced infarct volumes reduced sensory and motor deficits	
		Crab-eating macaque thrombotic internal carotid artery occlusion	Iv injection + 24 h-infusion after embolization	reduced infarct volume (when co-administered with tissue plasminogen activator) reduced neurological deficit	

Table 1. *Cont.*

No.	Compound Name and Structural Formula	Experimental Model	Mode of Administration	Effect(s)	Reference(s)
13	Mefenamic acid 2-(2,3-Dimethylphenyl)aminobenzoic acid 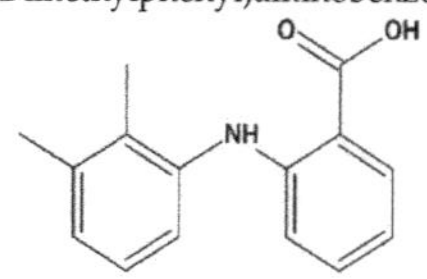	Glutamate toxicity in isolated rat embryonic hippocampal neurons	Co-incubation for 10 min	increased cell viability	[124]
		3xTg mice AD model	Administration by osmotic minipump over 28 days	reduced cognitive deficit	[125]
		Rat transient MCAO	Iv injection before MCAO	no effect on infarct and penumbra volumes and brain edema	[124]
			Iv injections at 1 h before + at 1, 2, and 3 h after MCAO	reduced infarct volume reduced brain edema	
			Icv 24 h-infusion starting at 1 h before MCAO		[119]
14	Meclofenamic acid 2-(2,6-Dichloro-3-methylanilino)benzoic acid 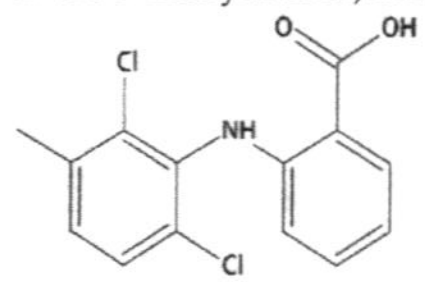	Glutamate toxicity in isolated rat embryonic hippocampal neurons	Co-incubation for 10 min	increased viability	[119]
15	Niflumic acid 2-{[3-(Trifluoromethyl)phenyl]amino}pyridine-3-carboxylic acid 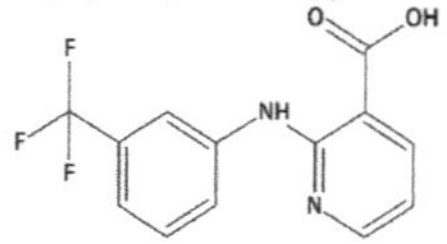				
16	SAR7334 4-[[(1R,2R)-2-[(3R)-3-Amino-1-piperidinyl]-2,3-dihydro-1H-inden-1-yl]oxy]-3-chlorobenzonitrile dihydrochloride 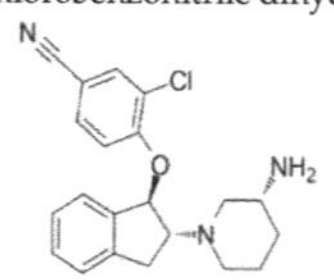	Primary cortical neurons	Treatment with 1 μM SAR7334 at the time of imaging	no effect on neuronal SOCE	[126]
17	EVP4593 4-N- [2- (4-phenoxyphenyl)ethyl]quinazoline-4,6-diamine 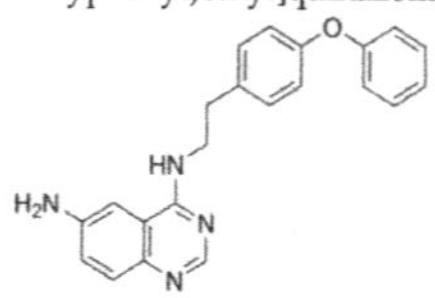	PSEN1ΔE9-hyperexpressing primary hippocampal neurons	Co-incubation for 16 h	reduced TRPC6-dependent neuronal SOCE in postsynaptic spines increased mushroom spines percentages	[24]

7.1.2. Hyperforin and Other Phytochemicals

Hyperforin

((1*R*,5*S*,6*R*,7*S*)-4-hydroxy-6-methyl-1,3,7-tris(3-methylbut-2-en-1-yl)-6-(4-methylpent-3-en-1-yl)-5-(2-methylpropanoyl)bicyclo[3.3.1]non-3-ene-2,9-dione) (Hyperforin, Table 1) is a phloroglucinol derivative and a major active constituent of St. John's wort (*Hypericum perforatum* L.). Hyperforin is a potent inhibitor of TRPC6 proteolysis and a positive modulator of TRPC6/CREB activity, acting in a manner similar to that of the brain-derived neurotrophic factor (BDNF) [110,127]. It is thought to bind to TRPC6 due to structural similarities to DAG and has higher selectivity because of the relative rigidity of the phloroglucinol pharmacophore moiety [128]. Neuroprotective and antidepressant-like properties of hyperforin and hyperforin-containing *H. perforatum* preparations involve the modulation of axonal growth, neurite growth and branching, dendritic spine formation, and the promotion of neuronal plasticity [106,127]. As proposed by Singer et al., the increase in Na^+ concentration resulting from TRPC6 activation by hyperforin might inhibit serotonin reuptake via the serotonin/Na^+ symporter, which, together with increased synaptic plasticity, could explain the antidepressant-like activity of *H. perforatum*-based drugs [129]. Confirming this hypothesis, larixyl acetate, a selective blocker of TRPC6, abolishes the antidepressant-like effects of hyperforin observed in mice in the tail suspension test [130].

In an ex vivo experiment, hyperforin (0.3 μM) promotes mature stubby spine formation and decreases the proportion of immature thin spine formation in rat hippocampal pyramidal neurons but does not affect mushroom spine density and morphology. Proper TRPC6 expression level and the presence of a fully functional TRPC6 channel are required for hyperforin to exert its effects, which suggests the key role of TRPC6 activation in its mechanism of action [106]. Using different rodent models of ischemic stroke, hyperforin has been shown to promote post-stroke neuro- and angiogenesis [103,109], inhibit microglial activation [108], attenuate brain edema [104], stimulate hippocampal neurogenesis, ameliorate post-stroke depression and anxiety, and restore memory function [107]. Chronic hyperforin treatment stimulates the expression of the tropomyosine receptor kinase B (TrkB) BDNF receptors as well as of TRPC6 in murine cortical neurons but has no effect on hippocampal neurogenesis [131]. When applied intracerebroventricularly to rats immediately after MCAO, hyperforin preserves TRPC6 activity, reduces infarct volumes, promotes functional recovery, and increases neurologic scores at 24 h after reperfusion [110].

There is a lot of evidence that hyperforin and its derivatives are highly selective towards the TRPC6 channel and do not exert similar effects on its closest relative, the TRPC3 channel [106,127,128,132]. Several studies have shown that hyperforin activates TRPC6 and increases its expression [106,133], leading to a decrease in the Aβ level and an improvement in cognitive performance in AD models [92,105,111].

The neuroprotective effect of hyperforin has been demonstrated in several rodent models of AD. In rats co-injected with amyloid fibrils and hyperforin in the hippocampus, hyperforin reduces amyloid deposit formation and, therefore, decreases the Aβ-induced neurotoxicity, reactive oxidative species formation, and attenuated behavioral impairments [105]. A more stable hyperforin derivative, tetrahydrohyperforin, also prevents the cognitive decline and synaptic impairment in double transgenic APPswe/PSEN1ΔE9 mice in a dose-dependent manner. It has been shown that the neuroprotective mechanism of tetrahydrohyperforin is associated with a reduced rate of proteolytic processing of APP, decreased the total amount of fibrillar and oligomeric forms of Aβ, reduced level of tau hyperphosphorylation, and attenuated astrogliosis [132]. Tetrahydrohyperforin has been shown to specifically target TRPC6 [92].

Hyperforin is also thought to be responsible for the induction of the cytochrome P450 enzyme CYP3A4 by binding to and activating the pregnane X receptor [134], indicating that it might have side effects and undesirable drug-to-drug interactions. Moreover, hyperforin is difficult to synthetize [135], unstable when exposed to light, and irritant to the gastrointestinal tract [136]. Such side effects might limit the use of hyperforin as a TRPC6 activator.

Resveratrol

Resveratrol (5-[(*E*)-2-(4-hydroxyphenyl)ethenyl]benzene-1,3-diol) (Table 1), which is found in grapes, berries, peanuts, and other plants, is among the best-known natural compounds with antioxidant and antihypoxic activity [66,137,138]. In the pioneering study of Wang et al. [116], resveratrol is shown to be able to cross the blood–brain barrier (BBB) and exert neuroprotective activity. Injected intraperitoneally either during or shortly after the induction of cerebral ischemia, it largely prevents delayed neuronal cell death and glial cell activation in a gerbil model of transient bilateral common carotid artery occlusion [116]. Based on the observed increase in TRPC6 and CREB activity, which has been prevented by PD98059 or KN62, inhibitors of MEK and CAMKIV/ CaMKII, respectively, it is suggested that resveratrol has exerted its effects via TRPC6 activation. Since its administration has been accompanied by a marked decrease in calpain activity, resveratrol is classified as an indirect positive modulator of TRPC6 activity [66]. When given to rats for 7 days before MCAO, resveratrol significantly reduces infarct volumes and enhances neurological scores at 24 h after reperfusion [66]. Low-dose oral resveratrol treatment for three consecutive days before and after an ischemic stroke induced in rats by middle cerebral artery clipping alleviates brain damage caused by the following recurrent stroke. Resveratrol normalizes BBB function and reduces cerebral edema without affecting regional cerebral blood flow and systemic blood pressure [112]. Resveratrol preconditioning (48 h before the induction of ischemia) effectively prevents neuronal cell loss in a mouse MCAO model of stroke [113]. In a rat model of global cerebral ischemia induced by asphyxial cardiac arrest, resveratrol (48 h before the induction of ischemia) is shown to protect the CA1 region of the hippocampus similarly to ischemic preconditioning [115].

Resveratrol is actively used in AD research [139–141]. Neuroprotective effects of resveratrol have been shown to be associated with the activation of silent mating type information regulation 2 homolog 1 (SIRT1) and vitagenes production [142]. In a phase II trial in AD patients, resveratrol is safe and well-tolerated, but its effectiveness is contradictory [143,144].

Although generally considered as a non-toxic therapeutic agent, high doses of resveratrol inhibit CYP3A4 activity in vitro [145] and in healthy volunteers [146], thus potentially inhibiting drug metabolic clearance, increasing bioavailability and toxicity of drugs taken concomitantly [147].

7.1.3. Synthetic Compounds

Flufenamic Acid

Flufenamic (2-[[3-(trifluoromethyl)phenyl]amino]benzoic) (Table 1) acid (FFA) is a member of the fenamate class of nonsteroidal anti-inflammatory drugs that have limited clinical applications due to their toxicity. FFA has been found to selectively activate TRPC6, at the same time, inhibiting TRPC3, 4, 5, and 7 [81]. Direct activation of TRPC6 by FFA has been confirmed in a number of in vitro studies [148], including those in glomerular podocytes [149] and ventricular cardiomyocytes [150]. Male (but not female) embryonic mice cortical neurons, which have been pre-treated with FFA 15 min before oxygen-glucose deprivation, have shown significantly higher viability, although this effect is not linked by the authors to TRPC6 activation [118]. Similar results are obtained in a recent in vitro glutamate toxicity assay using isolated rat embryonic hippocampal neurons [119].

Multiple experimental evidences suggest that FFA is a broad spectrum ion channel modulator, with a preference for non-selective cation channels and chloride channels (reviewed here [81]). Its activity seems to be dose-dependent since FFA inhibits TRPC6 with a half maximal inhibitory concentration (IC_{50}) of 17.1 μM [151] but activates the same channel at 100 μM [148]. TRPM8 is inhibited by 100 μM FFA but is slightly activated at higher concentrations [152]. A worse situation is reported for big calcium-activated potassium channels (BK_{Ca}) modulation since FFA activates the channel below 10 μM, inhibits the channel between 10 to 50 μM, and then activates the channel above 50 μM [153]. Such opposing effects on the same channels and a huge number of other ion channels that are modulated by FFA makes it an inappropriate drug for usage in humans.

Piperazines

Sawamura et al. discovered a group of piperazine-based potent TRPC3/6/7 agonists functioning in receptor-operated mode with varying selectivity for different channel subtypes [83]. Among that group, 2-[4-(2,3-dimethylphenyl)piperazin-1-yl]-N-(2-ethoxyphenyl)acetamide (PPZ2, Table 1) dose-dependently activates TRPC6 and TRPC6-like channels in HEK cells, vascular smooth muscle cells, and cultured rat cerebellar granule neurons. PPZ2 and PPZ1 ([4-(5-chloro-2-methylphenyl)piperazin-1-yl]-3-fluorophenylmethanone) (Table 1) promote neurite outgrowth in a manner similar to that of BDNF and provide protection against serum deprivation-induced neuronal death [83].

Later on, another piperazine derivative, N-(2-chlorophenyl)-2-(4-phenylpiperazin-1-yl)acetamide (51164, Table 1), has been shown to activate the TRPC6 channel in store-operated mode with DAG acting as a co-factor [21]. Nanomolar concentrations of 51164 protect mushroom spines from amyloid toxicity, induce TRPC6-dependent neuronal SOCE in postsynaptic spines, and restore the induction of long-term potentiation in hippocampal slices taken from 6 months old 5xFAD mice [21].

N-[3-[4-[3-[bis(2-methylpropyl)amino]propyl]piperazin-1-yl]propyl]-1*H*-benzimidazol-2-amine (AZP2006), another piperazine derivative, attenuates Aβ and tau toxicity and improves cognitive performance in various mouse models [154]. Currently, AZP2006 is in phase 2 clinical trial in patients with progressive supranuclear palsy [155].

Piperazine derivatives as the majority of TRPC6 agonists cross-react with TRPC3 and TRPC7 [83], limiting their use as specific TRPC6 modulators. Among other side effects of piperazines is their hepatotoxicity [137]; however, hepatotoxicity has not been predicted by bioinformatical analyses for a 51164 compound [21]. Gastrointestinal hemorrhage and multiple organ failure have been predicted by bioinformatical analyses; thus, there is a need to search for the lowest therapeutic dose for the 51164 compound, and most likely, there is a need to modify its structure in order to minimize the mentioned side effects [21].

Bis-{2-[(2*E*)-4-Hydroxy-4-Oxobut-2-Enoyloxy]-*N*,*N*-Diethylethanaminium} Butandioate

Bis-{2-[(2*E*)-4-hydroxy-4-oxobut-2-enoyloxy]-*N*,*N*-diethylethanaminium} butandioate (Table 1), abbreviated as FDES, is an ethanolamine derivative known to possess antihypoxic, anti-ischemic, and neuroprotective properties [88,89,120,156]. Chronic FDES administration decreases mortality and improves motor function and coordination following permanent bilateral common carotid artery ligation [120] and reduces spatial memory deficit following middle cerebral artery (MCA) occlusion/reperfusion [89] in rats. Later, FDES was demonstrated to ameliorate fore- and hindlimb motor disturbances and increase overall locomotor activity in rats with unilateral traumatic brain injury [88].

FDES is shown to potentiate neuronal SOCE into postsynaptic spines in mouse hippocampal neurons [89]. Since TRPC6 knockdown abolishes the effects of FDES on neuronal SOCE (similarly to hyperforin), TRPC6 activation is suggested to be the primary mechanism of FDES neuroprotective action. Nanomolar concentrations of FDES effectively protect mushroom dendritic spines from amyloid synaptotoxicity, stabilizing and enhancing synaptic transmission, and preserving synaptic contact density [89]. Similarly to hyperforin, FDES decreases the proportion of immature thin and stubby spines in hippocampal neurons. When administered intraperitoneally to rats subjected to MCAO for 7 consecutive days starting from 1 h after reperfusion, FDES improves short-term spatial memory retention, as observed in the Barnes maze [89].

FDES is a precursor of choline and has been shown to have nootropic and actoprotective properties [89]. We assume that FDES would cross-react with muscarinic acetylcholine receptors, causing phospholipase C activation and production of IP3 and DAG. This cross-reactivity of FDES could further enhance its TRPC6-agonistic properties, although this hypothesis remains to be experimentally proven.

N-[4-[2-[(6-Aminoquinazolin-4-yl)Amino]ethyl]phenyl]acetamide

N-[4-[2-[(6-aminoquinazolin-4-yl)amino]ethyl]phenyl]acetamide (NSN21778, Table 1) was proposed by Zhang et al. as a novel positive modulator of the TRPC6/neuronal SOCE pathway acting in a manner similar to that of 51164. Despite its effectiveness in terms of improving mushroom spine morphology and TRPC6-mediated SOCE in PS1-KI and APP-KI hippocampal neurons and rescuing long-term potentiation in the APP-KI mouse model of AD, NSN21778 is found to have a rather poor pharmacokinetic profile and a low penetration of the blood–brain barrier [14].

7.1.4. Other TRPC6 Agonists

Several compounds described below have been confirmed to activate the TRPC6 channel using in vitro assays. However, to the best of our knowledge, their specific neuroprotective properties remain unexplored. Given their ability to interact with TRPC6, these compounds can be considered as potential neuroprotective agents.

Pyrazolopyrimidines

A number of pyrazolopyrimidines obtained by Qu et al. are reported to be direct agonists of TRPC6, 3, and 7. Among the four pyrazolopyrimidines tested by Qu et al., ethyl 4-(7-hydroxy-2-methyl-3-(4-(trifluoromethyl)phenyl)-pyrazolo[1,5-a]pyrimidin-5-yl)piperidine-1-carboxylate (compound 4n) is most active towards TRPC6 (EC_{50} = 1.39 or 0.89 μM depending on the conditions). However, compound 4n has demonstrated a much higher affinity for TRPC3 and TRPC7 (EC_{50} = 0.019 and 0.090 μM, respectively) [82].

GSK1702934A and OptoBI-1

GSK1702934A (1,3-Dihydro-1-[1-[(5,6,7,8-tetrahydro-4H-cyclohepta[b]thien-2-yl)carbonyl]-4-piperidinyl]-2H-benzimidazol-2-one) has been reported by Xu et al. to activate TRPC3 and 6 (EC_{50} = 0.08 and 0.44 μM, respectively), acting directly and independent of protein lipase C signaling from the extracellular side [157]. OptoBI-1, an azobenzene moiety-containing photochromic derivative of GSK1702934A, is found to activate TRPC6 as well as TRPC3 and 7, although having a slightly higher affinity for TRPC3. Light treatment of cultured murine hippocampal neurons with OptoBI-1 suppresses action potential firing elicited by repetitive depolarizing current injections [84].

3-(6,7-Dimethoxy-3,3-Dimethyl-3,4-Dihydroisoquinolin-1-yl)-2H-Chromen-2-One

Recently, a novel small-molecule allosteric TRPC6 agent, 3-(6,7-dimethoxy-3,3-dimethyl-3,4-dihydroisoquinolin-1-yl)-2H-chromen-2-one (C20), has been reported by Häfner et al. [85]. C20 (EC_{50} = 2.37 μM) selectively activates TRPC6 channels in several HEK cell lines while only slightly reducing the basal activity of TRPC3 and increasing that of TRPC7 and not affecting TRPC4 and 5 activity at all. Higher concentrations of C20 (10 μM) potentiate the efficacy of OAG and GSK1702934A, low-selective TRPC6 agonists described above, in HEK cells and freshly prepared human platelets [85].

It can be assumed that the mechanism of action of C20 involves TRPC6 sensitization and not with its activation per se; that is, C20 allows TRPC6 to be activated at a low basal concentration of DAG [85].

7.2. TRPC6 Inhibitors

AD seems to be a multifactorial disease with different pathogenic cascades occurring in different patients. In terms of TRPC6 channel dysfunction, there are forms of fAD, which demonstrate

TRPC6 hyperfunction [24]. For those patients, TRPC6 inhibitors might be used in order to normalize intracellular Ca^{2+} homeostasis.

The pathogenesis of cerebral ischemia is not fully understood. Similarly to AD, cerebral ischemia involves several different pathological cascades. There are studies reporting that TRPC6-mediated Ca^{2+} and Na+ influx facilitates NMDAR activation and exacerbates excitotoxicity, while TRPC6 deletion attenuates neuronal damage and death following focal cerebral ischemia [25]. In such cases, where excessive TRPC6 activity seems to be present, the use of TRPC6 inhibitors might be beneficial.

Arachidonic acid, which is released following cerebral ischemia, can be metabolized to 20-hydroxyeicosatetraenoic acid (20-HETE). 20-HETE is a potent vasoconstrictor that may contribute to ischemic injury [67]. Synthetic 20-HETE has been shown to activate TRPC6 [77]. Thus, inhibition of 20-HETE production by HET0016 reduces TRPC6 activation [158]. Inhibition of 20-HETE synthesis by N-hydroxy-N'-(4-n-butyl-2-methylphenyl)formamidine (HET0016, Table 1) decreases infarct volumes and increases cortical cerebral blood flow in cerebral ischemia induced by asphyxia cardiac arrest in rat pups [69] and in transient MCAO-induced ischemia in adult rats [121]. In neonatal piglets subjected to 6 min of acute asphyxia, HET0016 potentiates the neuroprotective effects of delayed hypothermia, increasing neuronal viability, preventing seizure development, and reducing neurological deficit [122,123]. Another 20-HETE inhibitor known as N-(3-chloro-4-morpholin-4-yl)phenyl-N'-hydroxyimidoformamide (TS-011, Table 1) markedly decreases infarct volumes and improves functional recovery in rats and primates [67,68].

We are unaware of any direct investigations of neuroprotective effects of HET0016 and TS-011 (Table 1) in AD models. However, since patients with Alzheimer's disease show an accumulation of (2E)-4-hydroxy-2-nonenal (HNE) adducts [159], and HET0016 is a potent inhibitor of ω- and ω-1-hydroxylation of HNE/HNA (4-hydroxynonanoic acid) [160], HET0016 could be of interest regarding its potential neuroprotective properties in AD.

In mice with closed-head traumatic brain injury, larixyl acetate, a naturally occurring diterpene, ameliorates endothelial dysfunction [74], which is closely associated with cerebral ischemia as well [161]. In isolated mouse lungs, larixyl acetate prevents the development of the acute hypoxic ventilatory response [72]. TRPC6 inhibition is now considered to be the primary mechanism of larixyl's neuroprotective action [72,74].

Mefenamic (2-(2,3-dimethylphenyl)aminobenzoic acid) (MFA), meclofenamic (2-(2,6-dichloro-3-methylanilino)benzoic), and niflumic (2-{[3-(trifluoromethyl)phenyl]amino}pyridine-3-carboxylic) acids (Table 1), non-steroidal anti-inflammatory drugs structurally related to flufenamic acid, are potent inhibitors of TRPC6 and some other closely related ion channels [151]. These compounds have been shown to attenuate glutamate-evoked excitotoxicity in cultured rat embryonic hippocampal neurons similarly to flufenamic acid [119,124]. In a 3xTgAD mouse AD model, MFA ameliorates cognitive impairments [125].

Maier et al. discovered a novel TRPC3/6/7 inhibitor, the aminoindanol derivative 4-[[(1R,2R)-2-[(3R)-3-Amino-1-piperidinyl]-2,3-dihydro-1H-inden-1-yl]oxy]-3-chlorobenzonitrile dihydrochloride (SAR7334, Table 1), with a higher selectivity towards TRPC6 (IC_{50} of 7.9 nM, as indicated by patch-clamp data) [71]. Hou et al. found that TRPC6 knockout or inhibition by SAR7334 mitigates oxidative stress-induced apoptosis of renal proximal tubular cells, which is considered to play a major role in renal ischemia/reperfusion [73]. SAR7334 and the tryptoline derivative 8009-5364 are reported to diminish acute hypoxia-induced pulmonary vasoconstriction and pulmonary arterial pressure in isolated mouse lungs [70,71]. SAR7334 has no effect on SOCE in primary cortical neurons [126].

Some rare-earth metal ions, including La3+ and Gd3+, have been shown to inhibit TRPC6 activity [106,127,133]. But since those ions inhibit all channels of the TRP family (except TRPM2), they cannot be used as selective TRPC6 antagonists. Clotrimazole (1-[(2-chlorophenyl)diphenyl-methyl]-1*H*-imidazole) is an imidazole compound, which inhibits TRPM2, TRPM3, TRPV4, and TRPC6 channels [90]. In SOCE mechanism studies, 2-aminoethoxydiphenyl borate (2-APB) [90] and 1-[2-[3-(4-methoxyphenyl)propoxy]-2-(4-methoxyphenyl)ethyl]-1H-imidazole hydrochloride

(SKF-96365) [162] are identified as agents targeting TRPC6. 2-APB blocks TRPC6 [163] and was later found to impact Orai channel functioning [164]. 2-APB has also been shown to block Ca^{2+} influx induced by acetylcholine or thapsigargin application but not by DAG [163]. SKF-96365 is considered to be an inhibitor of receptor- and store-operated elevation of intracellular calcium levels via entry through voltage-independent channels [162,165]. Studies have demonstrated successful blocking of TRPC6 using SKF-96365 (IC_{50} = 2 μM), but a less pronounced effect on TRPC3 is also observed (IC_{50} = 12 μM) [90]. 8009-5364 is another highly specific TRPC6 antagonist, which has an IC_{50} of 3.2 μM, and is considered a promising agent for the treatment of pulmonary hypertension [70]. Investigation of neuronal SOCE mechanism in striatal neurons has revealed 4-N-[2-(4-phenoxyphenyl)ethyl]quinazoline-4,6-diamine (EVP4593, Table 1) (IC_{50} = 300 nM [126]) to be an inhibitor of TRPC1 channels [166]. EVP4593 has also been found to target heteromeric but not homomeric TRCP1 channels [166]. Later on, EVP4593 was demonstrated to block Orai channels at 300 nM concentration [126]. In cultured hippocampal neurons exhibiting PSEN1ΔE9 mutation, TRPC6 hyperactivation is blocked by 30 nM EVP4593 [24]. EVP4593 has been shown to inhibit the nuclear factor kappa-b (NF-Kb) [167]. It has been also observed that NF-Kb downregulates TRPC6 protein expression [168]; thus, EVP4593-mediated inhibition of the NF-Kb pathway might cause an increase in TRPC6 protein expression. Whether this increase in TRPC6 protein expression would compete with EVP4593-mediated blockade of TRPC6-dependent SOCE is an open question.

8. Conclusions

The present review summarizes current knowledge on the role of TRPC6 channels in the development of two neurological disorders: Alzheimer's disease and cerebral ischemia. Cerebral ischemia serves as a risk factor for AD, and vice versa. It is becoming evident that both diseases can be caused by either upregulation or downregulation of TRPC6 channels. Thus, understanding the nature of the disruption of this molecular pathway in each particular patient is extremely important for appropriate drug prescription.

TRPC6 is structurally similar to TRPC3 and 7, and therefore the majority of compounds do not act selectively on either of these three isoforms, making it difficult to develop selective TRPC6 pharmacological modulators. Moreover, a number of TRPC6 channel modulators are cross-reactive to other cellular targets, thus limiting their pharmacological potential. Toxicity profiles of some known TRPC6 modulators (such as FFA) require further structural optimization. The presence of a wide range of different chemical substances that are known to interact with TRPC6 channels as well as the availability of cryo-electron microscopy structures of TRPC6 and 3 [169] may allow determining the pharmacophore in order to design selective TRPC6 activators and inhibitors in the future. In turn, the development of selective TRPC6 channel modulators could help slow down the progression of AD, cerebral ischemia, and, most likely, other TRPC6-dependent diseases.

Author Contributions: D.C., V.P., Y.S., N.Z., and E.P. wrote the review; E.P. and S.O. edited the review. All authors have read and agreed to the published version of the manuscript.

Acknowledgments: Authors thank Anastasiya Bolshakova for administrative support.

References

1. Forabosco, P.; Ramasamy, A.; Trabzuni, D.; Walker, R.; Smith, C.; Bras, J.; Levine, A.P.; Hardy, J.; Pocock, J.M.; Guerreiro, R.; et al. Insights into TREM2 biology by network analysis of human brain gene expression data. *Neurobiol. Aging* **2013**, *34*, 2699–2714. [CrossRef] [PubMed]
2. Dirnagl, U.; Iadecola, C.; Moskowitz, M.A. Pathobiology of ischaemic stroke: An integrated view. *Trends Neurosci.* **1999**, *22*, 391–397. [CrossRef]

3. Lipton, P. Ischemic cell death in brain neurons. *Physiol. Rev.* **1999**, *79*, 1431–1568. [CrossRef] [PubMed]
4. Zhou, J.; Yu, J.; Wang, H.; Meng, X.; Tan, C.; Wang, J.; Wang, C.; Tan, L. Association between Stroke and Alzheimer's Disease: Systematic Review and Meta-Analysis. *J. Alzheimers Dis.* **2015**, *43*, 479–489. [CrossRef]
5. Chi, N.-F.; Chien, L.-N.; Ku, H.-L.; Hu, C.-J.; Chiou, H.-Y. Alzheimer disease and risk of stroke: A population-based cohort study. *Neurology* **2013**, *80*, 705–711. [CrossRef]
6. Tolppanen, A.; Lavikainen, P.; Solomon, A.; Kivipelto, M.; Esoininen, H.; Hartikainen, S. Incidence of stroke in people with Alzheimer disease: A national register-based approach. *Neurology* **2013**, *80*, 353–358. [CrossRef]
7. Wang, R.; Reddy, P.H. Role of Glutamate and NMDA Receptors in Alzheimer's Disease. *J. Alzheimers Dis.* **2017**, *57*, 1041–1048. [CrossRef]
8. Chen, M.; Lu, T.-J.; Chen, X.-J.; Zhou, Y.; Chen, Q.; Feng, X.-Y.; Xu, L.; Duan, W.-H.; Xiong, Z.-Q. Differential roles of NMDA receptor subtypes in ischemic neuronal cell death and ischemic tolerance. *Stroke* **2008**, *39*, 3042–3048. [CrossRef]
9. Grossberg, G.T.; Thomas, S.J. Memantine: A review of studies into its safety and efficacy in treating Alzheimer's disease and other dementias. *Clin. Interv. Aging* **2009**, *4*, 367–377. [CrossRef]
10. Schneider, L.S.; Dagerman, K.S.; Higgins, J.P.; McShane, R. Lack of Evidence for the Efficacy of Memantine in Mild Alzheimer Disease. *Arch. Neurol.* **2011**, *68*, 991. [CrossRef]
11. Hoyte, L.; Barber, P.A.; Buchan, A.M.; Hill, M.D. The rise and fall of NMDA antagonists for ischemic stroke. *Curr. Mol. Med.* **2004**, *4*, 131–136. [CrossRef] [PubMed]
12. Ginsberg, M.D. Neuroprotection for ischemic stroke: Past, present and future. *Neuropharmacology* **2008**, *55*, 363–389. [CrossRef] [PubMed]
13. Zhou, J.; Du, W.; Zhou, K.; Tai, Y.; Yao, H.; Jia, Y.; Ding, Y.; Wang, Y. Critical role of TRPC6 channels in the formation of excitatory synapses. *Nat. Neurosci.* **2008**, *11*, 741–743. [CrossRef]
14. Zhang, H.; Sun, S.; Wu, L.; Pchitskaya, E.; Zakharova, O.; Tacer, K.F.; Bezprozvanny, I. Store-Operated Calcium Channel Complex in Postsynaptic Spines: A New Therapeutic Target for Alzheimer's Disease Treatment. *J. Neurosci.* **2016**, *36*, 11837–11850. [CrossRef] [PubMed]
15. Shen, H.; Pan, J.; Pan, L.; Zhang, N. TRPC6 inhibited NMDA current in cultured hippocampal neurons. *Neuromol. Med.* **2013**, *15*, 389–395. [CrossRef]
16. Li, H.; Huang, J.; Du, W.; Jia, C.; Yao, H.; Wang, Y. TRPC6 inhibited NMDA receptor activities and protected neurons from ischemic excitotoxicity. *J. Neurochem.* **2012**, *123*, 1010–1018. [CrossRef]
17. Tai, Y.; Feng, S.; Ge, R.; Du, W.; Zhang, X.; He, Z.; Wang, Y. TRPC6 channels promote dendritic growth via the CaMKIV-CREB pathway. *J. Cell Sci.* **2008**, *121*, 2301–2307. [CrossRef]
18. Guilbert, A.; Dhennin-Duthille, I.; El Hiani, Y.; Haren, N.; Khorsi, H.; Sevestre, H.; Ahidouch, A.; Ouadid-Ahidouch, H. Expression of TRPC6 channels in human epithelial breast cancer cells. *BMC Cancer* **2008**, *8*, 125. [CrossRef]
19. Ramirez, G.A.; Coletto, L.A.; Sciorati, C.; Bozzolo, E.P.; Manunta, P.; Rovere-Querini, P.; Manfredi, A.A. Ion Channels and Transporters in Inflammation: Special Focus on TRP Channels and TRPC6. *Cells* **2018**, *7*, 70. [CrossRef]
20. Santín, S.; Ars, E.; Rossetti, S.; Salido, E.; Silva, I.; García-Maset, R.; Giménez, I.; Ruíz, P.; Mendizábal, S.; Nieto, J.L.; et al. TRPC6 mutational analysis in a large cohort of patients with focal segmental glomerulosclerosis. *Nephrol. Dial. Transplant.* **2009**, *24*, 3089–3096. [CrossRef]
21. Popugaeva, E.; Chernyuk, D.; Zhang, H.; Postnikova, T.Y.; Pats, K.; Fedorova, E.; Poroikov, V.; Zaitsev, A.V.; Bezprozvanny, I.; Cherniuk, D.; et al. Derivatives of Piperazines as Potential Therapeutic Agents for Alzheimer's Disease. *Mol. Pharmacol.* **2019**, *95*, 337–348. [CrossRef] [PubMed]
22. Lessard, C.B.; Lussier, M.P.; Cayouette, S.; Bourque, G.; Boulay, G. The overexpression of presenilin2 and Alzheimer's-disease-linked presenilin2 variants influences TRPC6-enhanced Ca^{2+} entry into HEK293 cells. *Cell. Signal.* **2005**, *17*, 437–445. [CrossRef]
23. Liu, L.; Gu, L.; Chen, M.; Zheng, Y.; Xiong, X.; Zhu, S. Novel Targets for Stroke Therapy: Special Focus on TRPC Channels and TRPC6. *Front. Aging Neurosci.* **2020**, *12*, 70. [CrossRef]
24. Chernyuk, D.; Zernov, N.; Kabirova, M.; Bezprozvanny, I.; Popugaeva, E. Antagonist of neuronal store-operated calcium entry exerts beneficial effects in neurons expressing PSEN1ΔE9 mutant linked to familial Alzheimer disease. *Neuroscience* **2019**, *410*, 118–127. [CrossRef] [PubMed]

25. Chen, J.; Li, Z.; Hatcher, J.T.; Chen, Q.-H.; Chen, L.; Wurster, R.D.; Chan, S.L.; Cheng, Z. Deletion of TRPC6 Attenuates NMDA Receptor-Mediated Ca(2+) Entry and Ca(2+)-Induced Neurotoxicity Following Cerebral Ischemia and Oxygen-Glucose Deprivation. *Front. Neurosci.* **2017**, *11*, 138. [CrossRef] [PubMed]
26. Chen, X.; Lu, M.; He, X.; Ma, L.; Birnbaumer, L.; Liao, Y. TRPC3/6/7 Knockdown Protects the Brain from Cerebral Ischemia Injury via Astrocyte Apoptosis Inhibition and Effects on NF-small ka, CyrillicB Translocation. *Mol. Neurobiol.* **2017**, *54*, 7555–7566. [CrossRef]
27. Wang, J.; Lu, R.; Yang, J.; Li, H.; He, Z.; Jing, N.; Wang, X.; Wang, Y. TRPC6 specifically interacts with APP to inhibit its cleavage by gamma-secretase and reduce Abeta production. *Nat. Commun.* **2015**, *6*, 8876. [CrossRef] [PubMed]
28. Venkatachalam, K.; Montell, C. TRP channels. *Annu. Rev. Biochem.* **2007**, *76*, 387–417. [CrossRef]
29. Sun, Y.; Sukumaran, P.; Bandyopadhyay, B.C.; Singh, B.B. Physiological Function and Characterization of TRPCs in Neurons. *Cells* **2014**, *3*, 455–475. [CrossRef]
30. Montell, C. The TRP superfamily of cation channels. *Sci. Signal.* **2005**, *2005*, re3. [CrossRef]
31. Dietrich, A.; Gudermann, T. TRPC6: Physiological function and pathophysiological relevance. *Handb. Exp. Pharmacol.* **2014**, *222*, 157–188. [PubMed]
32. Hofmann, T.; Obukhov, A.G.; Schaefer, M.; Harteneck, C.; Gudermann, T.; Schultz, G. Direct activation of human TRPC6 and TRPC3 channels by diacylglycerol. *Nature* **1999**, *397*, 259–263. [CrossRef] [PubMed]
33. Prakriya, M.; Lewis, R.S. Store-Operated Calcium Channels. *Physiol. Rev.* **2015**, *95*, 1383–1436. [CrossRef]
34. Roos, J.; Digregorio, P.J.; Yeromin, A.V.; Ohlsen, K.; Lioudyno, M.; Zhang, S.; Safrina, O.; Kozak, J.A.; Wagner, S.L.; Cahalan, M.D.; et al. STIM1, an essential and conserved component of store-operated Ca^{2+} channel function. *J. Cell Biol.* **2005**, *169*, 435–445. [CrossRef]
35. Zhang, S.L.; Yu, Y.; Roos, J.; Kozak, J.A.; Deerinck, T.J.; Ellisman, M.H.; Stauderman, K.A.; Cahalan, M.D. STIM1 is a Ca^{2+} sensor that activates CRAC channels and migrates from the Ca^{2+} store to the plasma membrane. *Nature* **2005**, *437*, 902–905. [CrossRef] [PubMed]
36. Liou, J.; Kim, M.L.; Heo, W.D.; Jones, J.T.; Myers, J.W.; Ferrell, J.E.; Meyer, T. STIM is a Ca^{2+} sensor essential for Ca^{2+}-store-depletion-triggered Ca^{2+} influx. *Curr. Biol.* **2005**, *15*, 1235–1241. [CrossRef]
37. Feske, S.; Gwack, Y.; Prakriya, M.; Srikanth, S.; Puppel, S.-H.; Tanasa, B.; Hogan, P.G.; Lewis, R.S.; Daly, M.J.; Rao, A. A mutation in Orai1 causes immune deficiency by abrogating CRAC channel function. *Nature* **2006**, *441*, 179–185. [CrossRef]
38. Sun, S.; Zhang, H.; Liu, J.; Popugaeva, E.; Xu, N.-J.; Feske, S.; White, C.L.; Bezprozvanny, I. Reduced synaptic STIM2 expression and impaired store-operated calcium entry cause destabilization of mature spines in mutant presenilin mice. *Neuron* **2014**, *82*, 79–93. [CrossRef]
39. Popugaeva, E.; Pchitskaya, E.; Speshilova, A.B.; Alexandrov, S.; Zhang, H.; Vlasova, O.L.; Bezprozvanny, I. STIM2 protects hippocampal mushroom spines from amyloid synaptotoxicity. *Mol. Neurodegener.* **2015**, *10*, 37. [CrossRef]
40. Qu, Z.; Wang, Y.; Li, X.; Wu, L.; Wang, Y. TRPC6 expression in neurons is differentially regulated by NR2A- and NR2B-containing NMDA receptors. *J. Neurochem.* **2017**, *143*, 282–293. [CrossRef]
41. Tu, H.; Nelson, O.; Bezprozvanny, A.; Wang, Z.; Lee, S.; Hao, Y.; Serneels, L.; de Strooper, B.; Yu, G.; Bezprozvanny, I. Presenilins form ER calcium leak channels, a function disrupted by mutations linked to familial Alzheimer's disease. *Cell* **2006**, *126*, 981–993. [CrossRef] [PubMed]
42. Zatti, G.; Burgo, A.; Giacomello, M.; Barbiero, L.; Ghidoni, R.; Sinigaglia, G.; Florean, C.; Bagnoli, S.; Binetti, G.; Sorbi, S.; et al. Presenilin mutations linked to familial Alzheimer's disease reduce endoplasmic reticulum and Golgi apparatus calcium levels. *Cell Calcium* **2006**, *39*, 539–550. [CrossRef] [PubMed]
43. Zhang, H.; Sun, S.; Herreman, A.; De Strooper, B.; Bezprozvanny, I. Role of presenilins in neuronal calcium homeostasis. *J. Neurosci.* **2010**, *30*, 8566–8580. [CrossRef] [PubMed]
44. Zhang, H.; Liu, J.; Sun, S.; Pchitskaya, E.; Popugaeva, E.; Bezprozvanny, I. Calcium signaling, excitability, and synaptic plasticity defects in a mouse model of Alzheimer's disease. *J. Alzheimers Dis.* **2015**, *45*, 561–580. [CrossRef]
45. Tong, B.C.; Lee, C.S.; Cheng, W.; Lai, K.; Foskett, J.K.; Cheung, K. Familial Alzheimer's disease-associated presenilin 1 mutants promote gamma-secretase cleavage of STIM1 to impair store-operated Ca^{2+} entry. *Sci. Signal.* **2016**, *9*, ra89. [CrossRef]

46. Bojarski, L.; Pomorski, P.; Szybinska, A.; Drab, M.; Skibinska-Kijek, A.; Gruszczynska-Biegala, J.; Kuznicki, J. Presenilin-dependent expression of STIM proteins and dysregulation of capacitative Ca^{2+} entry in familial Alzheimer's disease. *Biochim. Biophys. Acta* **2009**, *1793*, 1050–1057. [CrossRef]
47. Popugaeva, E.; Pchitskaya, E.; Bezprozvanny, I. Dysregulation of neuronal calcium homeostasis in Alzheimer's disease—A therapeutic opportunity? *Biochem. Biophys. Res. Commun.* **2017**, *483*, 998–1004. [CrossRef]
48. Pchitskaya, E.; Popugaeva, E.; Bezprozvanny, I. Calcium signaling and molecular mechanisms underlying neurodegenerative diseases. *Cell Calcium* **2018**, *70*, 87–94. [CrossRef]
49. Popugaeva, E.; Chernyuk, D.; Bezprozvanny, I. Correction of calcium dysregulation as potential approach for treating Alzheimer's disease. *Curr. Alzheimer Res.* **2019**, in press.
50. Ryazantseva, M.A.; Goncharova, A.; Skobeleva, K.; Erokhin, M.; Methner, A.; Georgiev, P.; Kaznacheyeva, E.V. Presenilin-1 Delta E9 Mutant Induces STIM1-Driven Store-Operated Calcium Channel Hyperactivation in Hippocampal Neurons. *Mol. Neurobiol.* **2017**, *55*, 4667–4680. [CrossRef]
51. Yoo, A.S.; Cheng, I.; Chung, S.; Grenfell, T.Z.; Lee, H.; Pack-Chung, E.; Handler, M.; Shen, J.; Xia, W.; Tesco, G.; et al. Presenilin-mediated modulation of capacitative calcium entry. *Neuron* **2000**, *27*, 561–572. [CrossRef]
52. Zhang, X.; Le, W. Pathological role of hypoxia in Alzheimer's disease. *Exp. Neurol.* **2010**, *223*, 299–303. [CrossRef]
53. Vijayan, M.; Reddy, P.H. Stroke, Vascular Dementia, and Alzheimer's Disease: Molecular Links. *J. Alzheimers Dis.* **2016**, *54*, 427–443. [CrossRef] [PubMed]
54. Olichney, J.M.; Hansen, L.A.; Galasko, D.; Saitoh, T.; Hofstetter, C.R.; Katzman, R.; Thal, L.J. The apolipoprotein E epsilon 4 allele is associated with increased neuritic plaques and cerebral amyloid angiopathy in Alzheimer's disease and Lewy body variant. *Neurology* **1996**, *47*, 190–196. [CrossRef] [PubMed]
55. Premkumar, D.R.; Cohen, D.L.; Hedera, P.; Friedland, R.P.; Kalaria, R.N. Apolipoprotein E-epsilon4 alleles in cerebral amyloid angiopathy and cerebrovascular pathology associated with Alzheimer's disease. *Am. J. Pathol.* **1996**, *148*, 2083–2095.
56. Xing, C.; Arai, K.; Lo, E.H.; Hommel, M. Pathophysiologic cascades in ischemic stroke. *Int. J. Stroke* **2012**, *7*, 378–385. [CrossRef] [PubMed]
57. Szydlowska, K.; Tymianski, M. Calcium, ischemia and excitotoxicity. *Cell Calcium* **2010**, *47*, 122–129. [CrossRef]
58. Wang, X.; Teng, L.; Li, A.; Ge, J.; Laties, A.M.; Zhang, X. TRPC6 channel protects retinal ganglion cells in a rat model of retinal ischemia/reperfusion-induced cell death. *Investig. Opthalmol. Vis. Sci.* **2010**, *51*, 5751–5758. [CrossRef]
59. Nakuluri, K.; Nishad, R.; Mukhi, D.; Kumar, S.; Nakka, V.P.; Kolligundla, L.P.; Narne, P.; Natuva, S.S.K.; Phanithi, P.B.; Pasupulati, A.K. Cerebral ischemia induces TRPC6 via HIF1alpha/ZEB2 axis in the glomerular podocytes and contributes to proteinuria. *Sci. Rep.* **2019**, *9*, 17897. [CrossRef]
60. Jia, Y.; Zhou, J.; Tai, Y.; Wang, Y. TRPC channels promote cerebellar granule neuron survival. *Nat. Neurosci.* **2007**, *10*, 559–567. [CrossRef]
61. Li, Y.; Jia, Y.; Cui, K.; Li, N.; Zheng, Z.-Y.; Wang, Y.; Yuan, X.-B. Essential role of TRPC channels in the guidance of nerve growth cones by brain-derived neurotrophic factor. *Nature* **2005**, *434*, 894–898. [CrossRef] [PubMed]
62. Caracciolo, L.; Marosi, M.; Mazzitelli, J.; Latifi, S.; Sano, Y.; Galvan, L.; Kawaguchi, R.; Holley, S.; Levine, M.S.; Coppola, G.; et al. CREB controls cortical circuit plasticity and functional recovery after stroke. *Nat. Commun.* **2018**, *9*, 2250. [CrossRef] [PubMed]
63. McCullough, L.D.; Tarabishy, S.; Liu, L.; Benashski, S.; Xu, Y.; Ribar, T.; Means, A.; Li, J. Inhibition of calcium/calmodulin-dependent protein kinase kinase beta and calcium/calmodulin-dependent protein kinase IV is detrimental in cerebral ischemia. *Stroke* **2013**, *44*, 2559–2566. [CrossRef] [PubMed]
64. Du, W.; Huang, J.; Yao, H.; Zhou, K.; Duan, B.; Wang, Y. Inhibition of TRPC6 degradation suppresses ischemic brain damage in rats. *J. Clin. Investig.* **2010**, *120*, 3480–3492. [CrossRef]
65. Fu, J.; Xue, R.; Gu, J.; Xiao, Y.; Zhong, H.; Pan, X.; Ran, R. Neuroprotective effect of calcitriol on ischemic/reperfusion injury through the NR3A/CREB pathways in the rat hippocampus. *Mol. Med. Rep.* **2013**, *8*, 1708–1714. [CrossRef]
66. Lin, Y.; Chen, F.; Zhang, J.; Wang, T.; Wei, X.; Wu, J.; Feng, Y.; Dai, Z.; Wu, Q. Neuroprotective effect of resveratrol on ischemia/reperfusion injury in rats through TRPC6/CREB pathways. *J. Mol. Neurosci.* **2013**, *50*, 504–513. [CrossRef]

67. Omura, T.; Tanaka, Y.; Miyata, N.; Koizumi, C.; Sakurai, T.; Fukasawa, M.; Hachiuma, K.; Minagawa, T.; Susumu, T.; Yoshida, S.; et al. Effect of a new inhibitor of the synthesis of 20-HETE on cerebral ischemia reperfusion injury. *Stroke* **2006**, *37*, 1307–1313. [CrossRef]
68. Renic, M.; Klaus, J.A.; Omura, T.; Kawashima, N.; Onishi, M.; Miyata, N.; Koehler, R.C.; Harder, D.R.; Roman, R.J. Effect of 20-HETE inhibition on infarct volume and cerebral blood flow after transient middle cerebral artery occlusion. *Br. J. Pharmacol.* **2008**, *29*, 629–639. [CrossRef]
69. Shaik, J.S.B.; Poloyac, S.M.; Kochanek, P.M.; Alexander, H.; Tudorascu, D.L.; Clark, R.S.; Manole, M.D. 20-Hydroxyeicosatetraenoic Acid Inhibition by HET0016 Offers Neuroprotection, Decreases Edema, and Increases Cortical Cerebral Blood Flow in a Pediatric Asphyxial Cardiac Arrest Model in Rats. *Br. J. Pharmacol.* **2015**, *35*, 1757–1763. [CrossRef]
70. Urban, N.; Hill, K.; Wang, L.; Kuebler, W.M.; Schaefer, M. Novel pharmacological TRPC inhibitors block hypoxia-induced vasoconstriction. *Cell Calcium* **2012**, *51*, 194–206. [CrossRef]
71. Maier, T.; Follmann, M.; Hessler, G.; Kleemann, H.-W.; Hachtel, S.; Fuchs, B.; Weissmann, N.; Linz, W.; Schmidt, T.; Löhn, M.; et al. Discovery and pharmacological characterization of a novel potent inhibitor of diacylglycerol-sensitive TRPC cation channels. *Br. J. Pharmacol.* **2015**, *172*, 3650–3660. [CrossRef] [PubMed]
72. Urban, N.; Wang, L.; Kwiek, S.; Rademann, J.; Kuebler, W.M.; Schaefer, M. Identification and Validation of Larixyl Acetate as a Potent TRPC6 Inhibitor. *Mol. Pharmacol.* **2015**, *89*, 197–213. [CrossRef] [PubMed]
73. Hou, X.; Xiao, H.; Zhang, Y.; Zeng, X.; Huang, M.; Chen, X.; Birnbaumer, L.; Liao, Y. Transient receptor potential channel 6 knockdown prevents apoptosis of renal tubular epithelial cells upon oxidative stress via autophagy activation. *Cell Death Dis.* **2018**, *9*, 1015. [CrossRef] [PubMed]
74. Chen, X.; Taylor-Nguyen, N.N.; Riley, A.M.; Herring, B.P.; White, F.A.; Obukhov, A.G. The TRPC6 inhibitor, larixyl acetate, is effective in protecting against traumatic brain injury-induced systemic endothelial dysfunction. *J. Neuroinflamm.* **2019**, *16*, 21. [CrossRef]
75. Cross, J.L.; Meloni, B.P.; Bakker, A.J.; Lee, S.; Knuckey, N.W. Modes of Neuronal Calcium Entry and Homeostasis following Cerebral Ischemia. *Stroke Res. Treat.* **2010**, *2010*, 316862. [CrossRef]
76. Wu, Q.J.; Tymianski, M. Targeting NMDA receptors in stroke: New hope in neuroprotection. *Mol. Brain* **2018**, *11*, 15. [CrossRef]
77. Basora, N.; Boulay, G.; Bilodeau, L.; Payet, M.D.; Rousseau, E. 20-hydroxyeicosatetraenoic acid (20-HETE) activates mouse TRPC6 channels expressed in HEK293 cells. *J. Biol. Chem.* **2003**, *278*, 31709–31716. [CrossRef]
78. Aires, V.; Hichami, A.; Boulay, G.; Khan, N.A. Activation of TRPC6 calcium channels by diacylglycerol (DAG)-containing arachidonic acid: A comparative study with DAG-containing docosahexaenoic acid. *Biochim.* **2007**, *89*, 926–937. [CrossRef]
79. Belayev, L.; Khoutorova, L.; Atkins, K.D.; Eady, T.N.; Hong, S.; Lu, Y.; Obenaus, A.; Bazan, N.G. Docosahexaenoic Acid therapy of experimental ischemic stroke. *Transl. Stroke Res.* **2010**, *2*, 33–41. [CrossRef]
80. Yao, C.; Zhang, J.; Chen, F.; Lin, Y. Neuroprotectin D1 attenuates brain damage induced by transient middle cerebral artery occlusion in rats through TRPC6/CREB pathways. *Mol. Med. Rep.* **2013**, *8*, 543–550. [CrossRef]
81. Guinamard, R.; Simard, C.; Del Negro, C. Flufenamic acid as an ion channel modulator. *Pharmacol. Ther.* **2013**, *138*, 272–284. [CrossRef] [PubMed]
82. Qu, C.; Ding, M.; Zhu, Y.; Lu, Y.; Du, J.; Miller, M.; Tian, J.; Zhu, J.; Xu, J.; Wen, M.; et al. Pyrazolopyrimidines as Potent Stimulators for Transient Receptor Potential Canonical 3/6/7 Channels. *J. Med. Chem.* **2017**, *60*, 4680–4692. [CrossRef] [PubMed]
83. Sawamura, S.; Hatano, M.; Takada, Y.; Hino, K.; Kawamura, T.; Tanikawa, J.; Nakagawa, H.; Hase, H.; Nakao, A.; Hirano, M.; et al. Screening of Transient Receptor Potential Canonical Channel Activators Identifies Novel Neurotrophic Piperazine Compounds. *Mol. Pharmacol.* **2016**, *89*, 348–363. [CrossRef] [PubMed]
84. Tiapko, O.; Shrestha, N.; Lindinger, S.; De La Cruz, G.G.; Graziani, A.; Klec, C.; Butorac, C.; Graier, W.F.; Kubista, H.; Freichel, M.; et al. Lipid-independent control of endothelial and neuronal TRPC3 channels by light. *Chem. Sci.* **2019**, *10*, 2837–2842. [CrossRef]
85. Häfner, S.; Urban, N.; Schaefer, M. Discovery and characterization of a positive allosteric modulator of transient receptor potential canonical 6 (TRPC6) channels. *Cell Calcium* **2019**, *78*, 26–34. [CrossRef]
86. Guo, C.; Tong, L.; Xi, M.; Yang, H.; Dong, H.; Wen, A. Neuroprotective effect of calycosin on cerebral ischemia and reperfusion injury in rats. *J. Ethnopharmacol.* **2012**, *144*, 768–774. [CrossRef]

87. Yao, C.; Zhang, J.; Liu, G.; Chen, F.; Lin, Y. Neuroprotection by (−)-epigallocatechin-3-gallate in a rat model of stroke is mediated through inhibition of endoplasmic reticulum stress. *Mol. Med. Rep.* **2014**, *9*, 69–76. [CrossRef]
88. Sysoev, Y.I.; Uzuegbunam, B.C.; Okovityi, S.V. Attenuation of neurological deficit by a novel ethanolamine derivative in rats after brain trauma. *J. Exp. Pharmacol.* **2019**, *11*, 53–63. [CrossRef]
89. Sysoev, Y.I.; Popugaeva, E.A.; Chernyuk, D.P.; Titovich, I.A.; Zagladkina, E.V.; Bolotova, V.C.; Bezprozvanny, I.; Okovityi, S.V. Mechanism of action of the new ethanolamine derivative bis{2-[(2E)-4-hydroxy-4-oxobut-2-enoyloxy]-N,N-diethylethanaminium}butanedioate. *Eksperimental'naya Klin. Farmakol.* **2019**, *82*, 3–10.
90. Harteneck, C.; Klose, C.; Krautwurst, D. Synthetic modulators of TRP channel activity. *Adv. Exp. Med. Biol.* **2011**, *704*, 87–106.
91. Tu, P.; Kunert-Keil, C.; Lucke, S.; Brinkmeier, H.; Bouron, A. Diacylglycerol analogues activate second messenger-operated calcium channels exhibiting TRPC-like properties in cortical neurons. *J. Neurochem.* **2009**, *108*, 126–138. [CrossRef] [PubMed]
92. Montecinos-Oliva, C.; Schuller, A.; Parodi, J.; Melo, F.; Inestrosa, N.C. Effects of tetrahydrohyperforin in mouse hippocampal slices: Neuroprotection, long-term potentiation and TRPC channels. *Curr. Med. Chem.* **2014**, *21*, 3494–3506. [CrossRef] [PubMed]
93. Law, S.-H.; Chan, M.-L.; Marathe, G.K.; Parveen, F.; Chen, C.-H.; Ke, L.-Y. An Updated Review of Lysophosphatidylcholine Metabolism in Human Diseases. *Int. J. Mol. Sci.* **2019**, *20*, 1149. [CrossRef] [PubMed]
94. Koizumi, S.; Yamamoto, S.; Hayasaka, T.; Konishi, Y.; Yamaguchi-Okada, M.; Goto-Inoue, N.; Sugiura, Y.; Setou, M.; Namba, H. Imaging mass spectrometry revealed the production of lyso-phosphatidylcholine in the injured ischemic rat brain. *Neuroscience* **2010**, *168*, 219–225. [CrossRef]
95. Sabogal-Guáqueta, A.M.; Posada-Duque, R.; Cortes, N.C.; Arias-Londoño, J.D.; Cardona-Gómez, G.P. Changes in the hippocampal and peripheral phospholipid profiles are associated with neurodegeneration hallmarks in a long-term global cerebral ischemia model: Attenuation by Linalool. *Neuropharmacology* **2018**, *135*, 555–571. [CrossRef]
96. Jickling, G.C.; Montaner, J. Lysophosphatidylcholine to stratify risk of ischemic stroke in TIA. *Neurology* **2014**, *84*, 17–18. [CrossRef]
97. Chaudhuri, P.; Colles, S.M.; Damron, D.S.; Graham, L.M. Lysophosphatidylcholine inhibits endothelial cell migration by increasing intracellular calcium and activating calpain. *Arter. Thromb. Vasc. Biol.* **2003**, *23*, 218–223. [CrossRef]
98. Chaudhuri, P.; Rosenbaum, M.A.; Birnbaumer, L.; Graham, L.M. Integration of TRPC6 and NADPH oxidase activation in lysophosphatidylcholine-induced TRPC5 externalization. *Am. J. Physiol. Physiol.* **2017**, *313*, C541–C555. [CrossRef]
99. Cloutier, M.; Campbell, S.; Basora, N.; Proteau, S.; Payet, M.D.; Rousseau, E. 20-HETE inotropic effects involve the activation of a nonselective cationic current in airway smooth muscle. *Am. J. Physiol. Cell. Mol. Physiol.* **2003**, *285*, L560–L568. [CrossRef]
100. Lu, L.; Wang, M.; Wei, X.; Li, W. Corrigendum: 20-HETE Inhibition by HET0016 Decreases the Blood-Brain Barrier Permeability and Brain Edema After Traumatic Brain Injury. *Front. Aging Neurosci.* **2018**, *10*, 207. [CrossRef]
101. Wen, H.; Östman, J.; Bubb, K.J.; Panayiotou, C.; Priestley, J.V.; Baker, M.D.; Ahluwalia, A. 20-Hydroxyeicosatetraenoic acid (20-HETE) is a novel activator of transient receptor potential vanilloid 1 (TRPV1) channel. *J. Biol. Chem.* **2012**, *287*, 13868–13876. [CrossRef] [PubMed]
102. Asatryan, A.; Bazan, N.G. Molecular mechanisms of signaling via the docosanoid neuroprotectin D1 for cellular homeostasis and neuroprotection. *J. Biol. Chem.* **2017**, *292*, 12390–12397. [CrossRef] [PubMed]
103. Yao, H.; Zhang, Y.; Shu, H.; Xie, B.; Tao, Y.; Yuan, Y.; Shang, Y.; Yuan, S.; Zhang, J. Hyperforin Promotes Post-stroke Neuroangiogenesis via Astrocytic IL-6-Mediated Negative Immune Regulation in the Ischemic Brain. *Front. Cell. Neurosci.* **2019**, *13*, 201. [CrossRef] [PubMed]
104. Kumar, V.; Mdzinarishvili, A.; Kiewert, C.; Abbruscato, T.; Bickel, U.; Van Der Schyf, C.J.; Klein, J. NMDA receptor-antagonistic properties of hyperforin, a constituent of St. John's Wort. *J. Pharmacol. Sci.* **2006**, *102*, 47–54. [CrossRef]

105. Dinamarca, M.C.; Cerpa, W.; Garrido, J.; Hancke, J.L.; Inestrosa, N.C. Hyperforin prevents beta-amyloid neurotoxicity and spatial memory impairments by disaggregation of Alzheimer's amyloid-beta-deposits. *Mol. Psychiatry* **2006**, *11*, 1032–1048. [CrossRef]
106. Leuner, K.; Li, W.; Amaral, M.D.; Rudolph, S.; Calfa, G.; Schuwald, A.M.; Harteneck, C.; Inoue, T.; Pozzo-Miller, L. Hyperforin modulates dendritic spine morphology in hippocampal pyramidal neurons by activating Ca(2+) -permeable TRPC6 channels. *Hippocampus* **2012**, *23*, 40–52. [CrossRef]
107. Zhang, Y.; Yu, P.; Liu, H.; Yao, H.; Yao, S.; Yuan, S.; Zhang, J.-C. Hyperforin improves post-stroke social isolation-induced exaggeration of PSD and PSA via TGF-β. *Int. J. Mol. Med.* **2018**, *43*, 413–425. [CrossRef]
108. Ma, L.; Pan, X.; Zhou, F.; Liu, K.; Wang, L. Hyperforin protects against acute cerebral ischemic injury through inhibition of interleukin-17A-mediated microglial activation. *Brain Res.* **2018**, *1678*, 254–261. [CrossRef]
109. Zhang, J.; Yao, C.; Chen, J.; Zhang, Y.; Yuan, S.; Lin, Y. Hyperforin promotes post-stroke functional recovery through interleukin (IL)−17A-mediated angiogenesis. *Brain Res.* **2016**, *1646*, 504–513. [CrossRef]
110. Lin, Y.; Zhang, J.-C.; Fu, J.; Chen, F.; Wang, J.; Wu, Z.-L.; Yuan, S.-Y. Hyperforin attenuates brain damage induced by transient middle cerebral artery occlusion (mcao) in rats via inhibition of TRPC6 channels degradation. *Br. J. Pharmacol.* **2012**, *33*, 253–262. [CrossRef]
111. Cerpa, W.; Hancke, J.L.; Morazzoni, P.; Bombardelli, E.; Riva, A.; Marin, P.P.; Inestrosa, N.C. The hyperforin derivative IDN5706 occludes spatial memory impairments and neuropathological changes in a double transgenic Alzheimer's mouse model. *Curr. Alzheimer Res.* **2010**, *7*, 126–133. [CrossRef] [PubMed]
112. Clark, D.; Tuor, U.I.; Thompson, R.; Institoris, A.; Kulynych, A.; Zhang, X.; Kinniburgh, D.W.; Bari, F.; Busija, D.W.; Barber, P.A. Protection against recurrent stroke with resveratrol: Endothelial protection. *PLoS ONE* **2012**, *7*, e47792. [CrossRef] [PubMed]
113. Narayanan, S.V.; Dave, K.R.; Saul, I.; Perez-Pinzon, M.A. Resveratrol Preconditioning Protects Against Cerebral Ischemic Injury via Nuclear Erythroid 2-Related Factor 2. *Stroke* **2015**, *46*, 1626–1632. [CrossRef] [PubMed]
114. Dong, W.; Li, N.; Gao, D.; Zhen, H.; Zhang, X.; Li, F. Resveratrol attenuates ischemic brain damage in the delayed phase after stroke and induces messenger RNA and protein express for angiogenic factors. *J. Vasc. Surg.* **2008**, *48*, 709–714. [CrossRef]
115. Della-Morte, D.; Dave, K.R.; DeFazio, R.A.; Bao, Y.C.; Raval, A.P.; Perez-Pinzon, M.A. Resveratrol pretreatment protects rat brain from cerebral ischemic damage via a sirtuin 1-uncoupling protein 2 pathway. *Neuroscience* **2009**, *159*, 993–1002. [CrossRef]
116. Wang, Q.; Xu, J.; Rottinghaus, G.E.; Simonyi, A.; Lubahn, D.; Sun, G.Y.; Sun, A.Y. Resveratrol protects against global cerebral ischemic injury in gerbils. *Brain Res.* **2002**, *958*, 439–447. [CrossRef]
117. Drygalski, K.; Fereniec, E.; Koryciński, K.; Chomentowski, A.; Kiełczewska, A.; Odrzygóźdź, C.; Modzelewska, B. Resveratrol and Alzheimer's disease. From molecular pathophysiology to clinical trials. *Exp. Gerontol.* **2018**, *113*, 36–47. [CrossRef]
118. Jia, J.; Verma, S.; Nakayama, S.; Quillinan, N.; Grafe, M.R.; Hurn, P.D.; Herson, P.S. Sex differences in neuroprotection provided by inhibition of TRPM2 channels following experimental stroke. *J. Cereb. Blood Flow Metab.* **2011**, *31*, 2160–2168. [CrossRef]
119. Khansari, P.S.; Halliwell, R.F. Mechanisms Underlying Neuroprotection by the NSAID Mefenamic Acid in an Experimental Model of Stroke. *Front. Neurosci.* **2019**, *13*, 64. [CrossRef]
120. Titovich, I.A.; Sysoev, Y.I.; Bolotova, V.C.; Okovityi, S.V. Neurotropic activity of a new aminoethanol derivative under conditions of experimental brain ischemia. *Exp. Clin. Pharmacol. (Rus)* **2017**, *80*, 3–6.
121. Poloyac, S.M.; Zhang, Y.; Bies, R.R.; Kochanek, P.M.; Graham, S.H. Protective effect of the 20-HETE inhibitor het0016 on brain damage after temporary focal ischemia. *J. Cereb. Blood Flow Metab.* **2006**, *26*, 1551–1561. [CrossRef] [PubMed]
122. Zhu, J.; Wang, B.; Lee, J.-H.; Armstrong, J.S.; Kulikowicz, E.; Bhalala, U.S.; Martin, L.J.; Koehler, R.C.; Yang, Z.-J. Additive Neuroprotection of a 20-HETE Inhibitor with Delayed Therapeutic Hypothermia after Hypoxia-Ischemia in Neonatal Piglets. *Dev. Neurosci.* **2015**, *37*, 376–389. [CrossRef] [PubMed]
123. Yang, Z.-J.; Carter, E.L.; Kibler, K.K.; Kwansa, H.; Crafa, D.; Martin, L.J.; Roman, R.J.; Harder, D.R.; Koehler, R.C. Attenuation of neonatal ischemic brain damage using a 20-HETE synthesis inhibitor. *J. Neurochem.* **2012**, *121*, 168–179. [CrossRef] [PubMed]
124. Khansari, P.S.; Halliwell, R.F. Evidence for neuroprotection by the fenamate NSAID, mefenamic acid. *Neurochem. Int.* **2009**, *55*, 683–688. [CrossRef] [PubMed]

125. Daniels, M.J.D.; Rivers-Auty, J.; Schilling, T.; Spencer, N.G.; Watremez, W.; Fasolino, V.; Booth, S.J.; White, C.S.; Baldwin, A.G.; Freeman, S.; et al. Fenamate NSAIDs inhibit the NLRP3 inflammasome and protect against Alzheimer's disease in rodent models. *Nat. Commun.* **2016**, *7*, 12504. [CrossRef]
126. Chauvet, S.; Jarvis, L.; Chevallet, M.; Shrestha, N.; Groschner, K.; Bouron, A. Pharmacological Characterization of the Native Store-Operated Calcium Channels of Cortical Neurons from Embryonic Mouse Brain. *Front. Pharmacol.* **2016**, *7*, 486. [CrossRef]
127. Leuner, K.; Kazanski, V.; Muller, M.; Essin, K.; Henke, B.; Gollasch, M.; Harteneck, C.; Müller, W.E. Hyperforin—A key constituent of St. John's wort specifically activates TRPC6 channels. *FASEB J.* **2007**, *21*, 4101–4111. [CrossRef]
128. Leuner, K.; Heiser, J.H.; Derksen, S.; Mladenov, M.I.; Fehske, C.J.; Schubert, R.; Gollasch, M.; Schneider, G.; Harteneck, C.; Chatterjee, S.S.; et al. Simple 2,4-diacylphloroglucinols as classic transient receptor potential-6 activators—Identification of a novel pharmacophore. *Mol. Pharmacol.* **2009**, *77*, 368–377. [CrossRef]
129. Singer, A.; Wonnemann, M.; Müller, W.E. Hyperforin, a major antidepressant constituent of St. John's Wort, inhibits serotonin uptake by elevating free intracellular Na+1. *J. Pharmacol. Exp. Ther.* **1999**, *290*, 1363–1368.
130. Pochwat, B.; Szewczyk, B.; Kotarska, K.; Rafało-Ulińska, A.; Siwiec, M.; Sowa, J.E.; Tokarski, K.; Siwek, A.; Bouron, A.; Friedland, K.; et al. Hyperforin Potentiates Antidepressant-Like Activity of Lanicemine in Mice. *Front. Mol. Neurosci.* **2018**, *11*, 456. [CrossRef]
131. Gibon, J.; Deloulme, J.C.; Chevallier, T.; Ladevèze, E.; Abrous, D.N.; Bouron, A. The antidepressant hyperforin increases the phosphorylation of CREB and the expression of TrkB in a tissue-specific manner. *Int. J. Neuropsychopharmacol.* **2013**, *16*, 189–198. [CrossRef]
132. Inestrosa, N.C.; Tapia-Rojas, C.; Griffith, T.N.; Carvajal, F.J.; Benito, M.J.; Rivera-Dictter, A.; Alvarez, A.R.; Serrano, F.G.; Hancke, J.L.; Burgos, P.V.; et al. Tetrahydrohyperforin prevents cognitive deficit, Abeta deposition, tau phosphorylation and synaptotoxicity in the APPswe/PSEN1DeltaE9 model of Alzheimer's disease: A possible effect on APP processing. *Transl. Psychiatry* **2011**, *1*, e20. [CrossRef] [PubMed]
133. Müller, M.; Essin, K.; Hill, K.; Beschmann, H.; Rubant, S.; Schempp, C.M.; Gollasch, M.; Boehncke, W.H.; Harteneck, C.; Müller, W.E.; et al. Specific TRPC6 channel activation, a novel approach to stimulate keratinocyte differentiation. *J. Biol. Chem.* **2008**, *283*, 33942–33954. [CrossRef] [PubMed]
134. Moore, L.B.; Goodwin, B.; Jones, S.A.; Wisely, G.B.; Serabjit-Singh, C.J.; Willson, T.M.; Collins, J.L.; Kliewer, S.A. St. John's wort induces hepatic drug metabolism through activation of the pregnane X receptor. *Proc. Natl. Acad. Sci. USA* **2000**, *97*, 7500–7502. [CrossRef] [PubMed]
135. Ting, C.P.; Maimone, T.J. Total Synthesis of Hyperforin. *J. Am. Chem. Soc.* **2015**, *137*, 10516–10519. [CrossRef] [PubMed]
136. Woelk, H.; Burkard, G.; Grünwald, J. Benefits and risks of the hypericum extract LI 160: Drug monitoring study with 3250 patients. *J. Geriatr. Psychiatry Neurol.* **1994**, *7*, 34–38. [CrossRef]
137. Da Silva, D.D.; Arbo, M.D.; Valente, M.J.; Bastos, M.D.L.; Carmo, H. Hepatotoxicity of piperazine designer drugs: Comparison of different in vitro models. *Toxicol. Vitr.* **2015**, *29*, 987–996. [CrossRef]
138. Singh, N.; Agrawal, M.; Doré, S. Neuroprotective properties and mechanisms of resveratrol in in vitro and in vivo experimental cerebral stroke models. *ACS Chem. Neurosci.* **2013**, *4*, 1151–1162. [CrossRef]
139. Sun, A.Y.; Wang, Q.; Simonyi, A.; Sun, G.Y. Resveratrol as a therapeutic agent for neurodegenerative diseases. *Mol. Neurobiol.* **2010**, *41*, 375–383. [CrossRef]
140. Albani, D.; Polito, L.; Forloni, G. Sirtuins as novel targets for Alzheimer's disease and other neurodegenerative disorders: Experimental and genetic evidence. *J. Alzheimers Dis.* **2010**, *19*, 11–26. [CrossRef]
141. Anekonda, T.S. Resveratrol—A boon for treating Alzheimer's disease? *Brain Res. Rev.* **2006**, *52*, 316–326. [CrossRef]
142. Rasouri, S.; Lagouge, M.; Auwerx, J. SIRT1/PGC-1: A neuroprotective axis? *Med. Sci (Paris)* **2007**, *23*, 840–844. [CrossRef] [PubMed]
143. Turner, R.S.; Thomas, R.G.; Craft, S.; Van Dyck, C.H.; Mintzer, J.; Reynolds, B.A.; Brewer, J.B.; Rissman, R.A.; Raman, R.; Aisen, P.S.; et al. A randomized, double-blind, placebo-controlled trial of resveratrol for Alzheimer disease. *Neurology* **2015**, *85*, 1383–1391. [CrossRef] [PubMed]
144. Sawda, C.; Moussa, C.; Turner, R.S. Resveratrol for Alzheimer's disease. *Ann. N. Y. Acad. Sci.* **2017**, *1403*, 142–149. [CrossRef] [PubMed]

145. Piver, B.; Berthou, F.; Dreano, Y.; Lucas, D. Inhibition of CYP3A, CYP1A and CYP2E1 activities by resveratrol and other non volatile red wine components. *Toxicol. Lett.* **2001**, *125*, 83–91. [CrossRef]
146. Chow, H.-H.S.; Garland, L.L.; Hsu, C.-H.; Vining, D.R.; Chew, W.M.; Miller, J.A.; Perloff, M.; Crowell, J.A.; Alberts, D.S. Resveratrol modulates drug- and carcinogen-metabolizing enzymes in a healthy volunteer study. *Cancer Prev. Res.* **2010**, *3*, 1168–1175. [CrossRef]
147. Salehi, B.; Mishra, A.P.; Nigam, M.; Sener, B.; Kilic, M.; Sharifi-Rad, M.; Fokou, P.V.T.; Martins, N.; Sharifi-Rad, J. Resveratrol: A Double-Edged Sword in Health Benefits. *Biomedicines* **2018**, *6*, 91. [CrossRef] [PubMed]
148. Inoue, R.; Okada, T.; Onoue, H.; Hara, Y.; Shimizu, S.; Naitoh, S.; Ito, Y.; Mori, Y. The transient receptor potential protein homologue TRP6 is the essential component of vascular α 1-adrenoceptor-activated ca 2+-permeable cation channel. *Circ. Res.* **2001**, *88*, 325–332. [CrossRef]
149. Foster, R.R.; Zadeh, M.A.; Welsh, G.I.; Satchell, S.C.; Ye, Y.; Mathieson, P.W.; Bates, D.O.; Saleem, M.A. Flufenamic acid is a tool for investigating TRPC6-mediated calcium signalling in human conditionally immortalised podocytes and HEK293 cells. *Cell Calcium* **2009**, *45*, 384–390. [CrossRef]
150. Macianskiene, R.; Gwanyanya, A.; Sipido, K.; Vereecke, J.; Mubagwa, D.K. Induction of a novel cation current in cardiac ventricular myocytes by flufenamic acid and related drugs. *Br. J. Pharmacol.* **2010**, *161*, 416–429. [CrossRef]
151. Klose, C.; Straub, I.; Riehle, M.; Ranta, F.; Krautwurst, D.; Ullrich, S.; Meyerhof, W.; Harteneck, C. Fenamates as TRP channel blockers: Mefenamic acid selectively blocks TRPM3. *Br. J. Pharmacol.* **2011**, *162*, 1757–1769. [CrossRef] [PubMed]
152. Hu, H.; Tian, J.; Zhu, Y.; Wang, C.; Xiao, R.; Herz, J.M.; Wood, J.D.; Zhu, M.X. Activation of TRPA1 channels by fenamate nonsteroidal anti-inflammatory drugs. *Pflug. Arch.* **2009**, *459*, 579–592. [CrossRef]
153. Kochetkov, K.V.; Kazachenko, V.N.; Marinov, B.S. Dose-dependent potentiation and inhibition of single Ca^{2+}-activated K+ channels by flufenamic acid. *Membr. cell Boil.* **2000**, *14*, 285–298.
154. Barrier, M.; Burlet, S.; Estrella, C.; Melnyk, P.; Sergeant, N.; Buee, L.; Verwaerde, P. Sulfate Salts of N-(3-(4-(3-(diisobutylamino)propyl)piperazin-1-yl)propyl)-1H-benzo [d]imidazol-2 Amine, Preparation Thereof and Use of the Same. U.S. Patent 9562018B2, 7 February 2017.
155. U.S. National Library of Medicine. A Study to Assess Tolerability, Safety, Pharmacokinetics and Effect of AZP2006 in Patients with PS. 2019. Available online: https://clinicaltrials.gov/ct2/show/study/NCT04008355?term=azp2006&draw=2&rank=1 (accessed on 1 August 2020).
156. Titovich, I.A.; Radko, S.V.; Lisitsky, D.S.; Okovity, S.V.; Bolotov, V.T.; Belsky, A.V.; Mikhailova, M.V.; Sysoev, I.Y. The study of a novel diethylaminoethanol derivative cognitive function in laboratory animals. *J. Biomed (Ru)* **2017**, *3*, 102–110.
157. Xu, X.; Lozinskaya, I.; Costell, M.; Lin, Z.; Ball, J.A.; Bernard, R.; Behm, D.J.; Marino, J.P.; Schnackenberg, C.G. Characterization of small molecule TRPC3 and TRPC6 agonist and antagonists. *Biophys. J.* **2013**, *104*, 454a. [CrossRef]
158. Inoue, R.; Jensen, L.J.; Jian, Z.; Shi, J.; Hai, L.; Lurie, A.I.; Henriksen, F.H.; Salomonsson, M.; Morita, H.; Kawarabayashi, Y.; et al. Synergistic activation of vascular TRPC6 channel by receptor and mechanical stimulation via phospholipase C/diacylglycerol and phospholipase A2/omega-hydroxylase/20-HETE pathways. *Circ. Res.* **2009**, *104*, 1399–1409. [CrossRef]
159. Butterfield, D.A.; Reed, T.; Sultana, R. Roles of 3-nitrotyrosine- and 4-hydroxynonenal-modified brain proteins in the progression and pathogenesis of Alzheimer's disease. *Free Radic Res.* **2011**, *45*, 59–72. [CrossRef]
160. Jin, Z.; Berthiaume, J.M.; Li, Q.; Henry, F.; Huang, Z.; Sadhukhan, S.; Gao, P.; Tochtrop, G.P.; Puchowicz, M.A.; Zhang, G. Catabolism of (2E)-4-hydroxy-2-nonenal via omega- and omega-1-oxidation stimulated by ketogenic diet. *J. Biol. Chem.* **2014**, *289*, 32327–32338. [CrossRef]
161. van Ierssel, S.H.; Conraads, V.M.; van Craenenbroeck, E.M.; Liu, Y.; Maas, A.I.; Parizel, P.M.; Hoymans, V.Y.; Vrints, C.J.; Jorens, P.G. Endothelial dysfunction in acute brain injury and the development of cerebral ischemia. *J. Neurosci. Res.* **2015**, *93*, 866–872. [CrossRef]
162. Clementi, E.; Meldolesi, J. Pharmacological and functional properties of voltagemi independent Ca^{2+} channels. *Cell Calcium* **1996**, *19*, 269–279. [CrossRef]
163. Tesfai, Y.; Brereton, H.M.; Barritt, G.J. A diacylglycerol-activated Ca^{2+} channel in PC12 cells (an adrenal chromaffin cell line) correlates with expression of the TRP-6 (transient receptor potential) protein. *Biochem. J.* **2001**, *358*, 717. [CrossRef]

164. Zhang, S.L.; Kozak, J.A.; Jiang, W.; Yeromin, A.V.; Chen, J.; Yu, Y.; Penna, A.; Shen, W.; Chi, V.; Cahalan, M.D. Store-dependent and -independent modes regulating Ca^{2+} release-activated Ca^{2+} channel activity of human Orai1 and Orai3. *J. Biol. Chem.* **2008**, *283*, 17662–17671. [CrossRef] [PubMed]
165. Nilius, B.; Flockerzi, V. Mammalian transient receptor potential (TRP) cation channels. In *Handbook of Experimental Pharmacology*; Springer: Heidelberg, Germany, 2014; Volume 223.
166. Wu, J.; Ryskamp, D.A.; Liang, X.; Egorova, P.; Zakharova, O.; Hung, G.; Bezprozvanny, I. Enhanced Store-Operated Calcium Entry Leads to Striatal Synaptic Loss in a Huntington's Disease Mouse Model. *J. Neurosci.* **2016**, *36*, 125–141. [CrossRef] [PubMed]
167. Tobe, M.; Yoshiaki Isobe, H.T.; Nagasaki, T.; Takahashi, H.; Fukazawa, T.; Hayashi, H. Discovery of quinazolines as a novel structural class of potent inhibitors of NF-kappa B activation. *Bioorg. Med. Chem.* **2003**, *11*, 383–391. [CrossRef]
168. Ma, R.; Wang, Y.X.; Ding, M. Nuclear transcription factor kappa B (NF-kB) mediates ROS and PKC-induced decrease in TRPC6 protein expression in human glomerular mesangial cells (HMCs). *Faseb. J.* **2012**, *26*, 687.
169. Tang, Q.; Guo, W.; Zheng, L.; Wu, J.-X.; Liu, M.; Zhou, X.; Zhang, X.; Chen, L. Structure of the receptor-activated human TRPC6 and TRPC3 ion channels. *Cell Res.* **2018**, *28*, 746–755. [CrossRef] [PubMed]

12

Sleep Disturbance as a Potential Modifiable Risk Factor for Alzheimer's Disease

Eiko N. Minakawa [1,*], Keiji Wada [1] and Yoshitaka Nagai [1,2,*]

[1] Department of Degenerative Neurological Diseases, National Institute of Neuroscience, National Center of Neurology and Psychiatry, Kodaira 187-8502, Japan; wada@ncnp.go.jp

[2] Department of Neurotherapeutics, Osaka University Graduate School of Medicine, Osaka 565-0871, Japan

* Correspondence: minakawa@ncnp.go.jp (E.N.M.); nagai@neurother.med.osaka-u.ac.jp (Y.N.)

Abstract: Sleep disturbance is a common symptom in patients with various neurodegenerative diseases, including Alzheimer's disease (AD), and it can manifest in the early stages of the disease. Impaired sleep in patients with AD has been attributed to AD pathology that affects brain regions regulating the sleep–wake or circadian rhythm. However, recent epidemiological and experimental studies have demonstrated an association between impaired sleep and an increased risk of AD. These studies have led to the idea of a bidirectional relationship between AD and impaired sleep; in addition to the conventional concept that impaired sleep is a consequence of AD pathology, various evidence strongly suggests that impaired sleep is a risk factor for the initiation and progression of AD. Despite this recent progress, much remains to be elucidated in order to establish the benefit of therapeutic interventions against impaired sleep to prevent or alleviate the disease course of AD. In this review, we provide an overview of previous studies that have linked AD and sleep. We then highlight the studies that have tested the causal relationship between impaired sleep and AD and will discuss the molecular and cellular mechanisms underlying this link. We also propose future works that will aid the development of a novel disease-modifying therapy and prevention of AD via targeting impaired sleep through non-pharmacological and pharmacological interventions.

Keywords: Alzheimer's disease; sleep disturbance; sleep fragmentation; slow-wave sleep; amyloid beta; tau; proteostasis; default-mode network; cognitive behavioral therapy for insomnia

---

1. Introduction

Sleep disturbance is a common symptom associated with Alzheimer's disease (AD), which is the leading cause of dementia worldwide [1]. More than 60% of patients with AD develop sleep disturbance, which often occurs at the early stages of the disease or even before the onset of major cognitive decline [2]. Impaired sleep in these patients has been attributed to the progression of AD pathology to brain regions that regulate the sleep–wake or circadian rhythm (Figure 1) [3]. However, various epidemiological studies have demonstrated the association between impaired sleep and an increased risk of AD or AD-related pathology [3]. Multiple studies using animal models of AD have also indicated that impaired sleep exacerbates memory decline and AD-related pathology (Figure 1) [4]. These recent findings suggest that sleep disturbance is a potential modifiable risk factor for AD and could be a novel target for disease-modifying therapies to prevent the development of AD and/or ameliorate the cognitive decline in patients with AD [3]. In this review, we will first provide an overview on the epidemiological and experimental studies that have linked AD and sleep. We will then describe experimental studies that have examined the causal relationship between impaired sleep and AD, and will discuss the molecular and cellular mechanisms that might underlie this link. Finally, we will propose future research directions, including the establishment of a novel disease-modifying therapy and the prevention of AD via targeting impaired sleep in patients with AD and cognitively normal people.

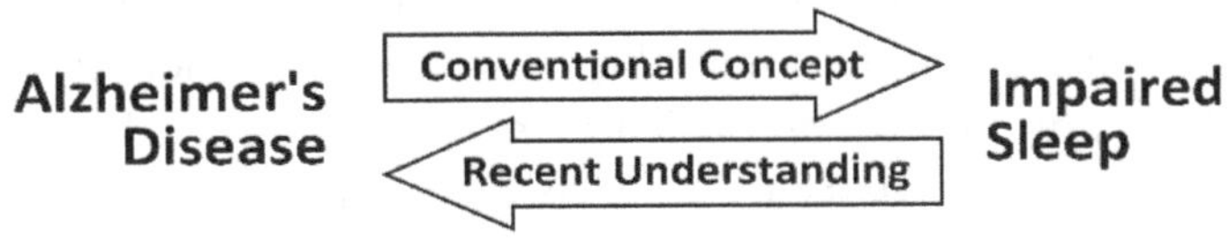

Figure 1. Bidirectional relationship between Alzheimer's disease (AD) and impaired sleep. Impaired sleep is prevalent in patients with AD. Both epidemiological and experimental studies have led to the recent concept of a bidirectional relationship between AD and impaired sleep. In addition to the conventional concept that impaired sleep is a consequence of AD pathology affecting brain regions regulating the sleep–wake or circadian rhythm, impaired sleep has been suggested as a risk factor for the initiation and progression of AD.

2. Age-Related Sleep Alterations

Physiological sleep in mammals, including humans, is composed of rapid eye movement (REM) sleep and non-REM (NREM) sleep. Human NREM sleep can be classified into three stages according to its depth, namely stage N1, N2, and N3, using electroencephalogram (EEG) findings that are characteristic of each stage [5]. Stage N3, the deepest NREM sleep, is characterized by a dominant EEG activity that consists of high-voltage slow waves with a frequency range of 1–4 Hz and is thus referred to as slow-wave sleep (SWS) [6].

The age-associated alterations in sleep architecture have been well characterized. The most prominent changes are increased sleep fragmentation by intermittent nocturnal arousals and a reduced amount of SWS, which is associated with shorter overall sleep duration and increased N1 and N2 duration [7]. Compared with these changes in NREM sleep, REM sleep is relatively spared except for a decreased REM latency with age [7] until around 80 years old, after which its duration is also reduced [8].

3. Sleep Disturbance in Alzheimer's Disease (AD)

3.1. Sleep Abnormalities in Patients with Alzheimer's Disease (AD)

Patients with AD often experience difficulty falling asleep, repeated nocturnal arousals, early arousals in the morning, and excessive sleepiness during daytime [9]. One or more sleep disorders, including insomnia, circadian rhythm sleep–wake disorders, sleep-related breathing disorders (SRBD), and sleep-related movement disorders, underlie these symptoms [10].

The most consistently reported changes in sleep architecture in patients with mild to moderate AD are sleep fragmentation, which is due to an increased number and duration of intermittent nocturnal arousals, a reduced amount of SWS, a resulting decrease in overall sleep duration, and an increase in N1 [11]. These AD-associated changes in NREM sleep seem to be an exaggeration of sleep alterations that are associated with normal aging, which become more pronounced with an increase in the severity of AD [12]. In addition, sleep spindles and K complexes, which are the EEG markers of stage N2, exhibit poorer formation, lower amplitude, shorter duration and smaller number [11]. These changes are mostly similar to the age-associated change in these stage N2 markers, except for the spindle formation, whose age-related change is still controversial [13]. Meanwhile, the total duration of REM sleep, which is relatively spared in normal aging, is reduced in patients with AD due to a reduced duration of each REM episode [14]. Other REM sleep variables, such as the number of REM episodes and REM latency, are usually spared in AD [14].

The alterations in the diurnal rhythm of activity and sleep due to circadian rhythm dysregulation are also present in patients with preclinical AD and symptomatic AD [15]. A disrupted circadian rhythm can cause sundowning syndrome or nocturnal delirium [16], in which patients often become agitated, restless or anxious in the early evening. These symptoms usually resolve during the daytime, but greatly impair the quality of life of patients, families and caregivers [16].

3.2. Sleep Disturbance as a Consequence of AD Pathology

Sleep alterations in patients with AD have been interpreted as a consequence of the progression of AD pathology to brain regions that are involved in the regulation of the sleep–wake or circadian rhythm [3]. AD pathology affects galaninergic neurons in the intermediate nucleus of the hypothalamus [17]. This area is a homolog of the ventrolateral preoptic nucleus of rodents, which is selectively active during sleep [18] and sends inhibitory projections to wake-promoting areas [19]. The number of remaining galaninergic neurons in the intermediate nucleus of autopsied AD brains has been found to be negatively correlated with the severity of ante-mortem sleep fragmentation evaluated within one year of death by actigraphy [17], which suggests that galaninergic neuronal loss due to AD pathology leads to sleep fragmentation in patients with AD.

AD pathology also affects the cholinergic neuronal network [14], which comprises the brainstem, thalamus, basal forebrain and cerebral cortex. This network regulates the initiation and maintenance of REM sleep [14]. The primary circadian pacemaker in the mammalian brain is the hypothalamic suprachiasmatic nucleus (SCN), which is also affected by AD pathology. AD is associated with a significant loss of vasopressin- and vasoactive intestinal peptide-expressing neurons, which are involved in the maintenance of circadian function in the SCN [20–22].

Various transgenic or knock-in mouse models of AD also develop sleep abnormalities, such as increased wakefulness [23–25], a decrease in NREM sleep [23,25] and REM sleep [23], circadian rhythm delay [24], or a reduced amplitude of the circadian rhythm [25]. The sleep–wake patterns of APPswe/PS1dE9 transgenic mice [26] are normal before Aβ deposition, but a tendency of increased wakefulness and decreased sleep starts at the age when Aβ deposition is initially observed. Furthermore, these sleep abnormalities exacerbte with age and increased Aβ deposition [23]. Furthermore, APPswe/PS1dE9 mice that are actively immunized with Aβ, which decreases Aβ deposition in the brain, showed a normal sleep–wake pattern [23]. Taken together, these findings suggest that sleep disturbance is caused not only by a neuronal loss in the brain regions regulating sleep or circadian rhythm, but also by Aβ accumulation in the brain.

4. Sleep Disturbance as a Risk Factor of AD

4.1. Epidemiological Studies

Contrary to the conventional understanding that impaired sleep in patients with AD is a consequence of AD-related pathology, multiple recent epidemiological studies have suggested that sleep disturbance could be a risk factor for cognitive decline and AD. According to a recent meta-analysis, sleep disturbance or sleep disorders, including short or long sleep duration, poor sleep quality (difficulty in falling asleep or increased intermittent nocturnal arousal), circadian rhythm abnormality, insomnia or SRBD, were associated with a significant increase in the risk ratio (RR) for cognitive impairment (RR: 1.64, 95% CI: 1.45–1.87), preclinical AD (RR: 3.78, 95% CI: 2.27–6.30) and AD diagnoses based on the ICD-9 (International Classification of Diseases, Ninth edition) or DSM-IV (Diagnostic Statistical Manual, Fourth edition) (RR: 1.55, 95% CI: 1.25–1.93) [27].

In a prospective study that used actigraphy to quantitatively assess the sleep of 737 community-dwelling older adults without dementia, a higher level of sleep fragmentation due to increased intermittent nocturnal arousal was associated with an increased risk of AD (hazard ratio = 1.22, 95% CI: 1.03–1.44) [28]. Individuals with high sleep fragmentation (in the 90th percentile) at baseline had a 1.5-fold higher risk of developing AD compared to those with low sleep fragmentation (in the 10th percentile) during the 6-year follow-up period (mean = 3.3 years) [28]. In addition, in a positron emission tomography (PET) study that examined the association between sleep variables and amyloid beta (Aβ) deposition in older people without dementia, a self-reported shorter sleep duration and poorer sleep quality were associated with significantly greater in vivo Aβ deposition in the precuneus [29], which is affected by Aβ pathology in preclinical AD [30].

Although these studies indicate an association between impaired sleep and AD, epidemiological observational studies conducted so far are limited in discerning the causal relationship between impaired sleep and AD, especially considering the relatively short follow-up periods compared to the long disease course of AD [3]. For example, a subgroup meta-analysis for the effect of sleep disturbance demonstrated that both short and long sleep duration were associated with a higher risk of cognitive decline or AD [27]. Additional studies are needed to determine whether both short and long sleep duration do indeed affect the disease course of AD, or whether either of these is a prodromal symptom of AD or reflecting the comorbidities of AD, such as depression.

4.2. The Causal Relationship between Sleep Disturbance and AD Pathology

Various animal models of AD and sleep disturbance have been used to assess the causal relationship between sleep disturbance and AD and the molecular or cellular mechanisms potentially underlying this link. Kang et al. (2009) were the first to report that chronic sleep restriction accelerates Aβ deposition in the brain using two transgenic AD mouse models (APPswe and APPswe/PS1dE9 mice) [31]. Other studies have also demonstrated that sleep deprivation or restriction in various AD models exacerbates AD-related biochemical or pathological changes in mice brains, such as an increase in Aβ or phosphorylated tau [32,33], an increase in insoluble phosphorylated tau and glial fibrillary acidic protein levels [34], and an increase in $A\beta_{40}$, $A\beta_{42}$ and β-site amyloid-precursor-protein-cleaving enzyme 1 (BACE1), which produce toxic Aβ species [35].

In these studies, sleep disturbance was induced in the mice either by intermittent gentle tactile stimuli, resulting in total deprivation of sleep [31], by the platform-over-water technique, resulting in elimination of REM sleep and a decrease in SWS [31–33,35], or by alteration of the light–dark cycle, resulting in a disrupted circadian rhythm [34]. The limitation of these studies is that the resultant sleep–wake patterns using the above methods are different from those observed in patients with AD or in normal aging. In addition, these methods induce relatively high levels of stress in mice. These acute or chronic behavioral stresses could aggravate the AD pathology via an increase in Aβ [36] and might therefore be a confounding factor. In a recent study, we took advantage of a novel device that induces impaired sleep closely resembling that of patients with AD (i.e., an increase in sleep fragmentation and a decrease in the amount of SWS) without severe stress [37] and found that chronic sleep fragmentation indeed aggravates Aβ deposition in the AD mice brain [38]. Notably, the severity of Aβ deposition showed a significant positive correlation with the severity of sleep fragmentation [38]. Since all mice were subjected to sleep impairment by a unified protocol, our results strongly suggest that the aggravation of Aβ pathology is more directly related to sleep impairment than the behavioral stress, if any, that was induced by the device we used to induce sleep impairment. Considering this point, our results are consistent with a previous epidemiological study that demonstrated an association between sleep fragmentation and an increased risk of AD [28]. Thus, our evidence supports the view that sleep disturbance in older people and patients with AD affects the disease course of AD.

5. Molecular/Cellular Mechanisms that Link AD and Sleep

5.1. Impaired Sleep Alters the Dynamics of Aβ and Tau in the Brain

The two major pathological hallmarks of AD are senile plaques, which are the extracellular deposits that are mainly composed of insoluble Aβ, and neurofibrillary tangles (NFT), which are the intracytoplasmic deposits that are mainly composed of hyperphosphorylated insoluble tau [39]. The dynamics of extracellular Aβ in relation to neuronal activity and the sleep–wake cycle have been extensively studied using various in vitro and in vivo animal and humans. Several recent studies have also examined the relationship between the dynamics of tau and sleep.

Extracellular Aβ in the central nervous system can be detected as a soluble form in cerebrospinal fluid (CSF) in humans as well as in CSF or interstitial fluid (ISF) in mice. The soluble Aβ shows diurnal fluctuation in both healthy young humans and mice, with an increase during wakefulness and a decrease during sleep [31,40]. The amplitude of this diurnal fluctuation is decreased in the CSF of older people without Aβ deposition and disappears in older people with Aβ deposition [40].

In APPswe/PS1dE9 mice, the diurnal Aβ fluctuation in ISF disappears when mice develop Aβ deposition [23]. These studies suggest that the dynamics of extracellular soluble Aβ is one of the potential mechanisms linking sleep and an increased risk of AD. Therefore, the mechanisms that affect the dynamics of soluble Aβ in ISF or CSF have been extensively studied.

Various studies have confirmed that Aβ production is regulated by neuronal action potential firing. An increase in neuronal firing leads to an increase in the extracellular secretion of soluble Aβ in an activity-dependent manner [41,42]. In vivo experiments have also demonstrated a direct relationship between increased neuronal activity and increased production of extracellular soluble Aβ in the brain, which was detected in the interstitial fluid (ISF) [43]. Furthermore, a sustained increase in the neuronal activity by optogenetic stimulation induces an increase in soluble Aβ in ISF followed by insoluble Aβ deposition in the projection area of the stimulated neurons [44]. Consistent with these studies, extended wakefulness by total sleep deprivation results in an increased level of soluble Aβ in the ISF or CSF [31,45]. Interestingly, specific disruption of SWS, but not sleep duration or sleep efficiency, induces an increase in CSF Aβ [46]. This suggests that each sleep component may influence the dynamics of extracellular Aβ in different ways.

The mechanism underlying the decrease in soluble Aβ during sleep is still controversial. The interchanging convective flow of ISF and CSF in the interstitial space of the brain has been reported to play a crucial role in the removal of the extracellular metabolites, including Aβ, in the brain [47]. Furthermore, Xie et al. reported that natural sleep is associated with a 60% increase in the interstitial space in the brain, which results in an increase in the clearance efficiency of interstitial metabolites, including Aβ, by the increased convective flow of CSF and ISF [48]. The removal of interstitial Aβ by this clearance system, named the glymphatic system, may be one of the mechanisms underlying the decrease in CSF and ISF Aβ during sleep. Meanwhile, recent human studies have analyzed Aβ turnover in CSF by radioactive labeling of Aβ [49,50]. These studies concluded that a decreased production of Aβ due to reduced neuronal activity rather than the increased clearance of Aβ is a necessary and critical factor for the decrease in CSF Aβ during sleep [49,50].

Extracellular soluble tau is another important component in ISF and CSF that is related to AD pathology, while intracellular aggregated tau is a pathological hallmark of AD. Recent studies have indicated that the total tau and phosphorylated tau in CSF are biomarkers that differentiate patients with AD from healthy controls as well as those with mild cognitive impairments due to preclinical AD from those due to other conditions [51,52].

Similarly to Aβ, neuronal activity has been found to induce the extracellular release of tau in an in vitro model [53]. Neuronal activity also induces the propagation of aggregated tau pathology in vivo via the extracellular release of tau and uptake of released tau by nearby neurons [54]. Extracellularly released tau is indeed detectable in the ISF of tau transgenic mouse models [55–58]. Multiple recent studies have examined the in vivo dynamics of the extracellular tau in ISF and CSF in relation to neuronal activity and the sleep–wake cycle. In tau transgenic mice with regulatable expression, the half-life of extracellular soluble ISF tau was revealed to be 17.3 days [56]. This is remarkably longer than that of Aβ, which shows diurnal fluctuation. Consistent with this finding, poorer sleep quality, which was measured for six consecutive nights before CSF collection, was found to have a significant negative correlation with an increase in CSF tau, while acute deprivation of SWS did not lead to CSF tau elevation [46]. Meanwhile, a very recent study demonstrated that acute sleep deprivation leads to a remarkable increase of tau in both mice ISF and human CSF [59]. Importantly, another recent study that used a combination of sleep monitoring by single-channel EEG with PET imaging and CSF analysis of both Aβ and tau revealed that a decrease in SWS, especially at the lowest frequencies of 1–2 Hz, was more associated with the accumulation of tau than that of Aβ [60].

Together, these studies suggest that impaired sleep affects the dynamics of both Aβ and tau, which may lead to the exacerbation of AD-related pathology. Further studies are awaitedto determine whether the dynamics of Aβ and tau are regulated via same mechanisms of production and clearance and via similar components of sleep.

5.2. Prolonged Wakefulness Induces Impaired Proteostasis, a Common Pathomechanism Underlying Neurodegenerative Diseases

Proteins with proper functions are indispensable for living organisms. Intracellular and in vivo protein quality is maintained in a homeostatic manner through the coordination of multiple intra- and extracellular systems that regulate protein synthesis, folding, disaggregation, and degradation [61]. The resultant homeostasis of protein quality (Figure 2; left), which is called proteostasis, is of general importance for maintaining human health.

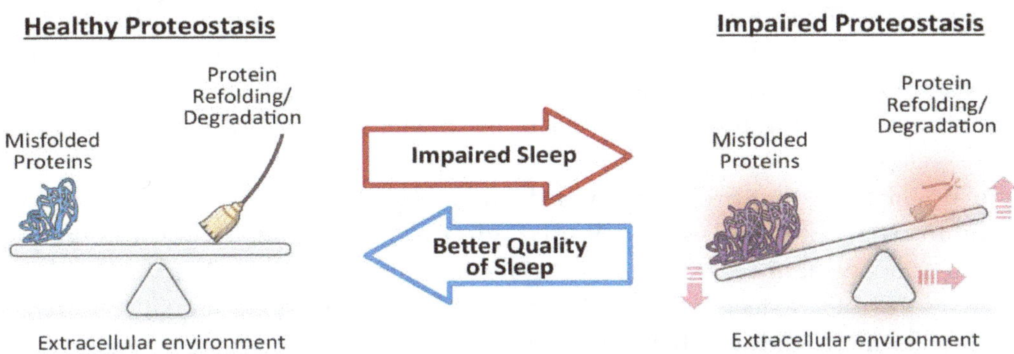

Figure 2. Impaired sleep as a potential therapeutic target to restore proteostasis. Healthy proteostasis is maintained through the coordination of various intra- and extracellular systems that regulate protein synthesis, folding, disaggregation, and degradation (left). Increased synthesis of misfolded proteins, dysfunction of protein refolding or degradation systems, or changes in extracellular environment can lead to impaired proteostasis and result in the accumulation of misfolded and aggregation-prone toxic proteins (right), which is a common pathomechanism underlying neurodegenerative diseases. Based on recent studies that have indicated that impaired sleep leads to impaired proteostasis (middle; red arrow), future studies that better examine the relationship between sleep and proteostasis could lead to the development of novel therapeutics that restore healthy proteostasis via better quality of sleep (middle; blue arrow).

Impaired proteostasis (Figure 2; right) is a common pathomechanism underlying neurodegenerative diseases, such as AD, Parkinson's disease (PD), dementia with Lewy bodies (DLB), amyotrophic lateral sclerosis and Huntington's disease [39]. Neurodegenerative diseases are characterized by selective and progressive neuronal degeneration, which is accompanied by abnormal protein aggregates in the regions of the central nervous system (CNS) that are characteristic of each disease [39]. Patients exhibit slowly progressive neurological or psychiatric symptoms of various types, such as cognitive or motor impairment, or involuntary movements, depending on the affected regions specific to each disease. Recent studies have reported that impaired proteostasis and the resultant accumulation of misfolded and aggregation-prone proteins (Figure 2; right) exhibit neurotoxicity and lead to neuronal dysfunction followed by neurodegeneration [61].

Sleep affects proteostasis in the brain. A detailed transcriptomic study revealed that the most abundant categories of genes that are upregulated in the mice brain during sleep are those involved in macromolecule biosynthesis, such as structural components of ribosomes, translation initiation and elongation factors and tRNA activators [62]. In addition, genes involved in intracellular transport, such as vesicle-mediated protein trafficking, are also upregulated during sleep [62].

Among the multiple molecules/pathways involved in the refolding or degradation of misfolded proteins to maintain proteostasis, such as chaperones, the ubiquitin–proteasome system and autophagy, the relationship between sleep and the unfolded protein response (UPR) pathway has been studied in detail. Prolonged wakefulness by sleep deprivation activates the UPR pathway, which is one of the major mechanisms that prevent the accumulation of misfolded proteins and maintains proteostasis [63]. When the endoplasmic reticulum (ER), a major site of protein folding and post-translational modification, is overloaded and stressed by the accumulation of misfolded and potentially toxic proteins, the UPR is activated and triggers different levels of downstream pathways according to the duration and the severity of the ER stress [64]. Mild or transient ER stress induces adaptive or protective pathways, such as increased transcription of chaperones for proper protein refolding, attenuation of general protein translation and removal of misfolded proteins for degradation at the proteasome. When ER stress is not alleviated by these pathways, the pro-apoptotic signaling pathway is activated, which leads to cellular injury or cell death [64]. Various studies have shown that prolonged wakefulness by sleep deprivation for six hours or longer leads to the upregulation of protective or adaptive pathways downstream of UPR activation in the rodent brain, such as the increased production of BiP/GRP78, a major ER chaperone and a marker of UPR activation [63,65–67]. However, in the aged mice brain, six hours of sleep deprivation failed to induce the protective pathways downstream of UPR activation, such as the upregulation of BiP/GRP78 or inhibition of general protein translation. On the contrary, six hours of sleep deprivation did activate pro-apoptotic signaling pathways [68].

These studies suggest that prolonged wakefulness by acute sleep deprivation is sufficient to at least transiently impair proteostasis in the brain (Figure 2, middle; red arrow), and that aging impairs the protective responses against impaired sleep, which could in turn lead to neurodegeneration. Further studies on the role of sleep in the maintenance of proteostasis via the UPR and other pathways could aid the development of novel therapeutics that can restore healthy proteostasis via better quality of sleep and could represent disease modification strategies for neurodegenerative diseases (Figure 2, middle; blue arrow).

5.3. Impaired Sleep May Aggravate the Propagation of AD-Related Pathology via Impaired Functional Connectivity in the Brain

Functional connectivity in the brain is defined as inter-regional correlations in the neuronal activation patterns of anatomically separate brain regions [69]. Functional connectivity reflects the integrity of communication between two functionally related brain regions [70]. Independent component analysis of the functional connectivity at the resting state, when individuals are awake but not focused on their external environment, has identified several functional resting-state networks (RSNs) in the cerebral cortex that exhibit increased activity, specifically at resting state [70]. The default mode network (DMN) is one of the major RSNs and underlies most of the baseline brain activity at rest [71]. The core regions of the DMN include the medial prefrontal cortex, posterior cingulate cortex, precuneus and parietal cortex, all of which have structural interconnections and functional connectivity [72].

Intriguingly, a recent study demonstrated that functional connectivity in the brain shows a diurnal patternand that nocturnal sleep restores morning-to-evening connectivity changes [73]. A lack of sleep has been associated with a deficit in the recovery of functional connectivity on the following morning within various networks, including the DMN [73]. Another study demonstrated that the significant functional correlations between frontal and posterior areas of the DMN become non-significant during SWS, which suggests that the integrity of the DMN is decreased during deep sleep [74]. These studies indicate the potential importance of sleep on the maintenance of the DMN during arousal.

It has also been well established that all regions of the DMN are vulnerable to AD-related pathology [75]. Indeed, DMN impairment is present in early symptomatic AD and progresses with the disease course [76]. DMN impairment is even observed in preclinical AD, when AD-related histopathology accumulates before overt clinical symptoms appear [76]. Furthermore, the carriers of the *ApoE ε4* allele, which is the most potent risk factor for AD, also show DMN impairment similar to that of preclinical AD, even in the absence of Aβ deposition in the brain [77].

The precise mechanism underlying the relationship between the DMN and the progression of AD pathology has yet to be fully elucidated. However, recent studies have strongly suggested that misfolded neurotoxic proteins, such as Aβ and tau in the case of AD, are transmitted along interconnected neural networks [78,79]. Consistent with this, it is plausible that misfolded toxic proteins can be propagated from the brain regions that are initially affected by AD pathology to adjacent healthy brain regions [76]. This protein propagation via interconnected brain regions could eventually lead to the gradual deterioration of the entire brain network from a semi-functional state to a dysfunctional state as misfolded proteins accumulate over the years [76]. From this point of view, the alterations in functional connectivity due to impaired sleep, especially at the preclinical or early stages of AD, might be an additional pathomechanism underlying the progression of AD-related pathology that results from impaired sleep.

5.4. Other Mechanisms that May Link Impaired Sleep and AD-Related Pathology

Inflammatory immune responses, blood–brain barrier (BBB) disruption, and oxidative stress are known to affect AD-related pathology, which can also be induced by impaired sleep [3,80].

Acute and chronic sleep loss in humans result in the induction of both cellular and humoral immunological responses. An increase in the number of circulating leukocytes (mainly monocytes and neutrophils) and increased levels of proinflammatory cytokines, such as interleukin-1β (IL-1β) and IL-6 and tumor necrosis factor-α (TNF-α), are observed after acute sleep deprivation or subacute sleep restriction [81]. The resulting low-grade systemic inflammation could facilitate neuroinflammation when sleep impairment is sustained, which could aggravate AD-related brain pathology [82]. Indeed, chronic sleep loss in rodents has been associated with microglial activation and astrocytic phagocytosis in the brain [83]. In addition, chronic low-grade inflammation has been proposed to underlie the BBB breakdown following sleep loss observed in rodent models [84], which could also worsen AD-related pathology [85]. Furthermore, sleep deprivation promotes oxidative stress in the rodent brain [86]. A recent prospective epidemiological study indicated that obstructive sleep apnea (OSA) in cognitively normal older people is associated with increased Aβ deposition [87]. Besides the sleep fragmentation itself due to OSA, which could affect Aβ dynamics (as discussed in Section 5.1), a combination of hypoxemia, neuroinflammation, and oxidative stress could be additional mechanisms underlying the exacerbation of AD pathology in patients with OSA.

6. Conclusions and Future Directions

Impaired sleep is prevalent in patients with AD, which often occurs in the early or even preclinical stages of AD. Both epidemiological and experimental studies have led to the recent concept of a bidirectional relationship between AD and impaired sleep (Figure 1). In addition to the conventional concept that impaired sleep is a consequence of AD-related pathology, impaired sleep has been suggested to be a risk factor for the initiation and progression of AD, at least in cognitively normal older people and in patients with AD. Despite this recent progress, much remains to be elucidated in future works that will aid the development of therapeutic interventions against impaired sleep to prevent or alleviate the disease course of AD.

First, the essential components of "better sleep" that reduce the risk for AD need to be determined. A recent study demonstrated that an acute inhibition of SWS is sufficient to affect Aβ dynamics in humans [46]. While the importance of REM sleep in regulating NREM sleep has been established [88], additional studies are crucial in obtaining a more comprehensive understanding of the roles and interactions between the different components of sleep, including REM sleep, light NREM sleep and SWS. Furthermore, the molecular and cellular mechanisms underlying the link between AD and these different components of sleep remain to be determined. It would also be necessary to determine the contribution of other sleep-related factors to AD-related pathology, such as the optimal duration of sleep that reduces the risk of AD.

Second, potential therapeutic methods to achieve "better sleep" need to be investigated. Recent meta-analyses have demonstrated the effect of non-pharmacological treatment by cognitive behavioral therapy for insomnia (CBT-I) on primary chronic insomnia [89,90]. In addition, several randomized control studies have shown that CBT-I is more effective than pharmacotherapy using conventional hypnotics that target γ-aminobutyric acid $(GABA)_A$ receptor-mediated systems [91]. CBT-I provided via cost-effective and accessible ways, such as computerized and online platforms or video conferencing, has also shown therapeutic benefits [91]. While these non-pharmacologic methods are recommended as first-line treatments for primary chronic insomnia [92], the recent development of novel hypnotics with different mechanisms of action and potentially better safety, especially in elderly patients, might provide better therapeutic opportunities compared to traditional hypnotics [93]. Whether these non-pharmacological and pharmacological treatments can also achieve "better sleep" that reduces the risk for AD development and progression remains to be determined.

Furthermore, chronic short sleep is highly prevalent in both healthy young adults and adolescents, especially in developed countries [94]. These people generally have insufficient sleep during weekdays and use weekends to catch up on sleep, which leads to the subjective normalization of sleepiness. However, several studies have demonstrated that weekend sleep is not sufficient to fully recover the cognitive performance deficit induced by sleep insufficiency during weekdays [95–97]. Whether the accumulation of sleep insufficiency that begins from adolescence or young adulthood affects the molecular or cellular links between sleep and AD and whether this could lead to an increased risk of AD development would be particularly important for the primary prevention of AD.

Last but not least, impaired sleep mainly due to sleep fragmentation and a decrease in SWS is also prevalent in patients with various neurodegenerative diseases other than AD. Considering that neurodegenerative diseases, including AD, share a common pathomechanism of misfolded protein accumulation and impaired proteostasis, "better sleep" that reduces the risk for AD might also alleviate the disease course of other neurodegenerative diseases. Elucidating the link between impaired sleep and the dynamics of misfolded proteins that accumulate in each disease, such as α-synuclein in PD and DLB as well as Aβ and tau in AD, could lead to the development of a novel disease-modifying therapy that has far-reaching implications for neurodegenerative diseases in general.

Acknowledgments: We thank Nia Cason from Edanz Group (www.edanzediting.com/ac) for editing a draft of this manuscript.

Abbreviations

AD	Alzheimer's disease
REM	Rapid Eye Movement
NREM	Non-Rapid Eye Movement
EEG	Electroencephalogram
SWS	Slow-wave Sleep
SRBD	Sleep-related breathing disorders
SCN	Suprachiasmatic Nucleus
RR	Risk Ratio
ICD-9	International Classification of Diseases, Ninth Edition
DSM-IV	Diagnostic Statistical Manual, Fourth Edition
Aβ	Amyloid β
BACE1	β-site amyloid precursor protein cleaving enzyme 1
NFT	Neurofibrillary Tangles
CSF	Cerebrospinal Fluid
ISF	Interstitial Fluid
PD	Parkinson's Disease
DLB	Dementia with Lewy Bodies
CNS	Central Nervous System
UPR	Unfolded Protein Response
ER	Endoplasmic Reticulum

RSN	Resting State Network
DMN	Default Mode Network
TNF-α	Tumor Necrosis Factor-α
OSA	Obstructive Sleep Apnea
CBT-I	Cognitive Behavioral Therapy for Insomnia
GABA	γ-aminobutyric Acid

References

1. Brzecka, A.; Leszek, J.; Ashraf, G.M.; Ejma, M.; Ávila-Rodriguez, M.F.; Yarla, N.S.; Tarasov, V.V.; Chubarev, V.N.; Samsonova, A.N.; Barreto, G.E.; et al. Sleep disorders associated with Alzheimer's disease: A perspective. *Front. Neurosci.* **2018**, *12*, 330. [CrossRef] [PubMed]
2. Guarnieri, B.; Adorni, F.; Musicco, M.; Appollonio, I.; Bonanni, E.; Caffarra, P.; Caltagirone, C.; Cerroni, G.; Concari, L.; Cosentino, F.I.I.; et al. Prevalence of sleep disturbances in mild cognitive impairment and dementing disorders: A multicenter italian clinical cross-sectional study on 431 patients. *Dement. Geriatr. Cogn. Disord.* **2012**, *33*, 50–58. [CrossRef] [PubMed]
3. Ju, Y.-E.S.; Lucey, B.P.; Holtzman, D.M. Sleep and Alzheimer disease pathology—A bidirectional relationship. *Nat. Rev. Neurol.* **2014**, *10*, 115–119. [CrossRef]
4. Dufort-Gervais, J.; Mongrain, V.; Brouillette, J. Bidirectional relationships between sleep and amyloid-beta in the hippocampus. *Neurobiol. Learn. Mem.* **2018**, (in press). [CrossRef] [PubMed]
5. Moser, D.; Anderer, P.; Gruber, G.; Parapatics, S.; Loretz, E.; Boeck, M.; Kloesch, G.; Heller, E.; Schmidt, A.; Danker-Hopfe, H.; et al. Sleep classification according to AASM and Rechtschaffen & Kales: Effects on sleep scoring parameters. *Sleep* **2009**, *32*, 139–149. [PubMed]
6. Léger, D.; Debellemaniere, E.; Rabat, A.; Bayon, V.; Benchenane, K.; Chennaoui, M. Slow-wave sleep: From the cell to the clinic. *Sleep Med. Rev.* **2018**, *41*, 113–132. [CrossRef] [PubMed]
7. Ohayon, M.M.; Carskadon, M.A.; Guilleminault, C.; Vitiello, M.V. Meta-analysis of quantitative sleep parameters from childhood to old age in healthy individuals: Developing normative sleep values across the human lifespan. *Sleep* **2004**, *27*, 1255–1273. [CrossRef]
8. Mander, B.A.; Winer, J.R.; Walker, M.P. Sleep and human aging. *Neuron* **2017**, *94*, 19–36. [CrossRef]
9. Peter-Derex, L.; Yammine, P.; Bastuji, H.; Croisile, B. Sleep and Alzheimer's disease. *Sleep Med. Rev.* **2015**, *19*, 29–38. [CrossRef]
10. Yaffe, K.; Falvey, C.M.; Hoang, T. Connections between sleep and cognition in older adults. *Lancet. Neurol.* **2014**, *13*, 1017–1028. [CrossRef]
11. Petit, D.; Gagnon, J.-F.; Fantini, M.L.; Ferini-Strambi, L.; Montplaisir, J. Sleep and quantitative EEG in neurodegenerative disorders. *J. Psychosom. Res.* **2004**, *56*, 487–496. [CrossRef] [PubMed]
12. Prinz, P.N.; Peskind, E.R.; Vitaliano, P.P.; Raskind, M.A.; Eisdorfer, C.; Zemcuznikov, H.N.; Gerber, C.J. Changes in the sleep and waking EEGs of nondemented and demented elderly subjects. *J. Am. Geriatr. Soc.* **1982**, *30*, 86–92. [CrossRef] [PubMed]
13. Crowley, K.; Trinder, J.; Kim, Y.; Carrington, M.; Colrain, I.M. The effects of normal aging on sleep spindle and K-complex production. *Clin. Neurophysiol.* **2002**, *113*, 1615–1622. [CrossRef]
14. Montplaisir, J.; Petit, D.; Lorrain, D.; Gauthier, S.; Nielsen, T. Sleep in Alzheimer's disease: Further considerations on the role of brainstem and forebrain cholinergic populations in sleep–wake mechanisms. *Sleep* **1995**, *18*, 145–148. [CrossRef] [PubMed]
15. Musiek, E.S.; Bhimasani, M.; Zangrilli, M.A.; Morris, J.C.; Holtzman, D.M.; Ju, Y.-E.S. Circadian rest-activity pattern changes in aging and preclinical alzheimer disease. *JAMA Neurol.* **2018**, *75*, 582–590. [CrossRef] [PubMed]
16. Bedrosian, T.A.; Nelson, R.J. Sundowning syndrome in aging and dementia: Research in mouse models. *Exp. Neurol.* **2013**, *243*, 67–73. [CrossRef] [PubMed]
17. Lim, A.S.P.; Ellison, B.A.; Wang, J.L.; Yu, L.; Schneider, J.A.; Buchman, A.S.; Bennett, D.A.; Saper, C.B. Sleep is related to neuron numbers in the ventrolateral preoptic/intermediate nucleus in older adults with and without Alzheimer's disease. *Brain* **2014**, *137*, 2847–2861. [CrossRef]

18. Sherin, J.E.; Shiromani, P.J.; McCarley, R.W.; Saper, C.B. Activation of ventrolateral preoptic neurons during sleep. *Science* **1996**, *271*, 216–219. [CrossRef]
19. Sherin, J.E.; Elmquist, J.K.; Torrealba, F.; Saper, C.B. Innervation of histaminergic tuberomammillary neurons by GABAergic and galaninergic neurons in the ventrolateral preoptic nucleus of the rat. *J. Neurosci.* **1998**, *18*, 4705–4721. [CrossRef]
20. Swaab, D.F.; Fliers, E.; Partiman, T.S. The suprachiasmatic nucleus of the human brain in relation to sex, age and senile dementia. *Brain Res.* **1985**, *342*, 37–44. [CrossRef]
21. Zhou, J.N.; Hofman, M.A.; Swaab, D.F. VIP neurons in the human SCN in relation to sex, age and Alzheimer's disease. *Neurobiol. Aging* **1995**, *16*, 571–576. [CrossRef]
22. Harper, D.G.; Stopa, E.G.; Kuo-Leblanc, V.; McKee, A.C.; Asayama, K.; Volicer, L.; Kowall, N.; Satlin, A. Dorsomedial SCN neuronal subpopulations subserve different functions in human dementia. *Brain* **2008**, *131*, 1609–1617. [CrossRef] [PubMed]
23. Roh, J.H.; Huang, Y.; Bero, A.W.; Kasten, T.; Stewart, F.R.; Bateman, R.J.; Holtzman, D.M. Disruption of the sleep–wake cycle and diurnal fluctuation of β-amyloid in mice with Alzheimer's disease pathology. *Sci. Transl. Med.* **2012**, *4*, 150ra122. [CrossRef] [PubMed]
24. Duncan, M.J.; Smith, J.T.; Franklin, K.M.; Beckett, T.L.; Murphy, M.P.; St Clair, D.K.; Donohue, K.D.; Striz, M.; O'Hara, B.F. Effects of aging and genotype on circadian rhythms, sleep and clock gene expression in APPxPS1 knock-in mice, a model for Alzheimer's disease. *Exp. Neurol.* **2012**, *236*, 249–258. [CrossRef] [PubMed]
25. Platt, B.; Drever, B.; Koss, D.; Stoppelkamp, S.; Jyoti, A.; Plano, A.; Utan, A.; Merrick, G.; Ryan, D.; Melis, V.; et al. Abnormal cognition, sleep, EEG and brain metabolism in a novel knock-in Alzheimer mouse, PLB1. *PLoS ONE* **2011**, *6*, e27068. [CrossRef]
26. Savonenko, A.; Xu, G.M.; Melnikova, T.; Morton, J.L.; Gonzales, V.; Wong, M.P.F.; Price, D.L.; Tang, F.; Markowska, A.L.; Borchelt, D.R. Episodic-like memory deficits in the APPswe/PS1dE9 mouse model of Alzheimer's disease: Relationships to β-amyloid deposition and neurotransmitter abnormalities. *Neurobiol. Dis.* **2005**, *18*, 602–617. [CrossRef] [PubMed]
27. Bubu, O.M.; Brannick, M.; Mortimer, J.; Umasabor-Bubu, O.; Sebastião, Y.V.; Wen, Y.; Schwartz, S.; Borenstein, A.R.; Wu, Y.; Morgan, D.; et al. Sleep, Cognitive impairment and Alzheimer's disease: A Systematic Review and Meta-Analysis. *Sleep* **2017**, *40*. [CrossRef]
28. Lim, A.S.P.; Kowgier, M.; Yu, L.; Buchman, A.S.; Bennett, D.A. Sleep fragmentation and the risk of incident Alzheimer's disease and cognitive decline in older persons. *Sleep* **2013**, *36*, 1027–1032. [CrossRef]
29. Spira, A.P.; Gamaldo, A.A.; An, Y.; Wu, M.N.; Simonsick, E.M.; Bilgel, M.; Zhou, Y.; Wong, D.F.; Ferrucci, L.; Resnick, S.M. Self-reported sleep and β-amyloid deposition in community-dwelling older adults. *JAMA Neurol.* **2013**, *70*, 1537–1543. [CrossRef]
30. Palmqvist, S.; Schöll, M.; Strandberg, O.; Mattsson, N.; Stomrud, E.; Zetterberg, H.; Blennow, K.; Landau, S.; Jagust, W.; Hansson, O. Earliest accumulation of β-amyloid occurs within the default-mode network and concurrently affects brain connectivity. *Nat. Commun.* **2017**, *8*, 1214. [CrossRef]
31. Kang, J.-E.; Lim, M.M.; Bateman, R.J.; Lee, J.J.; Smyth, L.P.; Cirrito, J.R.; Fujiki, N.; Nishino, S.; Holtzman, D.M. Amyloid-beta dynamics are regulated by orexin and the sleep–wake cycle. *Science* **2009**, *326*, 1005–1007. [CrossRef] [PubMed]
32. Rothman, S.M.; Herdener, N.; Frankola, K.A.; Mughal, M.R.; Mattson, M.P. Chronic mild sleep restriction accentuates contextual memory impairments and accumulations of cortical Aβ and pTau in a mouse model of Alzheimer's disease. *Brain Res.* **2013**, *1529*, 200–208. [CrossRef] [PubMed]
33. Qiu, H.; Zhong, R.; Liu, H.; Zhang, F.; Li, S.; Le, W. Chronic Sleep Deprivation Exacerbates Learning-Memory Disability and Alzheimer's Disease-Like Pathologies in AβPP(swe)/PS1(ΔE9) Mice. *J. Alzheimer's Dis.* **2016**, *50*, 669–685. [CrossRef] [PubMed]
34. Di Meco, A.; Joshi, Y.B.; Praticò, D. Sleep deprivation impairs memory, tau metabolism and synaptic integrity of a mouse model of Alzheimer's disease with plaques and tangles. *Neurobiol. Aging* **2014**, *35*, 1813–1820. [CrossRef] [PubMed]
35. Chen, L.; Huang, J.; Yang, L.; Zeng, X.-A.; Zhang, Y.; Wang, X.; Chen, M.; Li, X.; Zhang, Y.; Zhang, M. Sleep deprivation accelerates the progression of Alzheimer's disease by influencing Aβ-related metabolism. *Neurosci. Lett.* **2017**, *650*, 146–152. [CrossRef] [PubMed]
36. Kang, J.E.; Cirrito, J.R.; Dong, H.; Csernansky, J.G.; Holtzman, D.M. Acute stress increases interstitial fluid amyloid-beta via corticotropin-releasing factor and neuronal activity. *Proc. Natl. Acad. Sci. USA* **2007**, *104*, 10673–10678. [CrossRef] [PubMed]

37. Miyazaki, K.; Itoh, N.; Ohyama, S.; Kadota, K.; Oishi, K. Continuous exposure to a novel stressor based on water aversion induces abnormal circadian locomotor rhythms and sleep–wake cycles in mice. *PLoS ONE* **2013**, *8*, e55452. [CrossRef] [PubMed]
38. Minakawa, E.N.; Miyazaki, K.; Maruo, K.; Yagihara, H.; Fujita, H.; Wada, K.; Nagai, Y. Chronic sleep fragmentation exacerbates amyloid β deposition in Alzheimer's disease model mice. *Neurosci. Lett.* **2017**, *653*, 362–369. [CrossRef] [PubMed]
39. Nagai, Y.; Minakawa, E.N. Drug Development for Neurodegenerative Diseases. In *Neurodegenerative Disorders as Systemic Diseases*, 1st ed.; Wada, K., Ed.; Springer: Tokyo, Japan, 2015; ISBN 978-4-431-54541-5.
40. Huang, Y.; Potter, R.; Sigurdson, W.; Santacruz, A.; Shih, S.; Ju, Y.-E.; Kasten, T.; Morris, J.C.; Mintun, M.; Duntley, S.; et al. Effects of age and amyloid deposition on Aβ dynamics in the human central nervous system. *Arch. Neurol.* **2012**, *69*, 51–58. [CrossRef] [PubMed]
41. Nitsch, R.M.; Farber, S.A.; Growdon, J.H.; Wurtman, R.J. Release of amyloid beta-protein precursor derivatives by electrical depolarization of rat hippocampal slices. *Proc. Natl. Acad. Sci. USA* **1993**, *90*, 5191–5193. [CrossRef] [PubMed]
42. Kamenetz, F.; Tomita, T.; Hsieh, H.; Seabrook, G.; Borchelt, D.; Iwatsubo, T.; Sisodia, S.; Malinow, R. APP Processing and Synaptic Function. *Neuron* **2003**, *37*, 925–937. [CrossRef]
43. Cirrito, J.R.; Yamada, K.A.; Finn, M.B.; Sloviter, R.S.; Bales, K.R.; May, P.C.; Schoepp, D.D.; Paul, S.M.; Mennerick, S.; Holtzman, D.M. Synaptic activity regulates interstitial fluid amyloid-β levels in vivo. *Neuron* **2005**, *48*, 913–922. [CrossRef] [PubMed]
44. Yamamoto, K.; Tanei, Z.; Hashimoto, T.; Wakabayashi, T.; Okuno, H.; Naka, Y.; Yizhar, O.; Fenno, L.E.; Fukayama, M.; Bito, H.; et al. Chronic optogenetic activation augments aβ pathology in a mouse model of Alzheimer disease. *Cell Rep.* **2015**, *11*, 859–865. [CrossRef] [PubMed]
45. Ooms, S.; Overeem, S.; Besse, K.; Rikkert, M.O.; Verbeek, M.; Claassen, J.A.H.R. Effect of 1 night of total sleep deprivation on cerebrospinal fluid β-amyloid 42 in healthy middle-aged men: A randomized clinical trial. *JAMA Neurol.* **2014**, *71*, 971–977. [CrossRef] [PubMed]
46. Ju, Y.-E.S.; Ooms, S.J.; Sutphen, C.; Macauley, S.L.; Zangrilli, M.A.; Jerome, G.; Fagan, A.M.; Mignot, E.; Zempel, J.M.; Claassen, J.A.H.R.; et al. Slow wave sleep disruption increases cerebrospinal fluid amyloid-β levels. *Brain* **2017**, *140*, 2104–2111. [CrossRef] [PubMed]
47. Iliff, J.J.; Wang, M.; Liao, Y.; Plogg, B.A.; Peng, W.; Gundersen, G.A.; Benveniste, H.; Vates, G.E.; Deane, R.; Goldman, S.A.; et al. A paravascular pathway facilitates CSF flow through the brain parenchyma and the clearance of interstitial solutes, including amyloid β. *Sci. Transl. Med.* **2012**, *4*, 147ra111. [CrossRef]
48. Xie, L.; Kang, H.; Xu, Q.; Chen, M.J.; Liao, Y.; Thiyagarajan, M.; O'Donnell, J.; Christensen, D.J.; Nicholson, C.; Iliff, J.J.; et al. Sleep drives metabolite clearance from the adult brain. *Science* **2013**, *342*, 373–377. [CrossRef]
49. Lucey, B.P.; Mawuenyega, K.G.; Patterson, B.W.; Elbert, D.L.; Ovod, V.; Kasten, T.; Morris, J.C.; Bateman, R.J. Associations between β-amyloid kinetics and the β-amyloid diurnal pattern in the central nervous system. *JAMA Neurol.* **2017**, *74*, 207–215. [CrossRef] [PubMed]
50. Lucey, B.P.; Hicks, T.J.; McLeland, J.S.; Toedebusch, C.D.; Boyd, J.; Elbert, D.L.; Patterson, B.W.; Baty, J.; Morris, J.C.; Ovod, V.; et al. Effect of sleep on overnight cerebrospinal fluid amyloid β kinetics. *Ann. Neurol.* **2018**, *83*, 197–204. [CrossRef] [PubMed]
51. Polanco, J.C.; Li, C.; Bodea, L.-G.; Martinez-Marmol, R.; Meunier, F.A.; Götz, J. Amyloid-β and tau complexity—towards improved biomarkers and targeted therapies. *Nat. Rev. Neurol.* **2018**, *14*, 22–39. [CrossRef] [PubMed]
52. Olsson, B.; Lautner, R.; Andreasson, U.; Öhrfelt, A.; Portelius, E.; Bjerke, M.; Hölttä, M.; Rosén, C.; Olsson, C.; Strobel, G.; et al. CSF and blood biomarkers for the diagnosis of Alzheimer's disease: A systematic review and meta-analysis. *Lancet Neurol.* **2016**, *15*, 673–684. [CrossRef]
53. Pooler, A.M.; Phillips, E.C.; Lau, D.H.W.; Noble, W.; Hanger, D.P. Physiological release of endogenous tau is stimulated by neuronal activity. *EMBO Rep.* **2013**, *14*, 389–394. [CrossRef]
54. Wu, J.W.; Hussaini, S.A.; Bastille, I.M.; Rodriguez, G.A.; Mrejeru, A.; Rilett, K.; Sanders, D.W.; Cook, C.; Fu, H.; Boonen, R.A.C.M.; et al. Neuronal activity enhances tau propagation and tau pathology in vivo. *Nat. Neurosci.* **2016**, *19*, 1085–1092. [CrossRef] [PubMed]

55. Yamada, K.; Cirrito, J.R.; Stewart, F.R.; Jiang, H.; Finn, M.B.; Holmes, B.B.; Binder, L.I.; Mandelkow, E.-M.; Diamond, M.I.; Lee, V.M.-Y.; et al. In vivo microdialysis reveals age-dependent decrease of brain interstitial fluid tau levels in P301S human tau transgenic mice. *J. Neurosci.* **2011**, *31*, 13110–13117. [CrossRef] [PubMed]
56. Yamada, K.; Patel, T.K.; Hochgräfe, K.; Mahan, T.E.; Jiang, H.; Stewart, F.R.; Mandelkow, E.-M.; Holtzman, D.M. Analysis of in vivo turnover of tau in a mouse model of tauopathy. *Mol. Neurodegen.* **2015**, *10*, 55. [CrossRef] [PubMed]
57. Barten, D.M.; Cadelina, G.W.; Hoque, N.; DeCarr, L.B.; Guss, V.L.; Yang, L.; Sankaranarayanan, S.; Wes, P.D.; Flynn, M.E.; Meredith, J.E.; et al. Tau transgenic mice as models for cerebrospinal fluid tau biomarkers. *J. Alzheimer's Dis.* **2011**, *24*, 127–141. [CrossRef] [PubMed]
58. Takeda, S.; Wegmann, S.; Cho, H.; DeVos, S.L.; Commins, C.; Roe, A.D.; Nicholls, S.B.; Carlson, G.A.; Pitstick, R.; Nobuhara, C.K.; et al. Neuronal uptake and propagation of a rare phosphorylated high-molecular-weight tau derived from Alzheimer's disease brain. *Nat. Commun.* **2015**, *6*, 8490. [CrossRef] [PubMed]
59. Holth, J.K.; Fritschi, S.K.; Wang, C.; Pedersen, N.P.; Cirrito, J.R.; Mahan, T.E.; Finn, M.B.; Manis, M.; Geerling, J.C.; Fuller, P.M.; et al. The sleep–wake cycle regulates brain interstitial fluid tau in mice and CSF tau in humans. *Science* **2019**, in press. [CrossRef]
60. Lucey, B.P.; McCullough, A.; Landsness, E.C.; Toedebusch, C.D.; McLeland, J.S.; Zaza, A.M.; Fagan, A.M.; McCue, L.; Xiong, C.; Morris, J.C.; et al. Reduced non-rapid eye movement sleep is associated with tau pathology in early Alzheimer's disease. *Sci. Transl. Med.* **2019**, *11*. [CrossRef]
61. Labbadia, J.; Morimoto, R.I. The biology of proteostasis in aging and disease. *Annu. Rev. Biochem.* **2015**, *84*, 435–464. [CrossRef] [PubMed]
62. Mackiewicz, M.; Shockley, K.R.; Romer, M.A.; Galante, R.J.; Zimmerman, J.E.; Naidoo, N.; Baldwin, D.A.; Jensen, S.T.; Churchill, G.A.; Pack, A.I. Macromolecule biosynthesis: A key function of sleep. *Physiol. Genom.* **2007**, *31*, 441–457. [CrossRef] [PubMed]
63. Elliott, A.S.; Huber, J.D.; O'Callaghan, J.P.; Rosen, C.L.; Miller, D.B. A review of sleep deprivation studies evaluating the brain transcriptome. *SpringerPlus* **2014**, *3*, 728. [CrossRef] [PubMed]
64. Naidoo, N. Cellular stress/the unfolded protein response: Relevance to sleep and sleep disorders. *Sleep Med. Rev.* **2009**, *13*, 195–204. [CrossRef]
65. Naidoo, N.; Giang, W.; Galante, R.J.; Pack, A.I. Sleep deprivation induces the unfolded protein response in mouse cerebral cortex. *J. Neurochem.* **2005**, *92*, 1150–1157. [CrossRef] [PubMed]
66. Cirelli, C.; Gutierrez, C.M.; Tononi, G. Extensive and Divergent Effects of Sleep and Wakefulness on Brain Gene Expression. *Neuron* **2004**, *41*, 35–43. [CrossRef]
67. Cirelli, C.; Faraguna, U.; Tononi, G. Changes in brain gene expression after long-term sleep deprivation. *J. Neurochem.* **2006**, *98*, 1632–1645. [CrossRef]
68. Naidoo, N.; Ferber, M.; Master, M.; Zhu, Y.; Pack, A.I. Aging impairs the unfolded protein response to sleep deprivation and leads to proapoptotic signaling. *J. Neurosci.* **2008**, *28*, 6539–6548. [CrossRef]
69. Fox, M.D.; Raichle, M.E. Spontaneous fluctuations in brain activity observed with functional magnetic resonance imaging. *Nat. Rev. Neurosci.* **2007**, *8*, 700–711. [CrossRef]
70. Van den Heuvel, M.P.; Pol, H.E.H. Exploring the brain network: A review on resting-state fMRI functional connectivity. *Eur. Neuropsychopharmacol.* **2010**, *20*, 519–534. [CrossRef]
71. Raichle, M.E.; MacLeod, A.M.; Snyder, A.Z.; Powers, W.J.; Gusnard, D.A.; Shulman, G.L. A default mode of brain function. *Proc. Natl. Acad. Sci. USA* **2001**, *98*, 676–682. [CrossRef]
72. Buckner, R.L.; Andrews-Hanna, J.R.; Schacter, D.L. The brain's default network. *Ann. N. Y. Acad. Sci.* **2008**, *1124*, 1–38. [CrossRef] [PubMed]
73. Kaufmann, T.; Elvsåshagen, T.; Alnæs, D.; Zak, N.; Pedersen, P.Ø.; Norbom, L.B.; Quraishi, S.H.; Tagliazucchi, E.; Laufs, H.; Bjørnerud, A.; et al. The brain functional connectome is robustly altered by lack of sleep. *NeuroImage* **2016**, *127*, 324–332. [CrossRef] [PubMed]
74. Horovitz, S.G.; Braun, A.R.; Carr, W.S.; Picchioni, D.; Balkin, T.J.; Fukunaga, M.; Duyn, J.H. Decoupling of the brain's default mode network during deep sleep. *Proc. Natl. Acad. Sci. USA* **2009**, *106*, 11376–11381. [CrossRef] [PubMed]
75. Fjell, A.M.; McEvoy, L.; Holland, D.; Dale, A.M.; Walhovd, K.B. What is normal in normal aging? Effects of aging, amyloid and Alzheimer's disease on the cerebral cortex and the hippocampus. *Prog. Neurobiol.* **2014**, *117*, 20–40. [CrossRef] [PubMed]

76. Brier, M.R.; Thomas, J.B.; Ances, B.M. Network dysfunction in Alzheimer's disease: Refining the disconnection hypothesis. *Brain Connect.* **2014**, *4*, 299–311. [CrossRef]

77. Sheline, Y.I.; Morris, J.C.; Snyder, A.Z.; Price, J.L.; Yan, Z.; D'Angelo, G.; Liu, C.; Dixit, S.; Benzinger, T.; Fagan, A.; et al. APOE4 allele disrupts resting state fMRI connectivity in the absence of amyloid plaques or decreased CSF Aβ42. *J. Neurosci.* **2010**, *30*, 17035–17040. [CrossRef] [PubMed]

78. Walker, L.C.; Diamond, M.I.; Duff, K.E.; Hyman, B.T. Mechanisms of protein seeding in neurodegenerative diseases. *JAMA Neurol.* **2013**, *70*, 304–310. [CrossRef] [PubMed]

79. Zhou, J.; Gennatas, E.D.; Kramer, J.H.; Miller, B.L.; Seeley, W.W. Predicting regional neurodegeneration from the healthy brain functional connectome. *Neuron* **2012**, *73*, 1216–1227. [CrossRef]

80. Ingiosi, A.M.; Opp, M.R.; Krueger, J.M. Sleep and immune function: Glial contributions and consequences of aging. *Curr. Opin. Neurobiol.* **2013**, *23*, 806–811. [CrossRef]

81. Hurtado-Alvarado, G.; Pavón, L.; Castillo-García, S.A.; Hernández, M.E.; Domínguez-Salazar, E.; Velázquez-Moctezuma, J.; Gómez-González, B. Sleep loss as a factor to induce cellular and molecular inflammatory variations. *Clin. Dev. Immunol.* **2013**, *2013*, 801341. [CrossRef]

82. Heneka, M.T.; Carson, M.J.; El Khoury, J.; Landreth, G.E.; Brosseron, F.; Feinstein, D.L.; Jacobs, A.H.; Wyss-Coray, T.; Vitorica, J.; Ransohoff, R.M.; et al. Neuroinflammation in Alzheimer's disease. *Lancet Neurol.* **2015**, *14*, 388–405. [CrossRef]

83. Bellesi, M.; de Vivo, L.; Chini, M.; Gilli, F.; Tononi, G.; Cirelli, C. Sleep loss promotes astrocytic phagocytosis and microglial activation in mouse cerebral cortex. *J. Neurosci.* **2017**, *37*, 5263–5273. [CrossRef] [PubMed]

84. Hurtado-Alvarado, G.; Domínguez-Salazar, E.; Pavon, L.; Velazquez-Moctezuma, J.; Gomez-Gonzalez, B. Blood-brain barrier disruption induced by chronic sleep loss: Low-grade inflammation may be the link. *J. Immunol. Res.* **2016**, *2016*, e4576012. [CrossRef]

85. Sweeney, M.D.; Sagare, A.P.; Zlokovic, B.V. Blood–brain barrier breakdown in Alzheimer's disease and other neurodegenerative disorders. *Nat. Rev. Neurol.* **2018**, *14*, 133–150. [CrossRef] [PubMed]

86. Villafuerte, G.; Miguel-Puga, A.; Murillo Rodríguez, E.; Machado, S.; Manjarrez, E.; Arias-Carrión, O. Sleep deprivation and oxidative stress in animal models: A systematic review. *Oxid. Med. Cell. Longev.* **2015**, *2015*, 234952. [CrossRef]

87. Sharma, R.A.; Varga, A.W.; Bubu, O.M.; Pirraglia, E.; Kam, K.; Parekh, A.; Wohlleber, M.; Miller, M.D.; Andrade, A.; Lewis, C.; et al. Obstructive sleep apnea severity affects amyloid burden in cognitively normal elderly. A longitudinal study. *Am. J. Respir. Crit. Care. Med.* **2017**, *197*, 933–943. [CrossRef] [PubMed]

88. Hayashi, Y.; Kashiwagi, M.; Yasuda, K.; Ando, R.; Kanuka, M.; Sakai, K.; Itohara, S. Cells of a common developmental origin regulate REM/non-REM sleep and wakefulness in mice. *Science* **2015**, aad1023. [CrossRef]

89. Trauer, J.M.; Qian, M.Y.; Doyle, J.S.; Rajaratnam, S.M.W.; Cunnington, D. Cognitive behavioral therapy for chronic insomnia: A systematic review and meta-analysis. *Ann. Intern. Med.* **2015**, *163*, 191–204. [CrossRef]

90. Van Straten, A.; van der Zweerde, T.; Kleiboer, A.; Cuijpers, P.; Morin, C.M.; Lancee, J. Cognitive and behavioral therapies in the treatment of insomnia: A meta-analysis. *Sleep. Med. Rev.* **2018**, *38*, 3–16. [CrossRef]

91. Kay-Stacey, M.; Attarian, H. Advances in the management of chronic insomnia. *BMJ* **2016**, *354*, i2123. [CrossRef]

92. Wilson, S.; Nutt, D.; Alford, C.; Argyropoulos, S.; Baldwin, D.; Bateson, A.; Britton, T.; Crowe, C.; Dijk, D.-J.; Espie, C.; et al. British Association for Psychopharmacology consensus statement on evidence-based treatment of insomnia, parasomnias and circadian rhythm disorders. *J. Psychopharmacol.* **2010**, *24*, 1577–1601. [CrossRef] [PubMed]

93. Abad, V.C.; Guilleminault, C. Insomnia in elderly patients: Recommendations for pharmacological management. *Drugs Aging.* **2018**, *35*, 791–817. [CrossRef] [PubMed]

94. Zhao, Z.; Zhao, X.; Veasey, S.C. Neural consequences of chronic short sleep: Reversible or lasting? *Front. Neurol.* **2017**, *8*, 235. [CrossRef] [PubMed]

95. Van Dongen, H.P.A.; Maislin, G.; Mullington, J.M.; Dinges, D.F. The cumulative cost of additional wakefulness: Dose-response effects on neurobehavioral functions and sleep physiology from chronic sleep restriction and total sleep deprivation. *Sleep* **2003**, *26*, 117–126. [CrossRef]

96. Belenky, G.; Wesensten, N.J.; Thorne, D.R.; Thomas, M.L.; Sing, H.C.; Redmond, D.P.; Russo, M.B.; Balkin, T.J. Patterns of performance degradation and restoration during sleep restriction and subsequent recovery: A sleep dose-response study. *J. Sleep Res.* **2003**, *12*, 1–12. [CrossRef] [PubMed]
97. Pejovic, S.; Basta, M.; Vgontzas, A.N.; Kritikou, I.; Shaffer, M.L.; Tsaoussoglou, M.; Stiffler, D.; Stefanakis, Z.; Bixler, E.O.; Chrousos, G.P. Effects of recovery sleep after one work week of mild sleep restriction on interleukin-6 and cortisol secretion and daytime sleepiness and performance. *Am. J. Physiol. Endocrinol. Metab.* **2013**, *305*, E890–E896. [CrossRef] [PubMed]

13

Ca^{2+} Dyshomeostasis Disrupts Neuronal and Synaptic Function in Alzheimer's Disease

John McDaid [1,2], Sarah Mustaly-Kalimi [1,2] and Grace E. Stutzmann [1,2,3,*]

1 Center for Neurodegenerative Disease and Therapeutics, Rosalind Franklin University of Medicine and Science, 3333 Green Bay Rd., North Chicago, IL 60064, USA; john.mcdaid@rosalindfranklin.edu (J.M.); sarah.mustaly@my.rfums.org (S.M.-K.)

2 School of Graduate and Postdoctoral Studies, Rosalind Franklin University of Medicine and Science, 3333 Green Bay Rd., North Chicago, IL 60064, USA

3 Chicago Medical School, Rosalind Franklin University of Medicine and Science, 3333 Green Bay Rd., North Chicago, IL 60064, USA

* Correspondence: grace.stutzmann@rosalindfranklin.edu

Abstract: Ca^{2+} homeostasis is essential for multiple neuronal functions and thus, Ca^{2+} dyshomeostasis can lead to widespread impairment of cellular and synaptic signaling, subsequently contributing to dementia and Alzheimer's disease (AD). While numerous studies implicate Ca^{2+} mishandling in AD, the cellular basis for loss of cognitive function remains under investigation. The process of synaptic degradation and degeneration in AD is slow, and constitutes a series of maladaptive processes each contributing to a further destabilization of the Ca^{2+} homeostatic machinery. Ca^{2+} homeostasis involves precise maintenance of cytosolic Ca^{2+} levels, despite extracellular influx via multiple synaptic Ca^{2+} channels, and intracellular release via organelles such as the endoplasmic reticulum (ER) via ryanodine receptor (RyRs) and IP_3R, lysosomes via transient receptor potential mucolipin channel (TRPML) and two pore channel (TPC), and mitochondria via the permeability transition pore (PTP). Furthermore, functioning of these organelles relies upon regulated inter-organelle Ca^{2+} handling, with aberrant signaling resulting in synaptic dysfunction, protein mishandling, oxidative stress and defective bioenergetics, among other consequences consistent with AD. With few effective treatments currently available to mitigate AD, the past few years have seen a significant increase in the study of synaptic and cellular mechanisms as drivers of AD, including Ca^{2+} dyshomeostasis. Here, we detail some key findings and discuss implications for future AD treatments.

Keywords: calcium; synaptic; glutamate; nicotinic receptors; mitochondria; autophagy; lysosome

---

1. Ca^{2+} Dysregulation and Synaptic Defects in AD

The synapse, as the primary site of communication between neurons, plays a vital role in the transmission of neuronal impulses and information, and for encoding of learning and memory, all of which are affected in Alzheimer's disease (AD). AD, as a progressive neurodegenerative disease, is characterized by Ca^{2+} dysregulation i.e., a "calciumopathy" [1] and synapse loss, i.e., a "synaptopathy" [2], with emerging evidence for a causal link between the two. Synaptic density is decreased in post-mortem brain tissue from AD patients [3,4], and while amyloid plaques have been implicated in AD related synaptic loss, synaptic deficits occur prior to and in the absence of amyloid plaques [5], and may also be due to Ca^{2+} dysregulation, an effect which is exhibited in presymptomatic AD mouse models [6–9]. Ca^{2+} dysregulation is characterized by exaggerated Ca^{2+} responses to synaptic and other stimuli, as well as abnormal Ca^{2+} homeostasis [10,11], both of which may result in elevated resting cytosolic Ca^{2+}, an effect which is observed in AD and older non-AD rodent models [12–16].

1.1. Ca^{2+} Dysregulation Disrupts Synaptic Networks in AD

Synapses are unique Ca^{2+} entry points in the neuronal architecture, expressing both pre- and postsynaptic Ca^{2+} channels/receptors, including presynaptic RyRs, N/P/Q voltage gated Ca^{2+} channels (VGCCs), α7 nicotinic acetylcholine receptors (α7 nAChRs), and postsynaptic L-type VGCCs, RyRs and NMDA receptors (NMDARs). NMDARs in particular are one of the most well characterized postsynaptic glutamate receptors, with a high Ca^{2+} permeability and an established role in hippocampal synaptic plasticity [17]. At hyperpolarized potentials, NMDARs are blocked by Mg^{2+}, but postsynaptic depolarization results in removal of Mg^{2+} block, and receptor disinhibition. Repeated NMDAR activation enhances postsynaptic Ca^{2+} entry, an effect which is facilitated by RyRs through Ca^{2+}-induced-Ca^{2+} release (CICR), thus driving increased postsynaptic AMPA receptor (AMPAR) expression and subsequent synaptic long-term potentiation (LTP). This dual role of the NMDAR as coincidence detector and postsynaptic Ca^{2+} entry channel makes it uniquely positioned to mediate synaptic potentiation resulting from concurrent pre- and postsynaptic activation, thus forming a mechanistic basis for Hebbian plasticity and associative learning.

Paradoxically, NMDARS, as well as playing a role in synaptic plasticity, may also play a role in synaptic loss [18] and cell death [19]. The role of NMDARs in the deleterious effects of AD is further illustrated by the efficacy of the NMDAR antagonist memantine as a treatment for moderate to severe AD [20,21]. Interestingly, the clinical efficacy, or lack thereof, of specific Ca^{2+} channel antagonists could serve as a useful pointer for a role for those Ca^{2+} channels in the pathophysiology of AD, with the failure of large scale clinical trials for L-type VGCC antagonists in particular, contrasting with the positive effects of memantine [22]. AD is characterized by synaptic loss [2,4,23], including loss of synaptic terminals and dendritic spines [4], and similar dendritic spine loss is accompanied by impaired synaptic transmission and plasticity in animal models of AD [8,24–29]. Although the cause of synaptic loss in AD is not fully understood, it is thought to be associated with increased ER- Ca^{2+} release within spines [8,9,30,31], and at later disease states, toxic soluble Aβ species [32], resulting in hippocampal dendritic spine loss via NMDAR activation [33–35]. In contrast to Aβ, synaptic effects of abnormal tau expression have not been as extensively studied, however, a few recent studies have implicated effects of tau on VGCC function and synaptic signaling [36–38]. Specifically, tau accumulation may lead to synaptic loss and impairment of synaptic function via activation of calcineurin [39].

Hippocampal and cortical neurites in close proximity to amyloid plaques demonstrate Ca^{2+} hyperactivity in vivo, in presymptomatic AD mice, an effect which is blocked by AMPA receptor and NMDAR antagonists, suggesting that this hyperactivity is synaptically driven [6,7]. Although Ca^{2+} hyperactivity occurred mainly in the vicinity of insoluble dense core plaques, these plaques are also surrounded by soluble Aβ [40,41], which causes similar hyperactivity in WT mice [6]. Furthermore, plaque proximity has been reported to have no effect on evoked dendritic RyR and VGCC mediated Ca^{2+} signaling in AD mice [42], raising the possibility that some of the hyperactivity observed may be due to a presynaptic mechanism. Indeed, the presynaptic Ca^{2+} hyperactivity observed in an AD mouse model was inhibited by the sarcoplasmic endoplasmic Ca^{2+}-ATPase (SERCA) pump inhibitor cyclopiazonic acid, indicating that this Ca^{2+} hyperactivity is driven by activation of presynaptic Ca^{2+} stores [43]. In contrast to reports of synaptically driven hyperexcitability in vivo, studies carried out using acute brain slices from AD mice demonstrate decreased basal hippocampal synaptic transmission, sometimes accompanied by increased paired-pulse ratio of evoked field potentials, indicative of decreased presynaptic glutamate release probability [29,44,45]. In addition, the membrane afterhyperpolarization mediated by activation of postsynaptic Ca^{2+} activated SK2 channels is increased in a 3xTg AD mouse model [46], leading to decreased postsynaptic membrane excitability and possible decreased synaptic transmission. It should also be noted that the decreased hippocampal synaptic transmission recently observed in a 5xTg AD mouse model was coupled with increased postsynaptic membrane excitability, due to an RyR2 mediated decrease in A-type K^+ current (I_A) [47], thus further illustrating the complexity of synaptic effects observed in AD mouse models. It is also noteworthy that the in vivo hyperexcitability studies mentioned above were conducted in animals anesthetized using the volatile inhalational anesthetic isoflurane. As isoflurane has been shown to result in increased cytosolic Ca^{2+} in hippocampal neurons [48], possibly due to IP_3 receptor activation [49], effects which are exaggerated in AD mice [50], isoflurane anesthesia could be a potential mediator of the Ca^{2+} hyperexcitability observed in vivo in AD mice.

While the last two decades have seen a large increase in the number of studies using AD mouse models, a more recent development has been in the use of human induced neurons (HiNs), which are neurons derived from tissue samples taken from patients, to study synaptic transmission [51–53]. In a recent study, an increased frequency of spontaneous excitatory postsynaptic current (EPSC's) was observed in AD derived HiNs, indicating an impulse-independent spontaneous increase in presynaptic glutamate release probability which is consistent with findings in human and animal studies [52]. Studies in patients with mild cognitive impairment have demonstrated hippocampal hyperactivity and decreased hippocampal volume [54,55], indicating a possible correlation between increased hippocampal activity and neurodegeneration.

More recently, proteomics has emerged as a method that allows for high throughput analysis of protein expression in small tissue samples [56], including post-mortem brain tissue from AD patients [57,58], and which has allowed for the study of changes in the interaction between presynaptic proteins [59], including SNAP25 and syntaxin [60]. Increased SNAP25 and syntaxin interaction results in reduced glutamatergic synaptic transmission [61,62] and decreased interaction between these proteins has been observed in the brains of AD patients, along with decreased levels of Complexin II [63], effects which would be expected to result in increased excitatory synaptic transmission [64,65]. SNAP25 has also been shown to negatively interact with presynaptic VGCCs to control presynaptic Ca^{2+} and affect neurotransmitter release [66,67], and the demonstrated therapeutic efficacy of putative AD medications such as levetiracetam, which targets presynaptic VGCCs [68,69], suggests that presynaptic Ca^{2+} channels could serve as a therapeutic target for AD.

1.2. Acetylcholine Signaling and α7nAChR Function in AD

nAChRs are essential for normal cognitive function [70,71], and this family of receptors includes the highly Ca^{2+} permeable homomeric α7nAChR isoform [72,73]. α7nAChRs are expressed throughout the septo-hippocampal circuit, both on medial septal nucleus/diagonal band cholinergic neurons [74], and also in the hippocampus. Cholinergic neurons in particular show significant degeneration in the course of AD [75,76], and this has resulted in development of medications to enhance cholinergic transmission, presumably through the activation of postsynaptic nAChRs. Hippocampal α7nAChRs are expressed presynaptically on mossy fiber terminals [77], and postsynaptically on CA1 interneurons [78,79], with activation of both resulting in Ca^{2+} influx [79–83]. Nicotine enhances hippocampal excitatory synaptic transmission via activation of α7nAChRs on mossy fiber terminals in the hippocampal CA3 region [80,81,84] and activation of CA1 α7nAChRs facilitates hippocampal LTP [85].

Aβ binds with high affinity to α7nAChRs [86,87], resulting in noncompetitive block of α7nAChR function, including at presynaptic α7nAChRs [88]. Cortical and hippocampal α7nAChR expression is reduced in AD patients [89,90] and AD mice [91] and Aβ binding to α7nAChRs results in the endocytosis of the Aβ α7nAChR complex with resulting accumulation within the lysosomal compartment [92]. Aβ binding to α7nAChRs results in Ca^{2+} influx, both in oocytes and presynaptic terminals in hippocampus [93,94]. Low micromolar concentrations of Aβ trigger glutamate release in the hippocampal dentate gyrus, CA3 and CA1 subfields via α7nAChRs [95] and picomolar concentrations of Aβ enhance hippocampal LTP via α7nAChRs [96]. In addition, α7nAChR activation rescues LTP deficits in hippocampal slices taken from Aβ infused rat brains, and Aβ treated hippocampal slices [97,98] and chronic treatment with an α7nAChR agonist restores cognition in AD mice [99]. Cells treated with the acetylcholinesterase inhibitor donepezil, used clinically in the treatment of AD, also showed reduced glutamate NMDAR mediated Ca^{2+} influx, an effect which was blocked by an α7nAChR antagonist [100]. Galantamine, also an acetylcholinesterase inhibitor, has been shown to positively modulate human α7nAChRs expressed in xenopus oocytes, thus allowing for a dual effect of increased synaptic acetylcholine and α7nAChR potentiation [101].

Although a role for α7nAChRs in the etiology of AD has not been established, many animal studies have demonstrated cognitive enhancing effects of compounds targeting α7nAChRs [102], including the α7nAChR partial agonist EVP-6124, which has also been shown to enhance cognition in patients with mild to moderate AD [103]. EVP-6124 and the α7nAChR positive allosteric modulator AVL-3288 have been shown to be well tolerated in patients [104,105], but some concerns exist about effects of potentiation of α7nAChR mediated Ca^{2+} effects in AD. In addition to α7nAChR mediated Ca^{2+} influx, activation of α7nAChRs triggers CICR via ryanodine sensitive Ca^{2+} stores [106], including at presynaptic α7nAChRs on hippocampal mossy fiber terminals [107], which are known to have strong RyR expression [108]. As RyR mediated CICR may be increased in AD, positive allosteric modulation of α7nAChRs may facilitate pre- and postsynaptic Ca^{2+} overload via already increased RyR function [109], possibly exacerbating AD related synaptic deficits. Based on these studies, the use of α7nAChR compounds in the treatment of cognitive impairment and AD looks promising, but caution should be exercised regarding the use of drugs which result in overt α7nAChR potentiation.

1.3. *Potential Therapies for the Treatment of Synaptic Ca^{2+} Dysregulation in AD*

As of now, there are only two FDA-approved classes of drugs used in the symptomatic treatment of AD: the noncompetitive NMDA antagonist memantine, and the acetylcholinesterase inhibitors, donepezil, galantamine and rivastigmine, with both classes of drugs having a synaptic site of action. Although both memantine and donepezil have been shown to be moderately effective in the treatment of AD symptoms, there is an urgent need for disease-modifying approaches, which currently requires the identification of novel compounds and receptor targets at the pre- or postsynaptic level. While a number of studies have identified promising small molecules targeting NMDARs [19,51], α7nAChRs [85,99], RyRs [110] and SERCA [111], few have made it past the preclinical stage of testing. In addition, the smoking cessation medication varenicline, which is an agonist at the α7nAChR [112], has been tested as a treatment for AD, but without any observed beneficial effects in patients [113]. Despite its failure, the clinical trial for varenicline illustrates the use of existing FDA approved medications as a strategy in the treatment of AD, bypassing many of the arduous and expensive aspects of drug development. The RyR modulator dantrolene (Ryanodex) is an FDA approved medication that has been shown to be effective in reversing many of the synaptic and cognitive effects seen in mouse models of AD [8,114–116], and has good CNS penetration when given orally or by nasal administration [117]. In addition, the clinically used L-type VGCC inhibitor isradipine has been shown to be neuroprotective in an AD mouse model [22], as has the beta-blocker carvedilol [47], however results from a recent large clinical study suggested no benefit of the VGCC antagonist nilvadipine as a treatment for AD [118]. Although the failure of large scale clinical trials for VGCC inhibitors as a treatment for AD has resulted in diminished enthusiasm for their use, the antiepileptic drug levetiracetam, which inhibits presynaptic VGCCs [68], has been shown to be beneficial in AD patients [69] and clinical trials for its use in the treatment of AD are ongoing [119]. The relative success of levetiracetam, along with the well documented failure of clinical trials targeting amyloid, strengthens the case for the use of synaptically targeted drugs in the treatment of AD and argues for the testing of FDA-approved medications as an important therapeutic strategy in the treatment of AD.

1.4. *ER Ca^{2+} Channels in Synaptic Dysregulation in AD*

Cytosolic Ca^{2+} levels are tightly regulated and maintained at low nM concentrations, despite a much higher extracellular Ca^{2+} concentration, and similarly elevated Ca^{2+} levels within intracellular organelles such as the ER. The ER is located throughout the cell, including pre- and postsynaptically, at synaptic terminals and dendritic spines respectively. RyRs, as well as having a role in gating ER Ca^{2+}, are sensitive to changes in cytosolic Ca^{2+} through the process of CICR, with increases in postsynaptic Ca^{2+} resulting in RyR activation and release of ER Ca^{2+} into the cytosol. CICR has the effect of amplifying postsynaptic Ca^{2+} generated from influx via Ca^{2+} permeable receptors/ion channels such as NMDA receptors (NMDAR) and voltage gated Ca^{2+} channels (VGCCs), and RyR mediated CICR is upregulated in neurons in 3xTg AD mice [9]. Although RyR mediated amplification of postsynaptic Ca^{2+} allows for a large rapid increase in cytosolic Ca^{2+}, this increased Ca^{2+} is usually rapidly removed from the cytosol, against a concentration gradient, by Ca^{2+} ATPases including the SERCA pump, which is also located on the ER membrane. The ER membrane also expresses IP_3 receptors, although these are not thought to be synaptically expressed [120].

Mutations in the presenilin 1 (PS1) gene are linked to familial AD, an early onset form of the disease, and these mutations have specific functional implications for Ca^{2+} regulation. Although PS1 is a part of the γ-secretase complex which cleaves amyloid precursor protein (APP), it is also expressed on the ER membrane where it regulates RyR and IP_3R channel properties [121–124], and may serve as a Ca^{2+} leak channel [125,126]. Mutations or altered expression of PS1 also affect the expression and sensitivity of neighboring RyRs [124]. RyRs play an important role in Ca^{2+} regulation, and RyR dysfunction is implicated in the Ca^{2+} dysregulation observed in AD [1]. RyR expression and RyR mediated Ca^{2+} responses are increased in the soma and dendritic spines of hippocampal and cortical pyramidal neurons of AD mice expressing PS1 mutations (Figures 1 and 2) [9,30,127], effects which are normalized by acute or chronic treatment with dantrolene, a negative allosteric RyR modulator [50,114]. In particular, the RyR2 isoform, which is overexpressed in the hippocampus of AD mice [30,114], plays an important role in maintenance of synaptic function [128] and shortening of the RyR2 mean channel open time reverses the synaptic dysfunction and Ca^{2+} dyshomeostasis observed in an AD mouse model [47]. Human-induced neurons (HiN) derived from fibroblasts from AD patients expressing the PS1 mutation also display increased RyR expression and evoked RyR Ca^{2+} release [53], and RyR expression is also increased in post-mortem brains of AD patients, and patients with mild cognitive impairment [129,130]. Postsynaptic Ca^{2+} responses to high frequency stimulation (HFS) are increased in hippocampal and cortical neurons from several AD mouse models [8,9,131], effects which are mediated by RyR activation (Figure 1) [9]. Presynaptic RyR function is also increased in 3xTg AD mice and RyR activation by caffeine decreases the paired-pulse ratio of evoked CA1 field potentials to a greater extent in AD mice, as well as restoring normal frequency of spontaneously released vesicles, indicating increased facilitation of glutamate release by presynaptic RyRs [30]. Further indications of pathogenic synaptic effects resulting from altered RyR-Ca^{2+} signaling is the restoration of reduced presynaptic vesicle stores observed in AD mice back to normal levels upon treatment with Ryanodex [24].

In addition to effects on basal synaptic transmission, changes in RyR-Ca^{2+} signaling may also have implications for synaptic plasticity and LTP, which are impaired in AD mice [8,45]. High frequency stimulation (HFS) of hippocampal CA3-CA1 Schaffer collaterals, which generates LTP, initially results in a period of short-term, presynaptically mediated plasticity known as post tetanic potentiation (PTP), which results from an accumulation of presynaptic Ca^{2+} and is accompanied by an increased release probability of glutamate. This form of short term plasticity is necessary for the synaptic tagging processes involved in LTP [132], however in 3xTg AD mice, PTP is reduced, and this diminished short-term plasticity is followed by decreased LTP [8]. Chronic treatment with the RyR modulator dantrolene has been shown to restore PTP and LTP to control levels seen in non-AD mice, and this effect was accompanied by a restoration of presynaptic vesicles in the active zone, illustrating a role for aberrant presynaptic RyR-Ca^{2+} signaling in the impaired short and long-term synaptic plasticity observed in AD mice [8]. Presenilin deletion decreases Ca^{2+} effects of RyR activation, due to decreased RyR expression [121] and selective deletion of presynaptic presenilin decreases the release probability of glutamate, and LTP, an effect that is mimicked and occluded by RyR inhibition [133]. Thus, it would seem alterations in PS1 expression/function result in diminished LTP, either due to decreased or increased presynaptic RyR function, emphasizing the importance of RyR stabilization in maintenance of normal synaptic function.

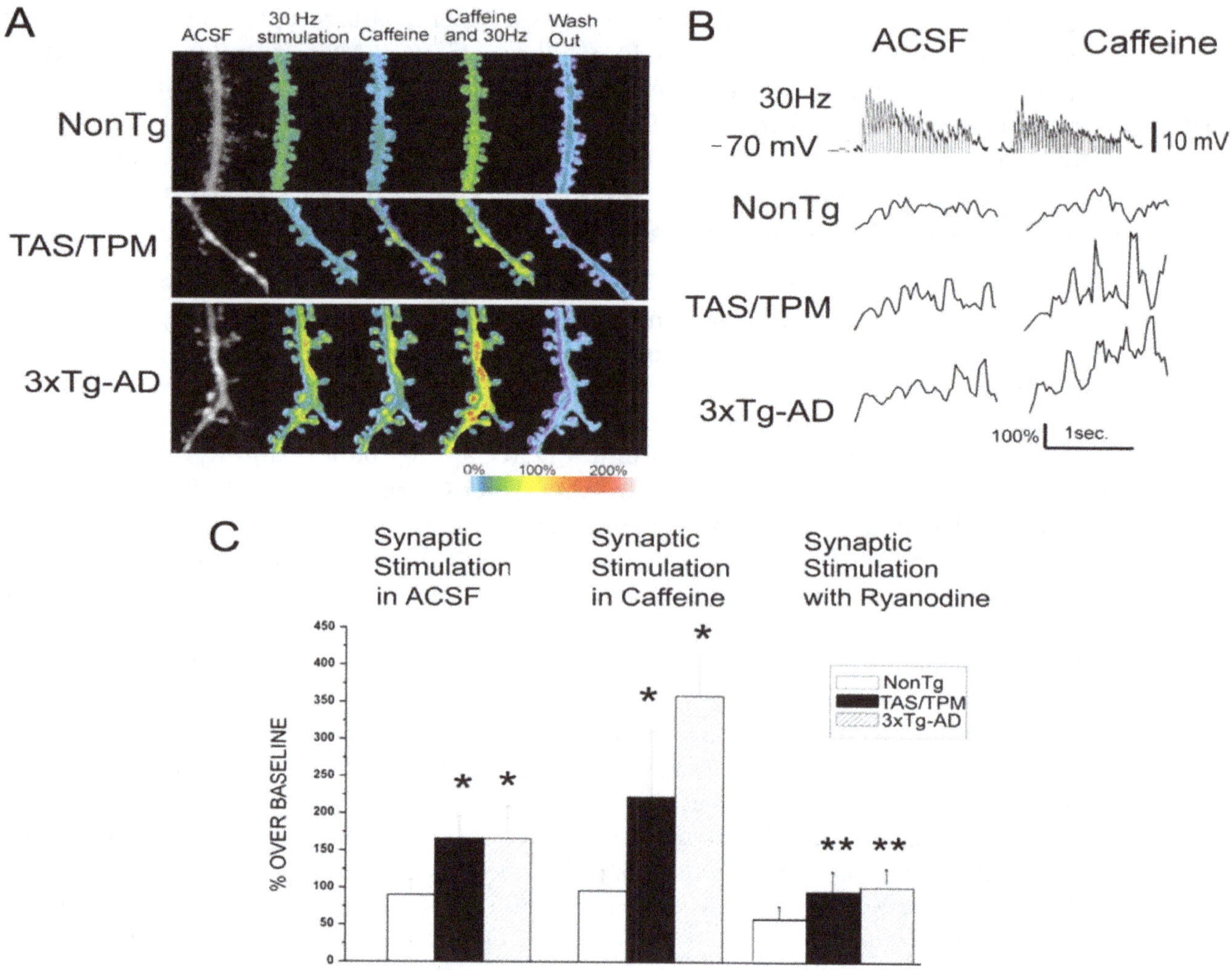

Figure 1. Synergistic Ca^{2+} interactions between RyR and glutamatergic synaptic transmission in AD mouse cortical neurons. (**A**) Pseudocolored images of relative Ca^{2+} changes in representative NonTg (top), TAS/TPM (a double transgenic AD mouse model) (middle), and 3xTg-AD (a triple transgenic AD mouse model) (bottom) neurons in the following conditions (from left to right): baseline 30 Hz synaptic stimulation (1.5 s), caffeine alone (10 mm), 30 Hz synaptic stimulation plus caffeine, and washout. (**B**) Representative Ca^{2+} response traces after 30 Hz synaptic stimulation (voltage trace shown in top) shown as percentage over baseline, in control aCSF (left panels) and in 10 mM caffeine (right panels) for NonTg (top), TAS/TPM (middle), and 3xTg-AD (bottom) neurons. (**C**) Bar graphs show averaged (mean ± SE) Ca^{2+} responses integrated over a 1.5 s time period of 30 Hz synaptic stimulation in control ACSF (left grouping), synaptic stimulation plus caffeine (center), and synaptic stimulation with ryanodine in the pipette (right grouping) for the NonTg, TAS/TPM, and 3xTg-AD neurons. Statistically significant differences are indicated by asterisks (one-way ANOVA, $p < 0.05$). * Significantly different from NonTg within treatment group; ** significantly different from synaptic stimulation in aCSF within transgenic strain (modified from [9]).

Low resting cytosolic Ca^{2+} is maintained in part due to the actions of Ca^{2+}-ATPases, which rapidly remove Ca^{2+} from the cell cytosol, against a concentration gradient. One of the major cellular Ca^{2+}-ATPases is the SERCA pump, located on the ER membrane. SERCA function is facilitated by presenilin, and knockdown of the genes for presenilin 1 and presenilin 2 results in elevated cytosolic Ca^{2+}, due to decreased SERCA mediated clearance of cytosolic Ca^{2+} [134]. Overexpression of the SERCA2b isoform typically found in neurons, and which physically interacts with the PS1 and PS2 Ca^{2+} channels on the ER membrane, results in increased Aβ [134]. Further evidence for presenilin's role in SERCA function comes from a study showing that cells expressing a PS1 mutation show an exaggerated cytosolic Ca^{2+} response to SERCA inhibition by thapsigargin, indicating increased SERCA function [135]. SERCA inhibition also mimics the effects of selective deletion of presynaptic presenilin, on synaptic transmission and LTP [133], and inhibition of presynaptic SERCA function by cyclopiazonic acid diminished the Ca^{2+} hyperactivity observed in cortical neurons of AD mice in vivo [43]. In addition to SERCA, STIM Ca^{2+} sensors and Orai Ca^{2+} channels facilitate ER Ca^{2+} filling through the process of store-operated-Ca^{2+} entry (SOCE), a process which is deficient in PS1 mutant expressing neurons [136,137]. As ER Ca^{2+} release is elevated in AD neurons (Figure 2), in parallel with diminished SOCE activity, this opens up the possibility of an increased role for SERCA in this maladaptive pathology.

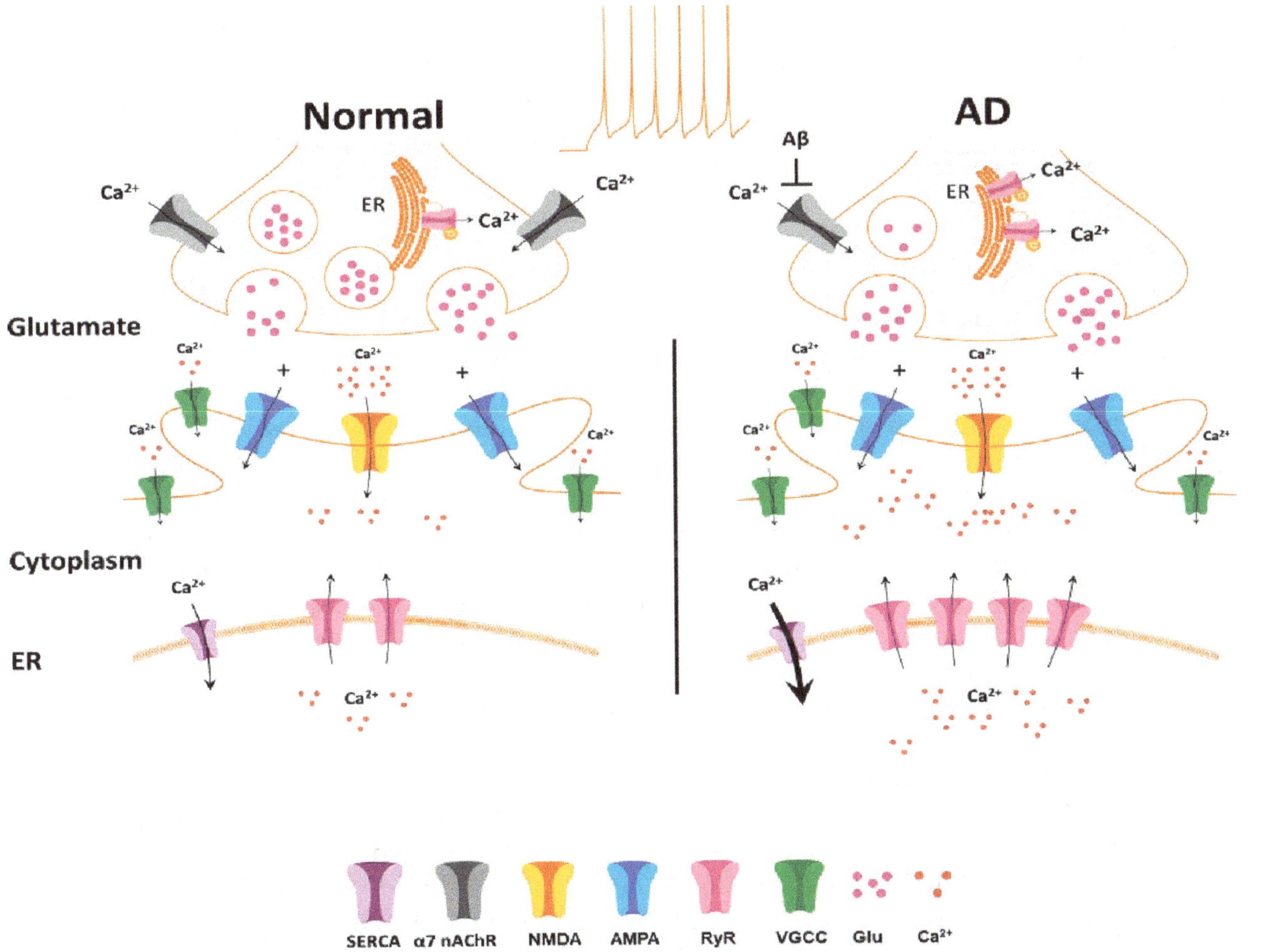

Figure 2. Schematic of synaptic Ca^{2+} dysregulation in AD. Under normal circumstances (left), impulse mediated increases in presynaptic Ca^{2+} result in neurotransmitter release via a ready releasable vesicular pool. In addition, activation of presynaptic α7nAChRs triggers further Ca^{2+} influx, thus facilitating impulse mediated release, and presynaptic effects may be further increased via presynaptic RyR mediated Ca^{2+}-induced-Ca^{2+} release (CICR). In mouse models of AD, although intrinsic cell excitability is not increased, presynaptic RyR mediated CICR may be increased, resulting in increased release probability of glutamate and depletion of vesicle stores. Aβ binding to presynaptic α7nAChRs may result in occlusion of the binding site, with decreased function and eventual decreased presynaptic α7nAChR expression due to endocytosis. In AD, increased ER Ca^{2+} stores, along with increased RyR expression results in increased postsynaptic CICR, which may facilitate stimulus-evoked postsynaptic Ca^{2+} increases.

The characteristic features of AD, including maladaptive protein accumulation, increased free radicals and metabolic disruptions, are concurrent with aberrant intracellular Ca^{2+} signaling and contributes to the activation of the ER stress response in cells [138]. In an attempt to restore ER homeostasis, the ER triggers the unfolded protein response (UPR) by increasing the expression of transcription factors (ATP6c, XBPIs, and ATF4) which provides tolerance to cellular stress [139]. If the UPR is incompetent in decreasing stress, the ER triggers cell death by apoptosis [140,141] or autophagy [142]. Several animal [143–145] and human studies [138,146] report that AD mutations cause alterations in the UPR, thus in AD, aberrant ER-Ca^{2+} release disrupts the neuron's compensatory mechanisms to restore cellular homeostasis and increases the vulnerability of neurons to stress and death.

2. Ca^{2+} Mishandling Impairs Cellular Organelle Functions in AD

In addition to synaptic signaling deficits, Ca^{2+} dyshomeostasis also has profound effects on the function of cell organelles, including the mitochondria and lysosomes, both of which play an important role in maintaining cellular and synaptic function. Like the ER, mitochondria and lysosomes act as intracellular Ca^{2+} stores, and dyshomeostasis of mitochondrial and lysosomal Ca^{2+} is emerging as a potential new source of cell dysfunction in AD, with profound implications for cellular and synaptic health.

2.1. Ca^{2+} Dysregulation Disrupts Mitochondrial Bioenergetics in AD

The mitochondria's ability to buffer intracellular Ca^{2+} signaling is critical for neuronal signal transductions, ATP synthesis, and coordination with other organelles in physiological and pathological conditions. Mitochondrial dysfunction is a well-established characteristic of AD manifesting as increased free radical production and rate of oxidative damage, decreased ATP/ADP ratio and impaired bioenergetics [147–150]. Numerous differentially expressed mitochondria regulatory genes (133 in total) have been identified in the AD cohort and found that genes coding for mitochondrial oxidative phosphorylation were downregulated in both early and late AD brain specimens–specifically, NADH ubiquinone oxidoreductase subunits and complex I components which transfer electrons to the respiratory chain [151,152]. Proteomic and protein expression studies also confirmed dysregulated mitochondrial oxidative phosphorylation complexes [153] and defective enzymatic activity in the citric acid cycle and electron transport chain (ETC) [154,155].

The main function of the mitochondria is the production of ATP. Unavoidably, the by-products of electron transport in aerobic respiration are reactive oxygen species (ROS), due to electron leaks at complex I and III. Ca^{2+} overload, as is the case in AD, hinders glucose metabolism by disrupting components of the ETC such as, mitochondria complex I and II, tricarboxylic acid cycle (TCA), pyruvate dehydrogenase complex (PDHC), α-ketoglutarate dehydrogenase complex (KGDHC), malate dehydrogenase (MDH), and increasing ROS production while decreasing ATP production [156]. Redox proteomics studies identify increased oxidatively modified proteins, specifically antioxidant enzymes such as glutathione-S-transferase Mu, peroxiredoxin 6, multidrug-resistant protein 1 or 3, and GSH, in various brain regions of MCI and AD patients [157]. Additionally, enzymes involved in respiration were oxidized, specifically ATP synthase, aconitase, and creatine kinase [157]. This suggests that increased oxidative stress, as a consequence of mitochondrial Ca^{2+} overload, contributed to mitochondrial dysfunction and impaired energy metabolism in AD.

The dynamic function of the mitochondria requires crosstalk between other major organelles, such as the ER (Figure 3). Mitochondria's physical coupling to the ER is crucial for efficient Ca^{2+} transfer and cellular homeostasis. Mitochondrial Ca^{2+} uptake controls the rate of energy production, regulates intracellular Ca^{2+} signaling, and mediates cell death. Ca^{2+} transfer between these organelles is facilitated via the mitochondrial-associated membrane proteins (MAM). Numerous molecular proteins have been identified to support this physical interaction. Of interest, the glucose-regulated protein 75 (GRP75) is linked to IP_3R and facilitates Ca^{2+} into the mitochondrial intermembrane space. From there, voltage-dependent anion-selective channel protein 1 (VDAC1) on the outer mitochondrial membrane, and the mitochondrial Ca^{2+} uniporter (MCU) on the inner mitochondrial membrane, transfer the

Ca^{2+} to the mitochondrial matrix to stimulate the mitochondrial dehydrogenase and increase ETC activity and ATP synthesis. [158–163]. These MAMs play a crucial role in regulating mitochondrial Ca^{2+} uptake. In AD, many genes involved in mitochondrial Ca^{2+} transport are altered [164–166]. Of note, genes encoding mitochondrial Ca^{2+} influx, such as MCU, are downregulated whereas genes encoding mitochondrial Ca^{2+} efflux, such as NCLX, are upregulated, suggesting a compensatory mechanism to avoid excessive Ca^{2+} uptake. Additionally, studies report that, soluble Aβ aggregations increase cytosolic Ca^{2+}, leading to mitochondrial Ca^{2+} overload via MCU. Excessive Ca^{2+} taken up by mitochondria leads to caspase activation and neuronal cell death [167].

In addition to Ca^{2+}, VDAC1 supports transport of superoxide anions [168] and since IP_3R and RyRs have been shown to be redox-sensitive, ROS and Ca^{2+} may play a regulatory role in ER-mitochondria communication. During AD- associated Ca^{2+} overload, mitochondrial Ca^{2+} influx elevates oxidative stress and increases ROS production. In AD, accumulated ROS has profound effects on cellular functions by oxidizing several proteins, such as the redox-sensitive RyR and IP_3R channels. Thus, Ca^{2+} induced ROS increase and ROS-mediated Ca^{2+} increase creates a self-amplifying loop that furthers neurotoxicity and cellular dyshomeostasis, and neuronal death [169–172]. In AD, MAM proteins are shown to be associated with presenilin 1 and 2, suggesting *PSEN1/2* may alter mitochondrial Ca^{2+} transport. Additionally, increased contact sites between ER and mitochondria, via MAM proteins in AD result in elevation in ER-mitochondrial Ca^{2+} signaling and increased mitochondrial superoxide production [173–178].

Ca^{2+} is released from the mitochondria through the Na^+/Ca^{2+} exchanger (NCLX) and the permeability transition pore [179]. The two functional states of the PTP regulates the amount of Ca^{2+} released; where the low conductance state amplifies Ca^{2+} waves and the high conductance state releases a surge of Ca^{2+} and apoptotic signals such as cytochrome C [180,181]. The biochemical signatures underlying apoptosis, rather than necrosis, indicates a choreographed and organized shutdown of the neuron. In AD, with continuous, prolonged increase in mitochondrial Ca^{2+} concentration, Ca^{2+} released from the mitochondria signals for apoptosis and increases AD pathology [172]. However the role of NCLX in AD needs further exploration as recent work suggests that impairment in glucose metabolism might reverse NCLX activity [182,183]. Additionally, impairment in NCLX accelerated memory declined and increased amyloidosis and tau pathology [184]. Mitochondrial calcium homeostasis may also rely on the activity of the plasma membrane NCLX, whose expression has been seen in differential patterns of mitochondrial expression dependent on cell type, and disruptions in expression may contribute to AD pathology [185–187].

Mitochondrial morphology and distribution are also crucial for neuronal homeostasis and synaptic function. Mitochondria undergo fusion and fission in the cytoplasm, which is a process to maintain a healthy pool of mitochondria with proper distribution. These mechanisms are controlled by DLP_1 for fission and Mfn_1, Mfn_2, and OPA_1 for fusion [188]. In AD, importantly, Aβ-induced and/or oxidative stress induced Ca^{2+} signaling led to increased DLP_1 activation, resulting in excessive mitochondrial translocation and fission [189,190]. Recent studies reported that mitochondrial fragmentation, along with extensive oxidative stress and neuroinflammation, lead to neuronal loss in the cortex and hippocampus [191,192]. Excessive mitochondrial fragmentation as a result of improper Ca^{2+} handling and increased oxidative stress disrupts mitochondrial function, advancing AD pathology. Disrupted DLP_1 and Mfn_2 function is also responsible for reduced mitochondrial distribution. In AD, mitochondria are less abundant in neuronal processes of susceptible pyramidal neurons [193,194]. Increased tau phosphorylation negatively regulates mitochondrial movement in neurons. Tau phosphorylated at the AT8 sites inhibited mitochondrial movement in neurite processes of PC12 cells and mouse cortical neurons due to impaired microtubule spacing [195,196].

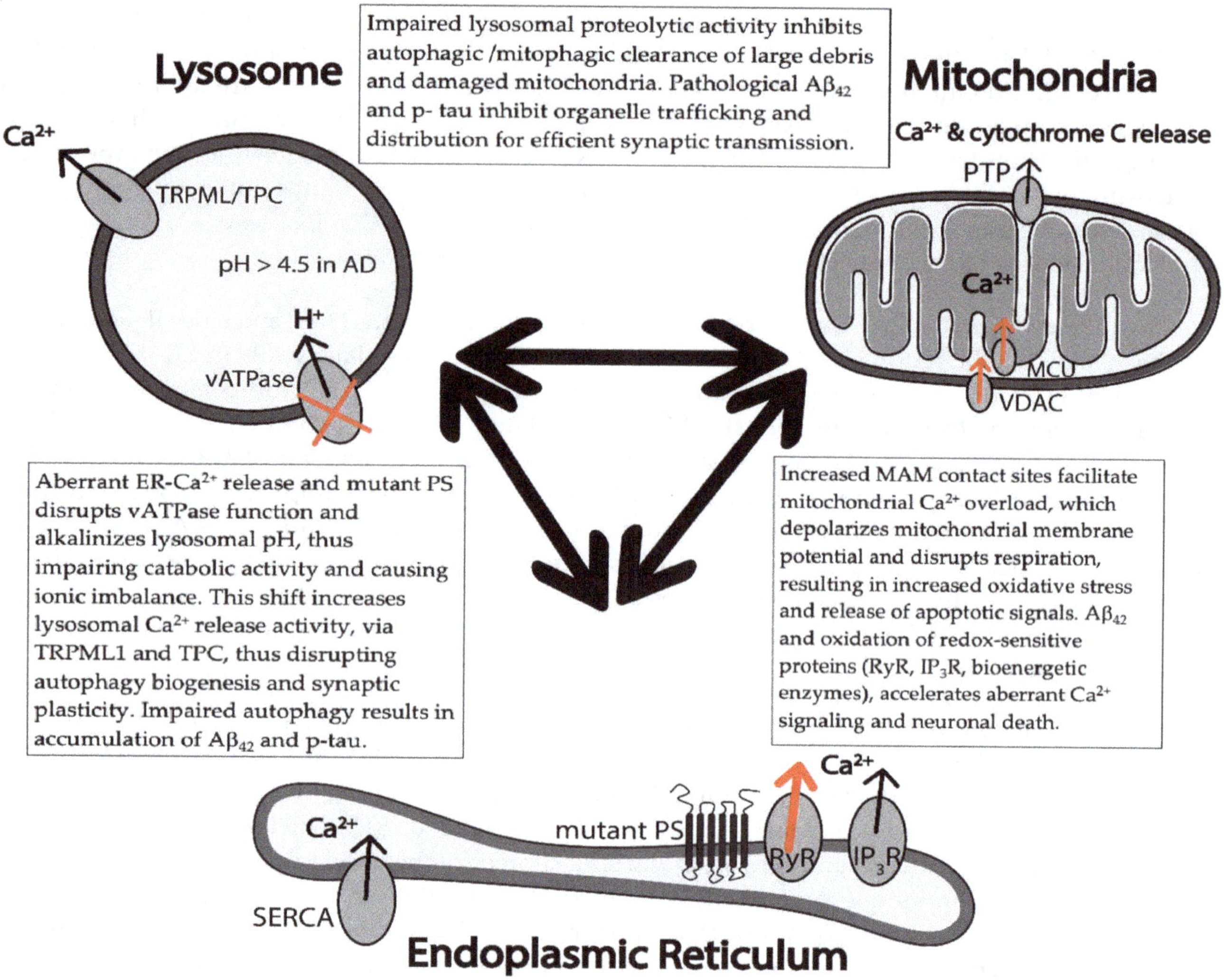

Figure 3. Aberrant Ca^{2+} disrupts inter-organelle functional relationships in early AD pathology. Schematic of feed-forward cascades among various neuronal Ca^{2+} handling organelles: Endoplasmic reticulutm (ER), lysosome, and mitochondria, in early AD pathology. Excess ER Ca^{2+} release through RyR and IP_3R cause mitochondrial Ca^{2+} overload that disrupts mitochondrial bioenergetics, resulting in increased oxidative stress and apoptosis. Additionally, ER Ca^{2+} disrupts lysosome-mediated clearance of maladaptive protein deposits and damaged organelle, such as Aβ, p-tau, and mitochondria, respectively. Aberrant intracellular Ca^{2+} signaling disrupts lysosomal Ca^{2+} release via TRPML and dysregulates autophagosome biosynthesis and impairs synaptic plasticity. Presenilin (PS) mutations disrupt vATPase trafficking resulting in alkaline lysosomes, thereby disrupting lysosomal ionic balance and lysosomal Ca^{2+} store. This alkaline environment impairs proteolysis and impairs autophagic clearance.

Damaged mitochondria are cleared through mitophagy, the selective degradation of mitochondria by autophagy following organelle damage or extreme cellular stress [197]. Mitophagy initiation involves the recruitment of PINK1 and PARKIN to the outer mitochondrial membrane, which tags the damaged mitochondria for degradation [198,199]. Additionally, mitophagy involves VDAC1 and MAM sensors, implicating the need for proper inter-organelle Ca^{2+} signaling and colocalization of the two organelles. Intracellular Ca^{2+} signaling relieves the inhibitory mammalian target of rapamycin (mTOR) block, thus activating mitophagy and initiating autophagosome biogenesis (ATG 32, 8, and 11) [200–202]. In AD patients, disruptions in mitophagy have been seen in the presence of Aβ, APP, and mutant PS1 expression. Aberrant inter-organelle Ca^{2+} signaling, as seen in AD, may disrupt degradation of damaged organelle via inactivation of lysosomal proteolysis and increase accumulation of cellular debris [198,199,203–205].

2.2. Ca^{2+} Dysregulation Impairs Lysosome-Autophagosome Mediated Protein Degradation

Lysosomal Ca^{2+} stores are responsible for regulating autophagy—a catabolic pathway utilizing the enzymatic activity of lysosomes to degrade and recycle large, bulky cellular debris, aggregated proteins, and damaged organelles. There are three types of autophagy: macroautophagy, microautophagy, and chaperone-mediated autophagy, however for simplicity, this review will focus on macroautophagy and be referred to as "autophagy". More detailed descriptions of the aforementioned can be found in these reviews [163,206]. Autophagy is a systematic, dynamic degradation process regulated by the fusion of cargo vesicles, autophagosomes, to degradative compartments, lysosomes, with active hydrolases and proteases. While other cells rely on division to dilute cellular debris, neurons are specialized, post-mitotic cells that require efficient basal autophagy regulation to prevent accumulation of misfolded proteins and damaged organelles. Autophagy depends on the close proximity and communication between lysosomes and ER [207,208], therefore disruptions in inter-organelle Ca^{2+} signaling hinders clearance of pathological protein deposits.

Transcriptomic profiles from the collective ongoing studies known as Rush Memory and Aging Project (ROSMAP), reveal clusters of genes that are associated with pathological protein handling. Specifically, higher expression of SORL1 and ABCA7 transcripts are associated with tau tangle pathology, while elevated BIN1 transcripts are associated with beta amyloid in AD brains [209]. PLXNB1 abundance is associated with increased amyloid load and higher paired helical filaments (PHF) tau tangle density. Notably, BIN1, ABCA7, and SORL1 have functions in endocytic transport, APP metabolism and lysosome recycling, and thus are ideally positioned to serve a role in AD proteinopathy [210]. Altered expression of protein handling genes is linked to blunted endosomal trafficking, diminished degradative potential of lysosomes, and reduced autophagy-mediated clearance [210].

The key, critical feature of lysosomes is the acidic lumen (pH ~4.5) necessary for protein degradation and autophagosome digestion. The acidic pH is maintained by an active vacuolar-ATPase H^+ pump (vATPase) driving the influx of H^+ into the lysosome [211–213]. Genetic evidence linking endosomal H^+ exchangers with AD suggest that proton leak pathways may regulate pathological Aβ generation and contribute to disease etiology [214]. In the ROSMAP AD population, there is downregulation of vATPase subunit (V1) genes, as well as the transcription factor "EB" (TFEB), a master regulator of lysosomal biogenesis that is associated with regulated autophagy [151]. Mutations in PS prevents the glycosylation, downstream maturation, and trafficking of the vATPase to the lysosome, resulting in an alkaline lysosomal lumen [215,216]. The alkaline environment inactivates protease activity, such as cathepsin B, which halts degradation of APP metabolites and dysregulates biogenesis of lysosomes and autophagosomes [217]. Additionally, cathepsins may also play a role in lysosomal trafficking along neuronal axons and dendrites, which is essential in mediating proper disposal of cellular debris. Studies showed that disrupting lysosomal proteolysis by inhibiting cathepsins or suppressing lysosomal acidification slowed axonal transport and caused selective accumulation within dystrophic neurites, a key feature of AD [218–220]. These are abnormally swollen regions of axons and dendrites filled mainly with autophagosomes and lysosomes, which implies improper transport of degradative organelles. Aberrant Ca^{2+} signaling, as seen in AD, can hinder lysosomal acidification and impair proteolytic enzymes in lysosomes, further AD proteinopathy and impair lysososmal trafficking, resulting in neuritic dystrophy.

Additionally, an increase in the lysosomal pH disrupts the homeostatic mechanisms to maintain the lysosomal membrane potential. The alkaline lumen depolarizes the lysosomal membrane via activation of lysosomal voltage-activated Na^+ channels (lysoNa_V). The Na^+ efflux potentiates the influx of protons by the vATPase to restore lysosomal acidity. However, lysoNa_V are also Ca^{2+} permeable, therefore aberrant Ca^{2+} increase and changes in the Ca^{2+} concentration gradient, as seen in early pathology of AD, can hinder lysosomal acidity by reducing the driving force of H^+ influx to restore lysosomal function [213,221,222].

This shift to a more alkaline lysosomal lumen causes hyperactivity of the lysosomal Ca^{2+} efflux channels, lysosomal transient receptor potential Ca^{2+} channel mucolipin subfamily member (TRPML1) and two-pore channel (TPC) [205,215,216,223–225] (although debated [226–228]). Lysosomal Ca^{2+} efflux through TRPML1, activates a calcineurin-dependent pathway that, via TFEB, enhances the transcription of genes involved in autophagy and lysosomal expression, such as LC3-II, ATG9B, UVRAG, WIPI, SQSTM1, MAPLC3B, GLA, GNS, HEXA, MCOLN1, TMEM55B, and ATP6V1H [229–231].

This lysosomal-mediated Ca^{2+} release is also responsible for fusion of autophagosomes to lysosomes. In a manner similar to neuronal vesicular fusion, lysosomal Ca^{2+} efflux channels such as, P/Q type VGCC, facilitate fusion between lysosomal tethering proteins, such as synaptogamin 7, SNAP29, and SNARE VAMP 7/8, to autophagosomal tethering proteins such as syntaxin 17 and possible SNARE proteins [232–235]. Aberrant Ca^{2+} concentration, as in AD, can influence fusion of autophagosomes to malfunctioned lysosome, resulting in accumulation of cargo vesicles with maladaptive proteins, furthering neurotoxicity.

Recent studies have shown that lysosomal functions go beyond their primary role as the degradative compartment within a neuron. Lysosomal Ca^{2+} stores are also involved in maintaining synaptic transmission. When mGluR1 is activated, NAADP-evoked lysosomal Ca^{2+} release from lysosomal Ca^{2+} channels, presumably through TPC, is amplified into Ca^{2+} waves via RyR activation [236]. This signal inactivates SK channels and prevents local hyperpolarization, which allows for greater Ca^{2+} entry through GluN receptors and facilitates the induction of LTP [237]. When VGCC is activated, NAADP-evoked lysosomal Ca^{2+} release facilitates fusion to the plasma membrane and release of cathepsin B. Cathepsin B then regulates structural plasticity and dendritic spine formation [238,239], however in pathological conditions, protease activity is inhibited and therefore synaptic dysfunctions occur. Recent work has shown that blocking endogenous cathepsin inhibitors, such as cystatin B, decreases Aβ accumulation, autophagic-lysosomal pathology, and cognitive improvement in AD mice [240].

The systemic destruction of collective organelles leads to the neuron's demise. The close proximity of the ER to the lysosome can enhance AD pathology (Figure 3) and PS mutations may alter the RyR-lysosomes trigger zone. In healthy neurons, RyR-mediated Ca^{2+} amplification suppresses autophagic flux [207] and induces LTP [237–239] however, increased Ca^{2+} signaling, as seen in neurodegenerative diseases, can alter this trigger zone and therefore disrupt autophagic clearance and synaptic plasticity.

Acknowledgments: The authors thank Nikki Barrington for editorial assistance in the preparation of this review.

References

1. Stutzmann, G.E. The pathogenesis of Alzheimers disease is it a lifelong "calciumopathy"? *Neuroscientist* **2007**, *13*, 546–559. [CrossRef] [PubMed]
2. Selkoe, D.J. Alzheimer's disease is a synaptic failure. *Science* **2002**, *298*, 789–791. [CrossRef] [PubMed]
3. DeKosky, S.T.; Scheff, S.W. Synapse loss in frontal cortex biopsies in Alzheimer's disease: Correlation with cognitive severity. *Ann. Neurol.* **1990**, *27*, 457–464. [CrossRef] [PubMed]
4. Terry, R.D.; Masliah, E.; Salmon, D.P.; Butters, N.; DeTeresa, R.; Hill, R.; Hansen, L.A.; Katzman, R. Physical basis of cognitive alterations in Alzheimer's disease: Synapse loss is the major correlate of cognitive impairment. *Ann. Neurol.* **1991**, *30*, 572–580. [CrossRef] [PubMed]
5. Hsia, A.Y.; Masliah, E.; McConlogue, L.; Yu, G.Q.; Tatsuno, G.; Hu, K.; Kholodenko, D.; Malenka, R.C.; Nicoll, R.A.; Mucke, L. Plaque-independent disruption of neural circuits in Alzheimer's disease mouse models. *Proc. Natl. Acad. Sci. USA* **1999**, *96*, 3228–3233. [CrossRef] [PubMed]
6. Busche, M.A.; Chen, X.; Henning, H.A.; Reichwald, J.; Staufenbiel, M.; Sakmann, B.; Konnerth, A. Critical role of soluble amyloid-β for early hippocampal hyperactivity in a mouse model of Alzheimer's disease. *Proc. Natl. Acad. Sci. USA* **2012**, *109*, 8740–8745. [CrossRef]

7. Busche, M.A.; Eichhoff, G.; Adelsberger, H.; Abramowski, D.; Wiederhold, K.-H.; Haass, C.; Staufenbiel, M.; Konnerth, A.; Garaschuk, O. Clusters of hyperactive neurons near amyloid plaques in a mouse model of Alzheimer's disease. *Science* **2008**, *321*, 1686–1689. [CrossRef]
8. Chakroborty, S.; Hill, E.S.; Christian, D.T.; Helfrich, R.; Riley, S.; Schneider, C.; Kapecki, N.; Mustaly-Kalimi, S.; Seiler, F.A.; Peterson, D.A.; et al. Reduced presynaptic vesicle stores mediate cellular and network plasticity defects in an early-stage mouse model of Alzheimer's disease. *Mol. Neurodegener.* **2019**, *14*, 7. [CrossRef]
9. Goussakov, I.; Miller, M.B.; Stutzmann, G.E. NMDA-mediated Ca^{2+} influx drives aberrant ryanodine receptor activation in dendrites of young Alzheimer's disease mice. *J. Neurosci.* **2010**, *30*, 12128–12137. [CrossRef]
10. Murchison, D.; McDermott, A.N.; LaSarge, C.L.; Peebles, K.A.; Bizon, J.L.; Griffith, W.H. Enhanced Calcium Buffering in F344 Rat Cholinergic Basal Forebrain Neurons Is Associated with Age-Related Cognitive Impairment. *J. Neurophysiol.* **2009**, *102*, 2194–2207. [CrossRef]
11. Moyer, J.R.; Furtak, S.C.; McGann, J.P.; Brown, T.H. Aging-related changes in calcium binding proteins in rat perirhinal cortex. *Neurobiol. Aging* **2011**, *32*, 1693–1706. [CrossRef] [PubMed]
12. Oh, M.M.; Oliveira, F.A.; Waters, J.; Disterhoft, J.F. Altered Calcium Metabolism in Aging CA1 Hippocampal Pyramidal Neurons. *J. Neurosci.* **2013**, *33*, 7905–7911. [CrossRef] [PubMed]
13. Kuchibhotla, K.V.; Goldman, S.T.; Lattarulo, C.R.; Wu, H.-Y.; Hyman, B.T.; Bacskai, B.J. Abeta plaques lead to aberrant regulation of calcium homeostasis in vivo resulting in structural and functional disruption of neuronal networks. *Neuron* **2008**, *59*, 214–225. [CrossRef] [PubMed]
14. Lopez, J.R.; Lyckman, A.; Oddo, S.; Laferla, F.M.; Querfurth, H.W.; Shtifman, A. Increased intraneuronal resting $[Ca^{2+}]$ in adult Alzheimer's disease mice. *J. Neurochem.* **2008**, *105*, 262–271. [CrossRef]
15. Uryash, A.; Flores, V.; Adams, J.A.; Allen, P.D.; Lopez, J.R. Memory and Learning Deficits Are Associated With Ca^{2+} Dyshomeostasis in Normal Aging. *Front. Aging Neurosci.* **2020**, *12*, 224. [CrossRef]
16. Thibault, O.; Hadley, R.; Landfield, P.W. Elevated postsynaptic $[Ca^{2+}]_i$ and L-type calcium channel activity in aged hippocampal neurons: Relationship to impaired synaptic plasticity. *J. Neurosci.* **2001**, *21*, 9744–9756. [CrossRef]
17. Bliss, T.V.; Collingridge, G.L. A synaptic model of memory: Long-term potentiation in the hippocampus. *Nature* **1993**, *361*, 31–39. [CrossRef]
18. Talantova, M.; Sanz-Blasco, S.; Zhang, X.; Xia, P.; Akhtar, M.W.; Okamoto, S.; Dziewczapolski, G.; Nakamura, T.; Cao, G.; Pratt, A.E.; et al. Aβ induces astrocytic glutamate release, extrasynaptic NMDA receptor activation, and synaptic loss. *Proc. Natl. Acad. Sci. USA* **2013**, *110*, E2518–E2527. [CrossRef]
19. Yan, J.; Bengtson, C.P.; Buchthal, B.; Hagenston, A.M.; Bading, H. Coupling of NMDA receptors and TRPM4 guides discovery of unconventional neuroprotectants. *Science* **2020**, *370*. [CrossRef]
20. Winblad, B.; Jones, R.W.; Wirth, Y.; Stöffler, A.; Möbius, H.J. Memantine in moderate to severe Alzheimer's disease: A meta-analysis of randomised clinical trials. *Dement. Geriatr. Cogn. Disord.* **2007**, *24*, 20–27. [CrossRef]
21. Gauthier, S.; Loft, H.; Cummings, J. Improvement in behavioural symptoms in patients with moderate to severe Alzheimer's disease by memantine: A pooled data analysis. *Int. J. Geriatr. Psychiatry* **2008**, *23*, 537–545. [CrossRef] [PubMed]
22. Copenhaver, P.F.; Anekonda, T.S.; Musashe, D.; Robinson, K.M.; Ramaker, J.M.; Swanson, T.L.; Wadsworth, T.L.; Kretzschmar, D.; Woltjer, R.L.; Quinn, J.F. A translational continuum of model systems for evaluating treatment strategies in Alzheimer's disease: Isradipine as a candidate drug. *Dis. Model. Mech.* **2011**, *4*, 634–648. [CrossRef] [PubMed]
23. Scheff, S.W.; Price, D.A.; Schmitt, F.A.; Mufson, E.J. Hippocampal synaptic loss in early Alzheimer's disease and mild cognitive impairment. *Neurobiol. Aging* **2006**, *27*, 1372–1384. [CrossRef] [PubMed]
24. Jacobsen, J.S.; Wu, C.-C.; Redwine, J.M.; Comery, T.A.; Arias, R.; Bowlby, M.; Martone, R.; Morrison, J.H.; Pangalos, M.N.; Reinhart, P.H.; et al. Early-onset behavioral and synaptic deficits in a mouse model of Alzheimer's disease. *Proc. Natl. Acad. Sci. USA* **2006**, *103*, 5161–5166. [CrossRef] [PubMed]
25. Spires, T.L.; Meyer-Luehmann, M.; Stern, E.A.; McLean, P.J.; Skoch, J.; Nguyen, P.T.; Bacskai, B.J.; Hyman, B.T. Dendritic spine abnormalities in amyloid precursor protein transgenic mice demonstrated by gene transfer and intravital multiphoton microscopy. *J. Neurosci.* **2005**, *25*, 7278–7287. [CrossRef]
26. Lanz, T.A.; Carter, D.B.; Merchant, K.M. Dendritic spine loss in the hippocampus of young PDAPP and Tg2576 mice and its prevention by the ApoE2 genotype. *Neurobiol. Dis.* **2003**, *13*, 246–253. [CrossRef]

27. Fitzjohn, S.M.; Morton, R.A.; Kuenzi, F.; Rosahl, T.W.; Shearman, M.; Lewis, H.; Smith, D.; Reynolds, D.S.; Davies, C.H.; Collingridge, G.L.; et al. Age-related impairment of synaptic transmission but normal long-term potentiation in transgenic mice that overexpress the human APP695SWE mutant form of amyloid precursor protein. *J. Neurosci.* **2001**, *21*, 4691–4698. [CrossRef]
28. Chapman, P.F.; White, G.L.; Jones, M.W.; Cooper-Blacketer, D.; Marshall, V.J.; Irizarry, M.; Younkin, L.; Good, M.A.; Bliss, T.V.; Hyman, B.T.; et al. Impaired synaptic plasticity and learning in aged amyloid precursor protein transgenic mice. *Nat. Neurosci.* **1999**, *2*, 271–276. [CrossRef]
29. Larson, J.; Lynch, G.; Games, D.; Seubert, P. Alterations in synaptic transmission and long-term potentiation in hippocampal slices from young and aged PDAPP mice. *Brain Res.* **1999**, *840*, 23–35. [CrossRef]
30. Chakroborty, S.; Goussakov, I.; Miller, M.B.; Stutzmann, G.E. Deviant ryanodine receptor-mediated calcium release resets synaptic homeostasis in presymptomatic 3xTg-AD mice. *J. Neurosci.* **2009**, *29*, 9458–9470. [CrossRef]
31. Zhang, H.; Wu, L.; Pchitskaya, E.; Zakharova, O.; Saito, T.; Saido, T.; Bezprozvanny, I. Neuronal Store-Operated Calcium Entry and Mushroom Spine Loss in Amyloid Precursor Protein Knock-In Mouse Model of Alzheimer's Disease. *J. Neurosci.* **2015**, *35*, 13275–13286. [CrossRef] [PubMed]
32. Lue, L.F.; Kuo, Y.M.; Roher, A.E.; Brachova, L.; Shen, Y.; Sue, L.; Beach, T.; Kurth, J.H.; Rydel, R.E.; Rogers, J. Soluble amyloid beta peptide concentration as a predictor of synaptic change in Alzheimer's disease. *Am. J. Pathol.* **1999**, *155*, 853–862. [CrossRef]
33. Arbel-Ornath, M.; Hudry, E.; Boivin, J.R.; Hashimoto, T.; Takeda, S.; Kuchibhotla, K.V.; Hou, S.; Lattarulo, C.R.; Belcher, A.M.; Shakerdge, N.; et al. Soluble oligomeric amyloid-β induces calcium dyshomeostasis that precedes synapse loss in the living mouse brain. *Mol. Neurodegener.* **2017**, *12*, 27. [CrossRef] [PubMed]
34. Calabrese, B.; Shaked, G.M.; Tabarean, I.V.; Braga, J.; Koo, E.H.; Halpain, S. Rapid, concurrent alterations in pre- and postsynaptic structure induced by naturally-secreted amyloid-β protein. *Mol. Cell. Neurosci.* **2007**, *35*, 183–193. [CrossRef] [PubMed]
35. Shankar, G.M.; Bloodgood, B.L.; Townsend, M.; Walsh, D.M.; Selkoe, D.J.; Sabatini, B.L. Natural oligomers of the Alzheimer amyloid-beta protein induce reversible synapse loss by modulating an NMDA-type glutamate receptor-dependent signaling pathway. *J. Neurosci.* **2007**, *27*, 2866–2875. [CrossRef]
36. Esteras, N.; Kundel, F.; Amodeo, G.F.; Pavlov, E.V.; Klenerman, D.; Abramov, A.Y. Insoluble tau aggregates induce neuronal death through modification of membrane ion conductance, activation of voltage-gated calcium channels and NADPH oxidase. *FEBS J.* **2020**. [CrossRef]
37. Zhou, L.; McInnes, J.; Wierda, K.; Holt, M.; Herrmann, A.G.; Jackson, R.J.; Wang, Y.-C.; Swerts, J.; Beyens, J.; Miskiewicz, K.; et al. Tau association with synaptic vesicles causes presynaptic dysfunction. *Nat. Commun.* **2017**, *8*, 15295. [CrossRef]
38. Gómez-Ramos, A.; Díaz-Hernández, M.; Cuadros, R.; Hernández, F.; Avila, J. Extracellular tau is toxic to neuronal cells. *FEBS Lett.* **2006**, *580*, 4842–4850. [CrossRef]
39. Yin, Y.; Gao, D.; Wang, Y.; Wang, Z.-H.; Wang, X.; Ye, J.; Wu, D.; Fang, L.; Pi, G.; Yang, Y.; et al. Tau accumulation induces synaptic impairment and memory deficit by calcineurin-mediated inactivation of nuclear CaMKIV/CREB signaling. *Proc. Natl. Acad. Sci. USA* **2016**, *113*, E3773–E3781. [CrossRef]
40. Keskin, A.D.; Kekuš, M.; Adelsberger, H.; Neumann, U.; Shimshek, D.R.; Song, B.; Zott, B.; Peng, T.; Förstl, H.; Staufenbiel, M.; et al. BACE inhibition-dependent repair of Alzheimer's pathophysiology. *Proc. Natl. Acad. Sci. USA* **2017**, *114*, 8631–8636. [CrossRef]
41. Koffie, R.M.; Meyer-Luehmann, M.; Hashimoto, T.; Adams, K.W.; Mielke, M.L.; Garcia-Alloza, M.; Micheva, K.D.; Smith, S.J.; Kim, M.L.; Lee, V.M.; et al. Oligomeric amyloid beta associates with postsynaptic densities and correlates with excitatory synapse loss near senile plaques. *Proc. Natl. Acad. Sci. USA* **2009**, *106*, 4012–4017. [CrossRef] [PubMed]
42. Briggs, C.A.; Schneider, C.; Richardson, J.C.; Stutzmann, G.E. β amyloid peptide plaques fail to alter evoked neuronal calcium signals in APP/PS1 Alzheimer's disease mice. *Neurobiol. Aging* **2013**, *34*, 1632–1643. [CrossRef] [PubMed]
43. Lerdkrai, C.; Asavapanumas, N.; Brawek, B.; Kovalchuk, Y.; Mojtahedi, N.; del Moral, M.O.; Garaschuk, O. Intracellular Ca^{2+} stores control in vivo neuronal hyperactivity in a mouse model of Alzheimer's disease. *Proc. Natl. Acad. Sci. USA* **2018**, *115*, E1279–E1288. [CrossRef] [PubMed]

44. He, Y.; Wei, M.; Wu, Y.; Qin, H.; Li, W.; Ma, X.; Cheng, J.; Ren, J.; Shen, Y.; Chen, Z.; et al. Amyloid β oligomers suppress excitatory transmitter release via presynaptic depletion of phosphatidylinositol-4,5-bisphosphate. *Nat. Commun.* **2019**, *10*, 1193. [CrossRef] [PubMed]
45. Oddo, S.; Caccamo, A.; Shepherd, J.D.; Murphy, M.P.; Golde, T.E.; Kayed, R.; Metherate, R.; Mattson, M.P.; Akbari, Y.; LaFerla, F.M. Triple-transgenic model of Alzheimer's disease with plaques and tangles: Intracellular Abeta and synaptic dysfunction. *Neuron* **2003**, *39*, 409–421. [CrossRef]
46. Chakroborty, S.; Kim, J.; Schneider, C.; Jacobson, C.; Molgó, J.; Stutzmann, G.E. Early presynaptic and postsynaptic calcium signaling abnormalities mask underlying synaptic depression in presymptomatic Alzheimer's disease mice. *J. Neurosci.* **2012**, *32*, 8341–8353. [CrossRef] [PubMed]
47. Yao, J.; Sun, B.; Institoris, A.; Zhan, X.; Guo, W.; Song, Z.; Liu, Y.; Hiess, F.; Boyce, A.K.J.; Ni, M.; et al. Limiting RyR2 Open Time Prevents Alzheimer's Disease-Related Neuronal Hyperactivity and Memory Loss but Not β-Amyloid Accumulation. *Cell Rep.* **2020**, *32*, 108169. [CrossRef] [PubMed]
48. Kindler, C.H.; Eilers, H.; Donohoe, P.; Ozer, S.; Bickler, P.E. Volatile anesthetics increase intracellular calcium in cerebrocortical and hippocampal neurons. *Anesthesiology* **1999**, *90*, 1137–1145. [CrossRef]
49. Wei, H.; Liang, G.; Yang, H.; Wang, Q.; Hawkins, B.; Madesh, M.; Wang, S.; Eckenhoff, R.G. The Common Inhalational Anesthetic Isoflurane Induces Apoptosis via Activation of Inositol 1,4,5-Trisphosphate Receptors. *Anesthesiol. J. Am. Soc. Anesthesiol.* **2008**, *108*, 251–260. [CrossRef]
50. Stutzmann, G.E.; Smith, I.; Caccamo, A.; Oddo, S.; Laferla, F.M.; Parker, I. Enhanced ryanodine receptor recruitment contributes to Ca^{2+} disruptions in young, adult, and aged Alzheimer's disease mice. *J. Neurosci.* **2006**, *26*, 5180–5189. [CrossRef]
51. Ghatak, S.; Dolatabadi, N.; Gao, R.; Wu, Y.; Scott, H.; Trudler, D.; Sultan, A.; Ambasudhan, R.; Nakamura, T.; Masliah, E.; et al. NitroSynapsin ameliorates hypersynchronous neural network activity in Alzheimer hiPSC models. *Mol. Psychiatry* **2020**. [CrossRef] [PubMed]
52. Ghatak, S.; Dolatabadi, N.; Trudler, D.; Zhang, X.; Wu, Y.; Mohata, M.; Ambasudhan, R.; Talantova, M.; Lipton, S.A. Mechanisms of hyperexcitability in Alzheimer's disease hiPSC-derived neurons and cerebral organoids vs. isogenic controls. *eLife* **2019**, *8*. [CrossRef] [PubMed]
53. Schrank, S.; McDaid, J.; Briggs, C.A.; Mustaly-Kalimi, S.; Brinks, D.; Houcek, A.; Singer, O.; Bottero, V.; Marr, R.A.; Stutzmann, G.E. Human-Induced Neurons from Presenilin 1 Mutant Patients Model Aspects of Alzheimer's Disease Pathology. *Int. J. Mol. Sci.* **2020**, *21*, 1030. [CrossRef] [PubMed]
54. Huijbers, W.; Mormino, E.C.; Schultz, A.P.; Wigman, S.; Ward, A.M.; Larvie, M.; Amariglio, R.E.; Marshall, G.A.; Rentz, D.M.; Johnson, K.A.; et al. Amyloid-β deposition in mild cognitive impairment is associated with increased hippocampal activity, atrophy and clinical progression. *Brain J. Neurol.* **2015**, *138*, 1023–1035. [CrossRef] [PubMed]
55. Hämäläinen, A.; Pihlajamäki, M.; Tanila, H.; Hänninen, T.; Niskanen, E.; Tervo, S.; Karjalainen, P.A.; Vanninen, R.L.; Soininen, H. Increased fMRI responses during encoding in mild cognitive impairment. *Neurobiol. Aging* **2007**, *28*, 1889–1903. [CrossRef] [PubMed]
56. Drummond, E.; Wisniewski, T. Using Proteomics to Understand Alzheimer's Disease Pathogenesis. In *Alzheimer's Disease*; Wisniewski, T., Ed.; Codon Publications: Brisbane, Australia, 2019; ISBN 978-0-646-80968-7.
57. Honer, W.G.; Ramos-Miguel, A.; Alamri, J.; Sawada, K.; Barr, A.M.; Schneider, J.A.; Bennett, D.A. The synaptic pathology of cognitive life. *Dialogues Clin. Neurosci.* **2019**, *21*, 271–279. [CrossRef] [PubMed]
58. Bennett, D.A.; Buchman, A.S.; Boyle, P.A.; Barnes, L.L.; Wilson, R.S.; Schneider, J.A. Religious Orders Study and Rush Memory and Aging Project. *J. Alzheimers Dis. JAD* **2018**, *64*, S161–S189. [CrossRef]
59. Dieterich, D.C.; Kreutz, M.R. Proteomics of the Synapse—A Quantitative Approach to Neuronal Plasticity. *Mol. Cell. Proteomics MCP* **2016**, *15*, 368–381. [CrossRef]
60. Honer, W.G.; Barr, A.M.; Sawada, K.; Thornton, A.E.; Morris, M.C.; Leurgans, S.E.; Schneider, J.A.; Bennett, D.A. Cognitive reserve, presynaptic proteins and dementia in the elderly. *Transl. Psychiatry* **2012**, *2*, e114. [CrossRef]
61. Jeans, A.F.; Oliver, P.L.; Johnson, R.; Capogna, M.; Vikman, J.; Molnár, Z.; Babbs, A.; Partridge, C.J.; Salehi, A.; Bengtsson, M.; et al. A dominant mutation in Snap25 causes impaired vesicle trafficking, sensorimotor gating, and ataxia in the blind-drunk mouse. *Proc. Natl. Acad. Sci. USA* **2007**, *104*, 2431–2436. [CrossRef]

62. Toft-Bertelsen, T.L.; Ziomkiewicz, I.; Houy, S.; Pinheiro, P.S.; Sørensen, J.B. Regulation of Ca^{2+} channels by SNAP-25 via recruitment of syntaxin-1 from plasma membrane clusters. *Mol. Biol. Cell* **2016**, *27*, 3329–3341. [CrossRef] [PubMed]
63. Ramos-Miguel, A.; Sawada, K.; Jones, A.A.; Thornton, A.E.; Barr, A.M.; Leurgans, S.E.; Schneider, J.A.; Bennett, D.A.; Honer, W.G. Presynaptic proteins complexin-I and complexin-II differentially influence cognitive function in early and late stages of Alzheimer's disease. *Acta Neuropathol.* **2017**, *133*, 395–407. [CrossRef] [PubMed]
64. Verderio, C.; Pozzi, D.; Pravettoni, E.; Inverardi, F.; Schenk, U.; Coco, S.; Proux-Gillardeaux, V.; Galli, T.; Rossetto, O.; Frassoni, C.; et al. SNAP-25 Modulation of Calcium Dynamics Underlies Differences in GABAergic and Glutamatergic Responsiveness to Depolarization. *Neuron* **2004**, *41*, 599–610. [CrossRef]
65. Malsam, J.; Bärfuss, S.; Trimbuch, T.; Zarebidaki, F.; Sonnen, A.F.-P.; Wild, K.; Scheutzow, A.; Rohland, L.; Mayer, M.P.; Sinning, I.; et al. Complexin Suppresses Spontaneous Exocytosis by Capturing the Membrane-Proximal Regions of VAMP2 and SNAP25. *Cell Rep.* **2020**, *32*, 107926. [CrossRef] [PubMed]
66. Rettig, J.; Sheng, Z.H.; Kim, D.K.; Hodson, C.D.; Snutch, T.P.; Catterall, W.A. Isoform-specific interaction of the alpha1A subunits of brain Ca^{2+} channels with the presynaptic proteins syntaxin and SNAP-25. *Proc. Natl. Acad. Sci. USA* **1996**, *93*, 7363–7368. [CrossRef] [PubMed]
67. Antonucci, F.; Corradini, I.; Morini, R.; Fossati, G.; Menna, E.; Pozzi, D.; Pacioni, S.; Verderio, C.; Bacci, A.; Matteoli, M. Reduced SNAP-25 alters short-term plasticity at developing glutamatergic synapses. *EMBO Rep.* **2013**, *14*, 645–651. [CrossRef] [PubMed]
68. Vogl, C.; Mochida, S.; Wolff, C.; Whalley, B.J.; Stephens, G.J. The synaptic vesicle glycoprotein 2A ligand levetiracetam inhibits presynaptic Ca^{2+} channels through an intracellular pathway. *Mol. Pharmacol.* **2012**, *82*, 199–208. [CrossRef]
69. Cumbo, E.; Ligori, L.D. Levetiracetam, lamotrigine, and phenobarbital in patients with epileptic seizures and Alzheimer's disease. *Epilepsy Behav. EB* **2010**, *17*, 461–466. [CrossRef]
70. Newhouse, P.A.; Potter, A.; Corwin, J.; Lenox, R. Acute nicotinic blockade produces cognitive impairment in normal humans. *Psychopharmacology* **1992**, *108*, 480–484. [CrossRef]
71. Kadir, A.; Almkvist, O.; Wall, A.; Långström, B.; Nordberg, A. PET imaging of cortical 11C-nicotine binding correlates with the cognitive function of attention in Alzheimer's disease. *Psychopharmacology* **2006**, *188*, 509–520. [CrossRef]
72. Fucile, S. Ca^{2+} permeability of nicotinic acetylcholine receptors. *Cell Calcium* **2004**, *35*, 1–8. [CrossRef] [PubMed]
73. Séguéla, P.; Wadiche, J.; Dineley-Miller, K.; Dani, J.A.; Patrick, J.W. Molecular cloning, functional properties, and distribution of rat brain alpha 7: A nicotinic cation channel highly permeable to calcium. *J. Neurosci.* **1993**, *13*, 596–604. [CrossRef] [PubMed]
74. Thinschmidt, J.S.; Frazier, C.J.; King, M.A.; Meyer, E.M.; Papke, R.L. Medial septal/diagonal band cells express multiple functional nicotinic receptor subtypes that are correlated with firing frequency. *Neurosci. Lett.* **2005**, *389*, 163–168. [CrossRef]
75. Davies, P.; Maloney, A.J. Selective loss of central cholinergic neurons in Alzheimer's disease. *Lancet Lond. Engl.* **1976**, *2*, 1403. [CrossRef]
76. Mufson, E.J.; Counts, S.E.; Perez, S.E.; Ginsberg, S.D. Cholinergic system during the progression of Alzheimer's disease: Therapeutic implications. *Expert Rev. Neurother.* **2008**, *8*, 1703–1718. [CrossRef] [PubMed]
77. Grybko, M.; Sharma, G.; Vijayaraghavan, S. Functional distribution of nicotinic receptors in CA3 region of the hippocampus. *J. Mol. Neurosci. MN* **2010**, *40*, 114–120. [CrossRef]
78. Frazier, C.J.; Rollins, Y.D.; Breese, C.R.; Leonard, S.; Freedman, R.; Dunwiddie, T.V. Acetylcholine activates an alpha-bungarotoxin-sensitive nicotinic current in rat hippocampal interneurons, but not pyramidal cells. *J. Neurosci.* **1998**, *18*, 1187–1195. [CrossRef]
79. Khiroug, L.; Giniatullin, R.; Klein, R.C.; Fayuk, D.; Yakel, J.L. Functional mapping and Ca^{2+} regulation of nicotinic acetylcholine receptor channels in rat hippocampal CA1 neurons. *J. Neurosci.* **2003**, *23*, 9024–9031. [CrossRef]
80. Gray, R.; Rajan, A.S.; Radcliffe, K.A.; Yakehiro, M.; Dani, J.A. Hippocampal synaptic transmission enhanced by low concentrations of nicotine. *Nature* **1996**, *383*, 713–716. [CrossRef]
81. Radcliffe, K.A.; Dani, J.A. Nicotinic stimulation produces multiple forms of increased glutamatergic synaptic transmission. *J. Neurosci.* **1998**, *18*, 7075–7083. [CrossRef]

82. Fayuk, D.; Yakel, J.L. Ca^{2+} permeability of nicotinic acetylcholine receptors in rat hippocampal CA1 interneurones. *J. Physiol.* **2005**, *566*, 759–768. [CrossRef] [PubMed]
83. Cheng, Q.; Yakel, J.L. Presynaptic α7 nicotinic acetylcholine receptors enhance hippocampal mossy fiber glutamatergic transmission via PKA activation. *J. Neurosci.* **2014**, *34*, 124–133. [CrossRef] [PubMed]
84. Sharma, G.; Grybko, M.; Vijayaraghavan, S. Action potential-independent and nicotinic receptor-mediated concerted release of multiple quanta at hippocampal CA3-mossy fiber synapses. *J. Neurosci.* **2008**, *28*, 2563–2575. [CrossRef] [PubMed]
85. Townsend, M.; Whyment, A.; Walczak, J.-S.; Jeggo, R.; van den Top, M.; Flood, D.G.; Leventhal, L.; Patzke, H.; Koenig, G. α7-nAChR agonist enhances neural plasticity in the hippocampus via a GABAergic circuit. *J. Neurophysiol.* **2016**, *116*, 2663–2675. [CrossRef] [PubMed]
86. Wang, H.Y.; Lee, D.H.; D'Andrea, M.R.; Peterson, P.A.; Shank, R.P.; Reitz, A.B. beta-Amyloid(1-42) binds to alpha7 nicotinic acetylcholine receptor with high affinity. Implications for Alzheimer's disease pathology. *J. Biol. Chem.* **2000**, *275*, 5626–5632. [CrossRef] [PubMed]
87. Wang, H.Y.; Lee, D.H.; Davis, C.B.; Shank, R.P. Amyloid peptide Abeta(1-42) binds selectively and with picomolar affinity to alpha7 nicotinic acetylcholine receptors. *J. Neurochem.* **2000**, *75*, 1155–1161. [CrossRef]
88. Liu, Q.; Kawai, H.; Berg, D.K. beta -Amyloid peptide blocks the response of alpha 7-containing nicotinic receptors on hippocampal neurons. *Proc. Natl. Acad. Sci. USA* **2001**, *98*, 4734–4739. [CrossRef]
89. Burghaus, L.; Schütz, U.; Krempel, U.; de Vos, R.A.; Jansen Steur, E.N.; Wevers, A.; Lindstrom, J.; Schröder, H. Quantitative assessment of nicotinic acetylcholine receptor proteins in the cerebral cortex of Alzheimer patients. *Brain Res. Mol. Brain Res.* **2000**, *76*, 385–388. [CrossRef]
90. Guan, Z.-Z.; Zhang, X.; Ravid, R.; Nordberg, A. Decreased Protein Levels of Nicotinic Receptor Subunits in the Hippocampus and Temporal Cortex of Patients with Alzheimer's Disease. *J. Neurochem.* **2000**, *74*, 237–243. [CrossRef]
91. Oddo, S.; Caccamo, A.; Green, K.N.; Liang, K.; Tran, L.; Chen, Y.; Leslie, F.M.; LaFerla, F.M. Chronic nicotine administration exacerbates tau pathology in a transgenic model of Alzheimer's disease. *Proc. Natl. Acad. Sci. USA* **2005**, *102*, 3046–3051. [CrossRef]
92. D'Andrea, M.R.; Nagele, R.G. Targeting the alpha 7 nicotinic acetylcholine receptor to reduce amyloid accumulation in Alzheimer's disease pyramidal neurons. *Curr. Pharm. Des.* **2006**, *12*, 677–684. [CrossRef] [PubMed]
93. Dougherty, J.J.; Wu, J.; Nichols, R.A. Beta-amyloid regulation of presynaptic nicotinic receptors in rat hippocampus and neocortex. *J. Neurosci.* **2003**, *23*, 6740–6747. [CrossRef] [PubMed]
94. Dineley, K.T.; Bell, K.A.; Bui, D.; Sweatt, J.D. beta-Amyloid peptide activates alpha 7 nicotinic acetylcholine receptors expressed in Xenopus oocytes. *J. Biol. Chem.* **2002**, *277*, 25056–25061. [CrossRef]
95. Hascup, K.N.; Hascup, E.R. Soluble Amyloid-β42 Stimulates Glutamate Release through Activation of the α7 Nicotinic Acetylcholine Receptor. *J. Alzheimers Dis. JAD* **2016**, *53*, 337–347. [CrossRef] [PubMed]
96. Puzzo, D.; Privitera, L.; Leznik, E.; Fà, M.; Staniszewski, A.; Palmeri, A.; Arancio, O. Picomolar Amyloid-β Positively Modulates Synaptic Plasticity and Memory in Hippocampus. *J. Neurosci.* **2008**, *28*, 14537–14545. [CrossRef]
97. Kroker, K.S.; Moreth, J.; Kussmaul, L.; Rast, G.; Rosenbrock, H. Restoring long-term potentiation impaired by amyloid-beta oligomers: Comparison of an acetylcholinesterase inhibitior and selective neuronal nicotinic receptor agonists. *Brain Res. Bull.* **2013**, *96*, 28–38. [CrossRef]
98. Ondrejcak, T.; Wang, Q.; Kew, J.N.C.; Virley, D.J.; Upton, N.; Anwyl, R.; Rowan, M.J. Activation of α7 nicotinic acetylcholine receptors persistently enhances hippocampal synaptic transmission and prevents Aß-mediated inhibition of LTP in the rat hippocampus. *Eur. J. Pharmacol.* **2012**, *677*, 63–70. [CrossRef]
99. Medeiros, R.; Castello, N.A.; Cheng, D.; Kitazawa, M.; Baglietto-Vargas, D.; Green, K.N.; Esbenshade, T.A.; Bitner, R.S.; Decker, M.W.; LaFerla, F.M. α7 Nicotinic receptor agonist enhances cognition in aged 3xTg-AD mice with robust plaques and tangles. *Am. J. Pathol.* **2014**, *184*, 520–529. [CrossRef]
100. Shen, H.; Kihara, T.; Hongo, H.; Wu, X.; Kem, W.R.; Shimohama, S.; Akaike, A.; Niidome, T.; Sugimoto, H. Neuroprotection by donepezil against glutamate excitotoxicity involves stimulation of alpha7 nicotinic receptors and internalization of NMDA receptors. *Br. J. Pharmacol.* **2010**, *161*, 127–139. [CrossRef]
101. Texidó, L.; Ros, E.; Martín-Satué, M.; López, S.; Aleu, J.; Marsal, J.; Solsona, C. Effect of galantamine on the human alpha7 neuronal nicotinic acetylcholine receptor, the Torpedo nicotinic acetylcholine receptor and spontaneous cholinergic synaptic activity. *Br. J. Pharmacol.* **2005**, *145*, 672–678. [CrossRef]

102. Yang, T.; Xiao, T.; Sun, Q.; Wang, K. The current agonists and positive allosteric modulators of α 7 nAChR for CNS indications in clinical trials. *Acta Pharm. Sin. B* **2017**, *7*, 611–622. [CrossRef] [PubMed]
103. Deardorff, W.J.; Shobassy, A.; Grossberg, G.T. Safety and clinical effects of EVP-6124 in subjects with Alzheimer's disease currently or previously receiving an acetylcholinesterase inhibitor medication. *Expert Rev. Neurother.* **2015**, *15*, 7–17. [CrossRef] [PubMed]
104. Barbier, A.J.; Hilhorst, M.; Van Vliet, A.; Snyder, P.; Palfreyman, M.G.; Gawryl, M.; Dgetluck, N.; Massaro, M.; Tiessen, R.; Timmerman, W.; et al. Pharmacodynamics, pharmacokinetics, safety, and tolerability of encenicline, a selective α7 nicotinic receptor partial agonist, in single ascending-dose and bioavailability studies. *Clin. Ther.* **2015**, *37*, 311–324. [CrossRef]
105. Gee, K.W.; Olincy, A.; Kanner, R.; Johnson, L.; Hogenkamp, D.; Harris, J.; Tran, M.; Edmonds, S.A.; Sauer, W.; Yoshimura, R.; et al. First in human trial of a type I positive allosteric modulator of alpha7-nicotinic acetylcholine receptors: Pharmacokinetics, safety, and evidence for neurocognitive effect of AVL-3288. *J. Psychopharmacol. Oxf. Engl.* **2017**, *31*, 434–441. [CrossRef]
106. Dajas-Bailador, F.A.; Mogg, A.J.; Wonnacott, S. Intracellular Ca^{2+} signals evoked by stimulation of nicotinic acetylcholine receptors in SH-SY5Y cells: Contribution of voltage-operated Ca^{2+} channels and Ca^{2+} stores. *J. Neurochem.* **2002**, *81*, 606–614. [CrossRef] [PubMed]
107. Sharma, G.; Vijayaraghavan, S. Modulation of presynaptic store calcium induces release of glutamate and postsynaptic firing. *Neuron* **2003**, *38*, 929–939. [CrossRef]
108. Padua, R.A.; Nagy, J.I.; Geiger, J.D. Subcellular localization of ryanodine receptors in rat brain. *Eur. J. Pharmacol.* **1996**, *298*, 185–189. [CrossRef]
109. Guerra-Álvarez, M.; Moreno-Ortega, A.J.; Navarro, E.; Fernández-Morales, J.C.; Egea, J.; López, M.G.; Cano-Abad, M.F. Positive allosteric modulation of alpha-7 nicotinic receptors promotes cell death by inducing Ca^{2+} release from the endoplasmic reticulum. *J. Neurochem.* **2015**, *133*, 309–319. [CrossRef]
110. Lacampagne, A.; Liu, X.; Reiken, S.; Bussiere, R.; Meli, A.C.; Lauritzen, I.; Teich, A.F.; Zalk, R.; Saint, N.; Arancio, O.; et al. Post-translational remodeling of ryanodine receptor induces calcium leak leading to Alzheimer's disease-like pathologies and cognitive deficits. *Acta Neuropathol.* **2017**, *134*, 749–767. [CrossRef]
111. Krajnak, K.; Dahl, R. A new target for Alzheimer's disease: A small molecule SERCA activator is neuroprotective in vitro and improves memory and cognition in APP/PS1 mice. *Bioorg. Med. Chem. Lett.* **2018**, *28*, 1591–1594. [CrossRef]
112. Mihalak, K.B.; Carroll, F.I.; Luetje, C.W. Varenicline is a partial agonist at alpha4beta2 and a full agonist at alpha7 neuronal nicotinic receptors. *Mol. Pharmacol.* **2006**, *70*, 801–805. [CrossRef] [PubMed]
113. Kim, S.Y.; Choi, S.H.; Rollema, H.; Schwam, E.M.; McRae, T.; Dubrava, S.; Jacobsen, J. Phase II crossover trial of varenicline in mild-to-moderate Alzheimer's disease. *Dement. Geriatr. Cogn. Disord.* **2014**, *37*, 232–245. [CrossRef]
114. Chakroborty, S.; Briggs, C.; Miller, M.B.; Goussakov, I.; Schneider, C.; Kim, J.; Wicks, J.; Richardson, J.C.; Conklin, V.; Cameransi, B.G.; et al. Stabilizing ER Ca^{2+} Channel Function as an Early Preventative Strategy for Alzheimer's Disease. *PLoS ONE* **2012**, *7*, e52056. [CrossRef] [PubMed]
115. Oulès, B.; Del Prete, D.; Greco, B.; Zhang, X.; Lauritzen, I.; Sevalle, J.; Moreno, S.; Paterlini-Bréchot, P.; Trebak, M.; Checler, F.; et al. Ryanodine Receptor Blockade Reduces Amyloid-β Load and Memory Impairments in Tg2576 Mouse Model of Alzheimer Disease. *J. Neurosci.* **2012**, *32*, 11820–11834. [CrossRef]
116. Peng, J.; Liang, G.; Inan, S.; Wu, Z.; Joseph, D.J.; Meng, Q.; Peng, Y.; Eckenhoff, M.F.; Wei, H. Dantrolene ameliorates cognitive decline and neuropathology in Alzheimer triple transgenic mice. *Neurosci. Lett.* **2012**, *516*, 274–279. [CrossRef]
117. Wang, J.; Shi, Y.; Yu, S.; Wang, Y.; Meng, Q.; Liang, G.; Eckenhoff, M.F.; Wei, H. Intranasal administration of dantrolene increased brain concentration and duration. *PLoS ONE* **2020**, *15*, e0229156. [CrossRef]
118. Lawlor, B.; Segurado, R.; Kennelly, S.; Olde Rikkert, M.G.M.; Howard, R.; Pasquier, F.; Börjesson-Hanson, A.; Tsolaki, M.; Lucca, U.; Molloy, D.W.; et al. Nilvadipine in mild to moderate Alzheimer disease: A randomised controlled trial. *PLoS Med.* **2018**, *15*, e1002660. [CrossRef]
119. Study of AGB101 in Mild Cognitive Impairment Due to Alzheimer's Disease—Full Text View—ClinicalTrials.gov. Available online: https://clinicaltrials.gov/ct2/show/NCT03486938 (accessed on 15 August 2020).

120. Sharp, A.H.; McPherson, P.S.; Dawson, T.M.; Aoki, C.; Campbell, K.P.; Snyder, S.H. Differential immunohistochemical localization of inositol 1,4,5-trisphosphate- and ryanodine-sensitive Ca^{2+} release channels in rat brain. *J. Neurosci.* **1993**, *13*, 3051–3063. [CrossRef]
121. Wu, B.; Yamaguchi, H.; Lai, F.A.; Shen, J. Presenilins regulate calcium homeostasis and presynaptic function via ryanodine receptors in hippocampal neurons. *Proc. Natl. Acad. Sci. USA* **2013**, *110*, 15091–15096. [CrossRef]
122. Payne, A.J.; Gerdes, B.C.; Naumchuk, Y.; McCalley, A.E.; Kaja, S.; Koulen, P. Presenilins regulate the cellular activity of ryanodine receptors differentially through isotype-specific N-terminal cysteines. *Exp. Neurol.* **2013**, *250*, 143–150. [CrossRef]
123. Cheung, K.-H.; Shineman, D.; Müller, M.; Cárdenas, C.; Mei, L.; Yang, J.; Tomita, T.; Iwatsubo, T.; Lee, V.M.-Y.; Foskett, J.K. Mechanism of Ca^{2+} disruption in Alzheimer's disease by presenilin regulation of InsP3 receptor channel gating. *Neuron* **2008**, *58*, 871–883. [CrossRef] [PubMed]
124. Chan, S.L.; Mayne, M.; Holden, C.P.; Geiger, J.D.; Mattson, M.P. Presenilin-1 mutations increase levels of ryanodine receptors and calcium release in PC12 cells and cortical neurons. *J. Biol. Chem.* **2000**, *275*, 18195–18200. [CrossRef] [PubMed]
125. Tu, H.; Nelson, O.; Bezprozvanny, A.; Wang, Z.; Lee, S.-F.; Hao, Y.-H.; Serneels, L.; De Strooper, B.; Yu, G.; Bezprozvanny, I. Presenilins form ER Ca^{2+} leak channels, a function disrupted by familial Alzheimer's disease-linked mutations. *Cell* **2006**, *126*, 981–993. [CrossRef] [PubMed]
126. Nelson, O.; Tu, H.; Lei, T.; Bentahir, M.; de Strooper, B.; Bezprozvanny, I. Familial Alzheimer disease-linked mutations specifically disrupt Ca^{2+} leak function of presenilin 1. *J. Clin. Investig.* **2007**, *117*, 1230–1239. [CrossRef] [PubMed]
127. Aloni, E.; Oni-Biton, E.; Tsoory, M.; Moallem, D.H.; Segal, M. Synaptopodin Deficiency Ameliorates Symptoms in the 3xTg Mouse Model of Alzheimer's Disease. *J. Neurosci.* **2019**, *39*, 3983–3992. [CrossRef] [PubMed]
128. Bertan, F.; Wischhof, L.; Sosulina, L.; Mittag, M.; Dalügge, D.; Fornarelli, A.; Gardoni, F.; Marcello, E.; Di Luca, M.; Fuhrmann, M.; et al. Loss of Ryanodine Receptor 2 impairs neuronal activity-dependent remodeling of dendritic spines and triggers compensatory neuronal hyperexcitability. *Cell Death Differ.* **2020**, 1–20. [CrossRef]
129. Kelliher, M.; Fastbom, J.; Cowburn, R.F.; Bonkale, W.; Ohm, T.G.; Ravid, R.; Sorrentino, V.; O'Neill, C. Alterations in the ryanodine receptor calcium release channel correlate with Alzheimer's disease neurofibrillary and beta-amyloid pathologies. *Neuroscience* **1999**, *92*, 499–513. [CrossRef]
130. Bruno, A.; Huang, J.; Bennett, D.A.; Marr, R.; Hastings, M.L.; Stutzmann, G.E. Altered Ryanodine Receptor Expression in Mild Cognitive Impairment and Alzheimer's Disease. *Neurobiol. Aging* **2012**, *33*, 1001.e1–1001.e6. [CrossRef]
131. Chakroborty, S.; Kim, J.; Schneider, C.; West, A.R.; Stutzmann, G.E. Nitric Oxide Signaling Is Recruited as a Compensatory Mechanism for Sustaining Synaptic Plasticity in Alzheimer's Disease Mice. *J. Neurosci.* **2015**, *35*, 6893–6902. [CrossRef]
132. Redondo, R.L.; Morris, R.G.M. Making memories last: The synaptic tagging and capture hypothesis. *Nat. Rev. Neurosci.* **2011**, *12*, 17–30. [CrossRef]
133. Zhang, C.; Wu, B.; Beglopoulos, V.; Wines-Samuelson, M.; Zhang, D.; Dragatsis, I.; Südhof, T.C.; Shen, J. Presenilins are essential for regulating neurotransmitter release. *Nature* **2009**, *460*, 632–636. [CrossRef] [PubMed]
134. Green, K.N.; Demuro, A.; Akbari, Y.; Hitt, B.D.; Smith, I.F.; Parker, I.; LaFerla, F.M. SERCA pump activity is physiologically regulated by presenilin and regulates amyloid beta production. *J. Cell Biol.* **2008**, *181*, 1107–1116. [CrossRef] [PubMed]
135. Guo, Q.; Sopher, B.L.; Furukawa, K.; Pham, D.G.; Robinson, N.; Martin, G.M.; Mattson, M.P. Alzheimer's presenilin mutation sensitizes neural cells to apoptosis induced by trophic factor withdrawal and amyloid beta-peptide: Involvement of calcium and oxyradicals. *J. Neurosci.* **1997**, *17*, 4212–4222. [CrossRef] [PubMed]
136. Leissring, M.A.; Akbari, Y.; Fanger, C.M.; Cahalan, M.D.; Mattson, M.P.; LaFerla, F.M. Capacitative Calcium Entry Deficits and Elevated Luminal Calcium Content in Mutant Presenilin-1 Knockin Mice. *J. Cell Biol.* **2000**, *149*, 793–798. [CrossRef]
137. Tong, B.C.-K.; Lee, C.S.-K.; Cheng, W.-H.; Lai, K.-O.; Foskett, J.K.; Cheung, K.-H. Familial Alzheimer's disease–associated presenilin 1 mutants promote γ-secretase cleavage of STIM1 to impair store-operated Ca^{2+} entry. *Sci. Signal.* **2016**, *9*, ra89. [CrossRef]

138. Hoozemans, J.J.M.; van Haastert, E.S.; Nijholt, D.A.T.; Rozemuller, A.J.M.; Eikelenboom, P.; Scheper, W. The Unfolded Protein Response Is Activated in Pretangle Neurons in Alzheimer's Disease Hippocampus. *Am. J. Pathol.* **2009**, *174*, 1241–1251. [CrossRef]
139. Uddin, M.S.; Tewari, D.; Sharma, G.; Kabir, M.T.; Barreto, G.E.; Bin-Jumah, M.N.; Perveen, A.; Abdel-Daim, M.M.; Ashraf, G.M. Molecular Mechanisms of ER Stress and UPR in the Pathogenesis of Alzheimer's Disease. *Mol. Neurobiol.* **2020**, *57*, 2902–2919. [CrossRef]
140. Szegezdi, E.; Logue, S.E.; Gorman, A.M.; Samali, A. Mediators of endoplasmic reticulum stress-induced apoptosis. *EMBO Rep.* **2006**, *7*, 880–885. [CrossRef]
141. Gorman, A.M.; Healy, S.J.M.; Jäger, R.; Samali, A. Stress management at the ER: Regulators of ER stress-induced apoptosis. *Pharmacol. Ther.* **2012**, *134*, 306–316. [CrossRef]
142. Ogata, M.; Hino, S.; Saito, A.; Morikawa, K.; Kondo, S.; Kanemoto, S.; Murakami, T.; Taniguchi, M.; Tanii, I.; Yoshinaga, K.; et al. Autophagy Is Activated for Cell Survival after Endoplasmic ReticulumStress. *Mol. Cell. Biol.* **2006**, *26*, 9220–9231. [CrossRef]
143. Cissé, M.; Duplan, E.; Lorivel, T.; Dunys, J.; Bauer, C.; Meckler, X.; Gerakis, Y.; Lauritzen, I.; Checler, F. The transcription factor XBP1s restores hippocampal synaptic plasticity and memory by control of the Kalirin-7 pathway in Alzheimer model. *Mol. Psychiatry* **2017**, *22*, 1562–1575. [CrossRef]
144. Ma, T.; Trinh, M.A.; Wexler, A.J.; Bourbon, C.; Gatti, E.; Pierre, P.; Cavener, D.R.; Klann, E. Suppression of eIF2α kinases alleviates Alzheimer's disease–related plasticity and memory deficits. *Nat. Neurosci.* **2013**, *16*, 1299–1305. [CrossRef] [PubMed]
145. Soejima, N.; Ohyagi, Y.; Nakamura, N.; Himeno, E.; Iinuma, K.M.; Sakae, N.; Yamasaki, R.; Tabira, T.; Murakami, K.; Irie, K.; et al. Intracellular accumulation of toxic turn amyloid-β is associated with endoplasmic reticulum stress in Alzheimer's disease. *Curr. Alzheimer Res.* **2013**, *10*, 11–20. [PubMed]
146. Katayama, T.; Imaizumi, K.; Sato, N.; Miyoshi, K.; Kudo, T.; Hitomi, J.; Morihara, T.; Yoneda, T.; Gomi, F.; Mori, Y.; et al. Presenilin-1 mutations downregulate the signalling pathway of the unfolded-protein response. *Nat. Cell Biol.* **1999**, *1*, 479–485. [CrossRef] [PubMed]
147. Hidalgo, C.; Arias-Cavieres, A. Calcium, Reactive Oxygen Species, and Synaptic Plasticity. *Physiology* **2016**, *31*, 201–215. [CrossRef] [PubMed]
148. Mostafavi, S.; Gaiteri, C.; Sullivan, S.E.; White, C.C.; Tasaki, S.; Xu, J.; Taga, M.; Klein, H.-U.; Patrick, E.; Komashko, V.; et al. A molecular network of the aging human brain provides insights into the pathology and cognitive decline of Alzheimer's disease. *Nat. Neurosci.* **2018**, *21*, 811–819. [CrossRef] [PubMed]
149. Tramutola, A.; Lanzillotta, C.; Perluigi, M.; Butterfield, D.A. Oxidative stress, protein modification and Alzheimer disease. *Brain Res. Bull.* **2017**, *133*, 88–96. [CrossRef]
150. Zhang, H.; Menzies, K.J.; Auwerx, J. The role of mitochondria in stem cell fate and aging. *Development* **2018**, *145*. [CrossRef]
151. Canchi, S.; Raao, B.; Masliah, D.; Rosenthal, S.B.; Sasik, R.; Fisch, K.M.; De Jager, P.L.; Bennett, D.A.; Rissman, R.A. Integrating Gene and Protein Expression Reveals Perturbed Functional Networks in Alzheimer's Disease. *Cell Rep.* **2019**, *28*, 1103–1116.e4. [CrossRef]
152. Manczak, M.; Park, B.S.; Jung, Y.; Reddy, P.H. Differential expression of oxidative phosphorylation genes in patients with Alzheimer's disease. *NeuroMolecular Med.* **2004**, *5*, 147–162. [CrossRef]
153. Adav, S.S.; Park, J.E.; Sze, S.K. Quantitative profiling brain proteomes revealed mitochondrial dysfunction in Alzheimer's disease. *Mol. Brain* **2019**, *12*. [CrossRef] [PubMed]
154. Bubber, P.; Haroutunian, V.; Fisch, G.; Blass, J.P.; Gibson, G.E. Mitochondrial abnormalities in Alzheimer brain: Mechanistic implications. *Ann. Neurol.* **2005**, *57*, 695–703. [CrossRef] [PubMed]
155. Parker, W.D.; Parks, J.; Filley, C.M.; Kleinschmidt-DeMasters, B.K. Electron transport chain defects in Alzheimer's disease brain. *Neurology* **1994**, *44*, 1090–1096. [CrossRef] [PubMed]
156. Gibson, G.E.; Thakkar, A. Interactions of Mitochondria/Metabolism and Calcium Regulation in Alzheimer's Disease: A Calcinist Point of View. *Neurochem. Res.* **2017**, *42*, 1636–1648. [CrossRef]
157. Swomley, A.M.; Butterfield, D.A. Oxidative stress in Alzheimer disease and mild cognitive impairment: Evidence from human data provided by redox proteomics. *Arch. Toxicol.* **2015**, *89*, 1669–1680. [CrossRef] [PubMed]
158. Duchen, M.R. Contributions of mitochondria to animal physiology: From homeostatic sensor to calcium signalling and cell death. *J. Physiol.* **1999**, *516*, 1–17. [CrossRef]

159. Hajnóczky, G.; Hager, R.; Thomas, A.P. Mitochondria suppress local feedback activation of inositol 1,4, 5-trisphosphate receptors by Ca^{2+}. *J. Biol. Chem.* **1999**, *274*, 14157–14162. [CrossRef]
160. Robb-Gaspers, L.D.; Burnett, P.; Rutter, G.A.; Denton, R.M.; Rizzuto, R.; Thomas, A.P. Integrating cytosolic calcium signals into mitochondrial metabolic responses. *EMBO J.* **1998**, *17*, 4987–5000. [CrossRef]
161. Rowland, A.A.; Voeltz, G.K. Endoplasmic reticulum-mitochondria contacts: Function of the junction. *Nat. Rev. Mol. Cell Biol.* **2012**, *13*, 607–615. [CrossRef]
162. Schon, E.A.; Area-Gomez, E. Mitochondria-associated ER membranes in Alzheimer disease. *Mol. Cell. Neurosci.* **2013**, *55*, 26–36. [CrossRef]
163. Szabadkai, G.; Bianchi, K.; Várnai, P.; De Stefani, D.; Wieckowski, M.R.; Cavagna, D.; Nagy, A.I.; Balla, T.; Rizzuto, R. Chaperone-mediated coupling of endoplasmic reticulum and mitochondrial Ca^{2+} channels. *J. Cell Biol.* **2006**, *175*, 901–911. [CrossRef]
164. Wang, M.; Beckmann, N.D.; Roussos, P.; Wang, E.; Zhou, X.; Wang, Q.; Ming, C.; Neff, R.; Ma, W.; Fullard, J.F.; et al. The Mount Sinai cohort of large-scale genomic, transcriptomic and proteomic data in Alzheimer's disease. *Sci. Data* **2018**, *5*, 180185. [CrossRef] [PubMed]
165. De Jager, P.L.; Ma, Y.; McCabe, C.; Xu, J.; Vardarajan, B.N.; Felsky, D.; Klein, H.-U.; White, C.C.; Peters, M.A.; Lodgson, B.; et al. A multi-omic atlas of the human frontal cortex for aging and Alzheimer's disease research. *Sci. Data* **2018**, *5*, 180142. [CrossRef] [PubMed]
166. Hodes, R.J.; Buckholtz, N. Accelerating Medicines Partnership: Alzheimer's Disease (AMP-AD) Knowledge Portal Aids Alzheimer's Drug Discovery through Open Data Sharing. *Expert Opin. Ther. Targets* **2016**, *20*, 389–391. [CrossRef] [PubMed]
167. Calvo-Rodriguez, M.; Hou, S.S.; Snyder, A.C.; Kharitonova, E.K.; Russ, A.N.; Das, S.; Fan, Z.; Muzikansky, A.; Garcia-Alloza, M.; Serrano-Pozo, A.; et al. Increased mitochondrial calcium levels associated with neuronal death in a mouse model of Alzheimer's disease. *Nat. Commun.* **2020**, *11*, 2146. [CrossRef] [PubMed]
168. Han, D.; Antunes, F.; Canali, R.; Rettori, D.; Cadenas, E. Voltage-dependent anion channels control the release of the superoxide anion from mitochondria to cytosol. *J. Biol. Chem.* **2003**, *278*, 5557–5563. [CrossRef]
169. Paula-Lima, A.C.; Adasme, T.; SanMartín, C.; Sebollela, A.; Hetz, C.; Carrasco, M.A.; Ferreira, S.T.; Hidalgo, C. Amyloid β-Peptide Oligomers Stimulate RyR-Mediated Ca^{2+} Release Inducing Mitochondrial Fragmentation in Hippocampal Neurons and Prevent RyR-Mediated Dendritic Spine Remodeling Produced by BDNF. *Antioxid. Redox Signal.* **2010**, *14*, 1209–1223. [CrossRef]
170. SanMartín, C.D.; Veloso, P.; Adasme, T.; Lobos, P.; Bruna, B.; Galaz, J.; García, A.; Hartel, S.; Hidalgo, C.; Paula-Lima, A.C. RyR2-Mediated Ca^{2+} Release and Mitochondrial ROS Generation Partake in the Synaptic Dysfunction Caused by Amyloid β Peptide Oligomers. *Front. Mol. Neurosci.* **2017**, *10*. [CrossRef]
171. Smaili, S.S.; Russell, J.T. Permeability transition pore regulates both mitochondrial membrane potential and agonist-evoked Ca^{2+} signals in oligodendrocyte progenitors. *Cell Calcium* **1999**, *26*, 121–130. [CrossRef]
172. Wang, W.; Zhao, F.; Ma, X.; Perry, G.; Zhu, X. Mitochondria dysfunction in the pathogenesis of Alzheimer's disease: Recent advances. *Mol. Neurodegener.* **2020**, *15*, 30. [CrossRef]
173. Area-Gomez, E.; del Carmen Lara Castillo, M.; Tambini, M.D.; Guardia-Laguarta, C.; de Groof, A.J.; Madra, M.; Ikenouchi, J.; Umeda, M.; Bird, T.D.; Sturley, S.L.; et al. Upregulated function of mitochondria-associated ER membranes in Alzheimer disease. *EMBO J.* **2012**, *31*, 4106–4123. [CrossRef] [PubMed]
174. Area-Gomez, E.; de Groof, A.; Bonilla, E.; Montesinos, J.; Tanji, K.; Boldogh, I.; Pon, L.; Schon, E.A. A key role for MAM in mediating mitochondrial dysfunction in Alzheimer disease. *Cell Death Dis.* **2018**, *9*, 1–10. [CrossRef] [PubMed]
175. Del Prete, D.; Suski, J.M.; Oulès, B.; Debayle, D.; Gay, A.S.; Lacas-Gervais, S.; Bussiere, R.; Bauer, C.; Pinton, P.; Paterlini-Bréchot, P.; et al. Localization and Processing of the Amyloid-β Protein Precursor in Mitochondria-Associated Membranes. *J. Alzheimers Dis. JAD* **2017**, *55*, 1549–1570. [CrossRef] [PubMed]
176. Hedskog, L.; Pinho, C.M.; Filadi, R.; Rönnbäck, A.; Hertwig, L.; Wiehager, B.; Larssen, P.; Gellhaar, S.; Sandebring, A.; Westerlund, M.; et al. Modulation of the endoplasmic reticulum-mitochondria interface in Alzheimer's disease and related models. *Proc. Natl. Acad. Sci. USA* **2013**, *110*, 7916–7921. [CrossRef]
177. Sarasija, S.; Laboy, J.T.; Ashkavand, Z.; Bonner, J.; Tang, Y.; Norman, K.R. Presenilin mutations deregulate mitochondrial Ca^{2+} homeostasis and metabolic activity causing neurodegeneration in Caenorhabditis elegans. *eLife* **2018**, *7*, e33052. [CrossRef]

178. Völgyi, K.; Badics, K.; Sialana, F.J.; Gulyássy, P.; Udvari, E.B.; Kis, V.; Drahos, L.; Lubec, G.; Kékesi, K.A.; Juhász, G. Early Presymptomatic Changes in the Proteome of Mitochondria-Associated Membrane in the APP/PS1 Mouse Model of Alzheimer's Disease. *Mol. Neurobiol.* **2018**, *55*, 7839–7857. [CrossRef]
179. Luongo, T.S.; Lambert, J.P.; Gross, P.; Nwokedi, M.; Lombardi, A.A.; Shanmughapriya, S.; Carpenter, A.C.; Kolmetzky, D.; Gao, E.; van Berlo, J.H.; et al. The Mitochondrial Na^+/Ca^{2+} Exchanger Is Essential for Ca^{2+} Homeostasis and Viability. Available online: https://pubmed.ncbi.nlm.nih.gov/28445457/ (accessed on 26 October 2020).
180. Kroemer, G.; Galluzzi, L.; Brenner, C. Mitochondrial membrane permeabilization in cell death. *Physiol. Rev.* **2007**, *87*, 99–163. [CrossRef]
181. Smaili, S.S.; Pereira, G.J.S.; Costa, M.M.; Rocha, K.K.; Rodrigues, L.; do Carmo, L.G.; Hirata, H.; Hsu, Y.-T. The Role of Calcium Stores in Apoptosis and Autophagy. *Curr. Mol. Med.* **2013**, *13*, 252–265. [CrossRef]
182. Magi, S.; Piccirillo, S.; Maiolino, M.; Lariccia, V.; Amoroso, S. NCX1 and EAAC1 transporters are involved in the protective action of glutamate in an in vitro Alzheimer's disease-like model. *Cell Calcium* **2020**, *91*, 102268. [CrossRef]
183. Zilberter, Y.; Zilberter, M. The vicious circle of hypometabolism in neurodegenerative diseases: Ways and mechanisms of metabolic correction. *J. Neurosci. Res.* **2017**, *95*, 2217–2235. [CrossRef]
184. Jadiya, P.; Kolmetzky, D.W.; Tomar, D.; Di Meco, A.; Lombardi, A.A.; Lambert, J.P.; Luongo, T.S.; Ludtmann, M.H.; Praticò, D.; Elrod, J.W. Impaired mitochondrial calcium efflux contributes to disease progression in models of Alzheimer's disease. *Nat. Commun.* **2019**, *10*, 3885. [CrossRef] [PubMed]
185. Piccirillo, S.; Magi, S.; Castaldo, P.; Preziuso, A.; Lariccia, V.; Amoroso, S. NCX and EAAT transporters in ischemia: At the crossroad between glutamate metabolism and cell survival. *Cell Calcium* **2020**, *86*, 102160. [CrossRef] [PubMed]
186. Magi, S.; Piccirillo, S.; Preziuso, A.; Amoroso, S.; Lariccia, V. Mitochondrial localization of NCXs: Balancing calcium and energy homeostasis. *Cell Calcium* **2020**, *86*, 102162. [CrossRef] [PubMed]
187. Gobbi, P.; Castaldo, P.; Minelli, A.; Salucci, S.; Magi, S.; Corcione, E.; Amoroso, S. Mitochondrial localization of Na^+/Ca^{2+} exchangers NCX1-3 in neurons and astrocytes of adult rat brain in situ. *Pharmacol. Res.* **2007**, *56*, 556–565. [CrossRef] [PubMed]
188. Mishra, P.; Chan, D.C. Mitochondrial dynamics and inheritance during cell division, development and disease. *Nat. Rev. Mol. Cell Biol.* **2014**, *15*, 634–646. [CrossRef]
189. Kim, B.; Park, J.; Chang, K.-T.; Lee, D.-S. Peroxiredoxin 5 prevents amyloid-beta oligomer-induced neuronal cell death by inhibiting ERK-Drp1-mediated mitochondrial fragmentation. *Free Radic. Biol. Med.* **2016**, *90*, 184–194. [CrossRef]
190. Kim, D.I.; Lee, K.H.; Gabr, A.A.; Choi, G.E.; Kim, J.S.; Ko, S.H.; Han, H.J. Aβ-Induced Drp1 phosphorylation through Akt activation promotes excessive mitochondrial fission leading to neuronal apoptosis. *Biochim. Biophys. Acta* **2016**, *1863*, 2820–2834. [CrossRef]
191. Han, S.; Nandy, P.; Austria, Q.; Siedlak, S.L.; Torres, S.; Fujioka, H.; Wang, W.; Zhu, X. Mfn2 Ablation in the Adult Mouse Hippocampus and Cortex Causes Neuronal Death. *Cells* **2020**, *9*, 116. [CrossRef]
192. Jiang, S.; Nandy, P.; Wang, W.; Ma, X.; Hsia, J.; Wang, C.; Wang, Z.; Niu, M.; Siedlak, S.L.; Torres, S.; et al. Mfn2 ablation causes an oxidative stress response and eventual neuronal death in the hippocampus and cortex. *Mol. Neurodegener.* **2018**, *13*, 5. [CrossRef]
193. Pickett, E.K.; Rose, J.; McCrory, C.; McKenzie, C.-A.; King, D.; Smith, C.; Gillingwater, T.H.; Henstridge, C.M.; Spires-Jones, T.L. Region-specific depletion of synaptic mitochondria in the brains of patients with Alzheimer's disease. *Acta Neuropathol. (Berl.)* **2018**, *136*, 747–757. [CrossRef]
194. Sheng, Z.-H.; Cai, Q. Mitochondrial transport in neurons: Impact on synaptic homeostasis and neurodegeneration. *Nat. Rev. Neurosci.* **2012**, *13*, 77–93. [CrossRef] [PubMed]
195. Ebneth, A.; Godemann, R.; Stamer, K.; Illenberger, S.; Trinczek, B.; Mandelkow, E. Overexpression of tau protein inhibits kinesin-dependent trafficking of vesicles, mitochondria, and endoplasmic reticulum: Implications for Alzheimer's disease. *J. Cell Biol.* **1998**, *143*, 777–794. [CrossRef] [PubMed]
196. Shahpasand, K.; Uemura, I.; Saito, T.; Asano, T.; Hata, K.; Shibata, K.; Toyoshima, Y.; Hasegawa, M.; Hisanaga, S. Regulation of Mitochondrial Transport and Inter-Microtubule Spacing by Tau Phosphorylation at the Sites Hyperphosphorylated in Alzheimer's Disease. *J. Neurosci.* **2012**, *32*, 2430–2441. [CrossRef]
197. Lemasters, J.J. Selective Mitochondrial Autophagy, or Mitophagy, as a Targeted Defense Against Oxidative Stress, Mitochondrial Dysfunction, and Aging. *Rejuvenation Res.* **2005**, *8*, 3–5. [CrossRef] [PubMed]

198. Kerr, J.S.; Adriaanse, B.A.; Greig, N.H.; Mattson, M.P.; Cader, M.Z.; Bohr, V.A.; Fang, E.F. Mitophagy and Alzheimer's Disease: Cellular and Molecular Mechanisms. *Trends Neurosci.* **2017**, *40*, 151–166. [CrossRef] [PubMed]
199. Martín-Maestro, P.; Gargini, R.; Perry, G.; Avila, J.; García-Escudero, V. PARK2 enhancement is able to compensate mitophagy alterations found in sporadic Alzheimer's disease. *Hum. Mol. Genet.* **2016**, *25*, 792–806. [CrossRef]
200. Cárdenas, C.; Foskett, J.K. Mitochondrial Ca^{2+} signals in autophagy. *Cell Calcium* **2012**, *52*, 44–51. [CrossRef]
201. Ding, W.X.; Yin, X.M. Mitophagy: Mechanisms, pathophysiological roles, and analysis. *Biol. Chem.* **2012**, *393*, 547–564. [CrossRef]
202. Okamoto, K.; Kondo-Okamoto, N.; Ohsumi, Y. Mitochondria-anchored receptor Atg32 mediates degradation of mitochondria via selective autophagy. *Dev. Cell* **2009**, *17*, 87–97. [CrossRef]
203. Martín-Maestro, P.; Gargini, R.; A Sproul, A.; García, E.; Antón, L.C.; Noggle, S.; Arancio, O.; Avila, J.; García-Escudero, V. Mitophagy Failure in Fibroblasts and iPSC-Derived Neurons of Alzheimer's Disease-Associated Presenilin 1 Mutation. *Front. Mol. Neurosci.* **2017**, *10*, 291. [CrossRef]
204. Nguyen, T.N.; Padman, B.S.; Lazarou, M. Deciphering the Molecular Signals of PINK1/Parkin Mitophagy. *Trends Cell Biol.* **2016**, *26*, 733–744. [CrossRef] [PubMed]
205. Mustaly, S.; Littlefield, A.; Stutzmann, G.E. Calcium Signaling Deficits in Glia and Autophagic Pathways Contributing to Neurodegenerative Disease. *Antioxid. Redox Signal.* **2018**, *29*, 1158–1175. [CrossRef] [PubMed]
206. Li, W.; Li, J.; Bao, J. Microautophagy: Lesser-known self-eating. *Cell. Mol. Life Sci.* **2012**, *69*, 1125–1136. [CrossRef]
207. Vervliet, T.; Pintelon, I.; Welkenhuyzen, K.; Bootman, M.D.; Bannai, H.; Mikoshiba, K.; Martinet, W.; Nadif Kasri, N.; Parys, J.B.; Bultynck, G. Basal ryanodine receptor activity suppresses autophagic flux. *Biochem. Pharmacol.* **2017**, *132*, 133–142. [CrossRef] [PubMed]
208. Wu, Y.; Whiteus, C.; Xu, C.S.; Hayworth, K.J.; Weinberg, R.J.; Hess, H.F.; De Camilli, P. Contacts between the endoplasmic reticulum and other membranes in neurons. *Proc. Natl. Acad. Sci. USA* **2017**, *114*, E4859–E4867. [CrossRef] [PubMed]
209. Yu, L.; Chibnik, L.B.; Srivastava, G.P.; Pochet, N.; Yang, J.; Xu, J.; Kozubek, J.; Obholzer, N.; Leurgans, S.E.; Schneider, J.A.; et al. Association of Brain DNA methylation in SORL1, ABCA7, HLA-DRB5, SLC24A4, and BIN1 with pathological diagnosis of Alzheimer disease. *JAMA Neurol.* **2015**, *72*, 15–24. [CrossRef]
210. Van Acker, Z.P.; Bretou, M.; Annaert, W. Endo-lysosomal dysregulations and late-onset Alzheimer's disease: Impact of genetic risk factors. *Mol. Neurodegener.* **2019**, *14*, 20. [CrossRef]
211. De Duve, C.; Wattiaux, R. Functions of Lysosomes. *Annu. Rev. Physiol.* **1966**, *28*, 435–492. [CrossRef]
212. Nakamura, N.; Matsuura, A.; Wada, Y.; Ohsumi, Y. Acidification of vacuoles is required for autophagic degradation in the yeast, Saccharomyces cerevisiae. *J. Biochem.* **1997**, *121*, 338–344. [CrossRef]
213. Xu, H.; Ren, D. Lysosomal Physiology. *Annu. Rev. Physiol.* **2015**, *77*, 57–80. [CrossRef]
214. Prasad, H.; Rao, R. The Na^+/H^+ Exchanger NHE6 Modulates Endosomal pH to Control Processing of Amyloid Precursor Protein in a Cell Culture Model of Alzheimer Disease. *J. Biol. Chem.* **2015**, *290*, 5311–5327. [CrossRef] [PubMed]
215. Lee, J.H.; Yu, W.H.; Kumar, A.; Lee, S.; Mohan, P.S.; Peterhoff, C.M.; Wolfe, D.M.; Martinez-Vicente, M.; Massey, A.C.; Sovak, G.; et al. Lysosomal proteolysis and autophagy require presenilin 1 and are disrupted by Alzheimer-related PS1 mutations. *Cell* **2010**, *141*, 1146–1158. [CrossRef] [PubMed]
216. Lee, J.H.; McBrayer, M.K.; Wolfe, D.M.; Haslett, L.J.; Kumar, A.; Sato, Y.; Lie, P.P.Y.; Mohan, P.; Coffey, E.E.; Kompella, U.; et al. Presenilin 1 Maintains Lysosomal Ca^{2+} Homeostasis via TRPML1 by Regulating vATPase-Mediated Lysosome Acidification. *Cell Rep.* **2015**, *12*, 1430–1444. [CrossRef] [PubMed]
217. Man, S.M.; Kanneganti, T.-D. Regulation of lysosomal dynamics and autophagy by CTSB/cathepsin B. *Autophagy* **2016**, *12*, 2504–2505. [CrossRef] [PubMed]
218. Lee, S.; Sato, Y.; Nixon, R.A. Lysosomal Proteolysis Inhibition Selectively Disrupts Axonal Transport of Degradative Organelles and Causes an Alzheimer's-Like Axonal Dystrophy. *J. Neurosci.* **2011**, *31*, 7817–7830. [CrossRef] [PubMed]
219. Lee, S.; Sato, Y.; Nixon, R.A. Primary lysosomal dysfunction causes cargo-specific deficits of axonal transport leading to Alzheimer-like neuritic dystrophy. *Autophagy* **2011**, *7*, 1562–1563. [CrossRef] [PubMed]

220. Torres, M.; Jimenez, S.; Sanchez-Varo, R.; Navarro, V.; Trujillo-Estrada, L.; Sanchez-Mejias, E.; Carmona, I.; Davila, J.C.; Vizuete, M.; Gutierrez, A.; et al. Defective lysosomal proteolysis and axonal transport are early pathogenic events that worsen with age leading to increased APP metabolism and synaptic Abeta in transgenic APP/PS1 hippocampus. *Mol. Neurodegener.* **2012**, *7*, 59. [CrossRef]
221. Calcraft, P.J.; Ruas, M.; Pan, Z.; Cheng, X.; Arredouani, A.; Hao, X.; Tang, J.; Rietdorf, K.; Teboul, L.; Chuang, K.-T.; et al. NAADP mobilizes calcium from acidic organelles through two-pore channels. *Nature* **2009**, *459*, 596–600. [CrossRef]
222. Cang, C.; Bekele, B.; Ren, D. The voltage-gated sodium channel TPC1 confers endolysosomal excitability. *Nat. Chem. Biol.* **2014**, *10*, 463–469. [CrossRef]
223. Carmona-Gutierrez, D.; Hughes, A.L.; Madeo, F.; Ruckenstuhl, C. The crucial impact of lysosomes in aging and longevity. *Ageing Res. Rev.* **2016**, *32*, 2–12. [CrossRef]
224. Colacurcio, D.J.; Nixon, R.A. Disorders of lysosomal acidificstion-The emerging role of v-ATPase in aging and neurodegenerative disease. *Ageing Res. Rev.* **2016**, *32*, 75–88. [CrossRef] [PubMed]
225. Neely Kayala, K.M.; Dickinson, G.D.; Minassian, A.; Walls, K.C.; Green, K.N.; Laferla, F.M. Presenilin-null cells have altered two-pore calcium channel expression and lysosomal calcium: Implications for lysosomal function. *Brain Res.* **2012**, *1489*, 8–16. [CrossRef] [PubMed]
226. Coen, K.; Flannagan, R.S.; Baron, S.; Carraro-Lacroix, L.R.; Wang, D.; Vermeire, W.; Michiels, C.; Munck, S.; Baert, V.; Sugita, S.; et al. Lysosomal calcium homeostasis defects, not proton pump defects, cause endo-lysosomal dysfunction in PSEN-deficient cells. *J. Cell Biol.* **2012**, *198*, 23–35. [CrossRef] [PubMed]
227. Mauvezin, C.; Nagy, P.; Juhász, G.; Neufeld, T.P. Autophagosome–lysosome fusion is independent of V-ATPase-mediated acidification. *Nat. Commun.* **2015**, *6*, 7007. [CrossRef]
228. Zhang, X.; Garbett, K.; Veeraraghavalu, K.; Wilburn, B.; Gilmore, R.; Mirnics, K.; Sisodia, S.S. A Role for Presenilins in Autophagy Revisited: Normal Acidification of Lysosomes in Cells Lacking PSEN1 and PSEN2. *J. Neurosci.* **2012**, *32*, 8633–8648. [CrossRef]
229. Medina, D.L.; Di Paola, S.; Peluso, I.; Armani, A.; De Stefani, D.; Venditti, R.; Montefusco, S.; Scotto-Rosato, A.; Prezioso, C.; Forrester, A.; et al. Lysosomal calcium signalling regulates autophagy through calcineurin and TFEB. *Nat. Cell Biol.* **2015**, *17*, 288–299. [CrossRef]
230. Sardiello, M.; Palmieri, M.; di Ronza, A.; Medina, D.L.; Valenza, M.; Gennarino, V.A.; Malta, C.D.; Donaudy, F.; Embrione, V.; Polishchuk, R.S.; et al. A Gene Network Regulating Lysosomal Biogenesis and Function. *Science* **2009**, *325*, 473–477. [CrossRef]
231. Settembre, C.; Zoncu, R.; Medina, D.L.; Vetrini, F.; Erdin, S.; Erdin, S.; Huynh, T.; Ferron, M.; Karsenty, G.; Vellard, M.C.; et al. A lysosome-to-nucleus signalling mechanism senses and regulates the lysosome via mTOR and TFEB. *EMBO J.* **2012**, *31*, 1095–1108. [CrossRef]
232. Glavan, G.; Schliebs, R.; Živin, M. Synaptotagmins in neurodegeneration. *Anat. Rec.* **2009**, *292*, 1849–1862. [CrossRef]
233. Jun, K.; Piedras-Rentería, E.S.; Smith, S.M.; Wheeler, D.B.; Lee, S.B.; Lee, T.G.; Chin, H.; Adams, M.E.; Scheller, R.H.; Tsien, R.W.; et al. Ablation of P/Q-type Ca^{2+} channel currents, altered synaptic transmission, and progressive ataxia in mice lacking the α1A-subunit. *Proc. Natl. Acad. Sci. USA* **1999**, *96*, 15245–15250. [CrossRef]
234. Saftig, P.; Klumperman, J. Lysosome biogenesis and lysosomal membrane proteins: Trafficking meets function. *Nat. Rev. Mol. Cell Biol.* **2009**, *10*, 623–635. [CrossRef] [PubMed]
235. Tian, X.; Gala, U.; Zhang, Y.; Shang, W.; Jaiswal, S.N.; di Ronza, A.; Jaiswal, M.; Yamamoto, S.; Sandoval, H.; Duraine, L.; et al. A voltage-gated calcium channel regulates lysosomal fusion with endosomes and autophagosomes and is required for neuronal homeostasis. *PLoS Biol.* **2015**, *13*. [CrossRef] [PubMed]
236. Kinnear, N.P.; Wyatt, C.N.; Clark, J.H.; Calcraft, P.J.; Fleischer, S.; Jeyakumar, L.H.; Nixon, G.F.; Evans, A.M. Lysosomes co-localize with ryanodine receptor subtype 3 to form a trigger zone for calcium signalling by NAADP in rat pulmonary arterial smooth muscle. *Cell Calcium* **2008**, *44*, 190–201. [CrossRef] [PubMed]
237. Foster, W.J.; Taylor, H.B.C.; Padamsey, Z.; Jeans, A.F.; Galione, A.; Emptage, N.J. Hippocampal mGluR1-dependent long-term potentiation requires NAADP-mediated acidic store Ca^{2+} signaling. *Sci. Signal.* **2018**, *11*. [CrossRef]
238. Padamsey, Z.; McGuinness, L.; Bardo, S.J.; Reinhart, M.; Tong, R.; Hedegaard, A.; Hart, M.L.; Emptage, N.J. Activity-Dependent Exocytosis of Lysosomes Regulates the Structural Plasticity of Dendritic Spines. *Neuron* **2017**, *93*, 132–146. [CrossRef]

239. Padamsey, Z.; McGuinness, L.; Emptage, N.J. Inhibition of lysosomal Ca^{2+} signalling disrupts dendritic spine structure and impairs wound healing in neurons. *Commun. Integr. Biol.* **2017**, *10*, e1344802. [CrossRef]
240. Yang, D.S.; Stavrides, P.; Mohan, P.S.; Kaushik, S.; Kumar, A.; Ohno, M.; Schmidt, S.D.; Wesson, D.; Bandyopadhyay, U.; Jiang, Y.; et al. Reversal of autophagy dysfunction in the TgCRND8 mouse model of Alzheimer's disease ameliorates amyloid pathologies and memory deficits. *Brain* **2011**, *134*, 258–277. [CrossRef]

Permissions

All chapters in this book were first published by MDPI; hereby published with permission under the Creative Commons Attribution License or equivalent. Every chapter published in this book has been scrutinized by our experts. Their significance has been extensively debated. The topics covered herein carry significant findings which will fuel the growth of the discipline. They may even be implemented as practical applications or may be referred to as a beginning point for another development.

The contributors of this book come from diverse backgrounds, making this book a truly international effort. This book will bring forth new frontiers with its revolutionizing research information and detailed analysis of the nascent developments around the world.

We would like to thank all the contributing authors for lending their expertise to make the book truly unique. They have played a crucial role in the development of this book. Without their invaluable contributions this book wouldn't have been possible. They have made vital efforts to compile up to date information on the varied aspects of this subject to make this book a valuable addition to the collection of many professionals and students.

This book was conceptualized with the vision of imparting up-to-date information and advanced data in this field. To ensure the same, a matchless editorial board was set up. Every individual on the board went through rigorous rounds of assessment to prove their worth. After which they invested a large part of their time researching and compiling the most relevant data for our readers.

The editorial board has been involved in producing this book since its inception. They have spent rigorous hours researching and exploring the diverse topics which have resulted in the successful publishing of this book. They have passed on their knowledge of decades through this book. To expedite this challenging task, the publisher supported the team at every step. A small team of assistant editors was also appointed to further simplify the editing procedure and attain best results for the readers.

Apart from the editorial board, the designing team has also invested a significant amount of their time in understanding the subject and creating the most relevant covers. They scrutinized every image to scout for the most suitable representation of the subject and create an appropriate cover for the book.

The publishing team has been an ardent support to the editorial, designing and production team. Their endless efforts to recruit the best for this project, has resulted in the accomplishment of this book. They are a veteran in the field of academics and their pool of knowledge is as vast as their experience in printing. Their expertise and guidance has proved useful at every step. Their uncompromising quality standards have made this book an exceptional effort. Their encouragement from time to time has been an inspiration for everyone.

The publisher and the editorial board hope that this book will prove to be a valuable piece of knowledge for researchers, students, practitioners and scholars across the globe.

List of Contributors

Gustavo C. Román
Department of Neurology, Methodist Neurological Institute, Institute for Academic Medicine Houston Methodist Research Institute, Houston Methodist Hospital, Houston, TX 77030, USA
Weill Cornell Medical College, Department of Neurology, Cornell University, New York, NY 10065, USA

Oscar Mancera-Páez
Universidad Nacional de Colombia, Hospital Universitario Nacional, Faculty of Medicine, Department of Neurology, Bogotá ZC 57, Colombia
David Cabello International Alzheimer Disease Scholarship Fund, Houston Methodist Hospital, Houston, TX77030, USA

Camilo Bernal
Universidad Nacional de Colombia, Hospital Universitario Nacional, Faculty of Medicine, Department of Neurology, Bogotá ZC 57, Colombia

Valeria D'Argenio
CEINGE-Biotecnologie Avanzate scarl, via G. Salvatore 486, 80145 Naples, Italy
Department of Human Sciences and Quality of Life Promotion, San Raffaele Open University, via di val Cannuta 247, 00166 Rome, Italy

Daniela Sarnataro
Department of Molecular Medicine and Medical Biotechnology, Federico II University, via S. Pansini 5, 80131 Naples, Italy

Agostino Chiaravalloti and Orazio Schillaci
Department of Biomedicine and Prevention, University Tor Vergata, 00133 Rome, Italy
IRCCS Neuromed, 86077 Pozzilli, Italy

Maria Ricci
Department of Biomedicine and Prevention, University Tor Vergata, 00133 Rome, Italy

Daniele Di Biagio
UOC Nuclear Medicine, Policlinico Tor Vergata, 00133 Rome, Italy

Luca Filippi
UOC Nuclear Medicine, Santa Maria Goretti Hospital, 04100 Latina, Italy

Alessandro Martorana
UOSD Centro Demenze Policlinico Tor Vergata, 00133 Rome, Italy
Department of System Medicine, University Tor Vergata, 00133 Rome, Italy

Anna Picca, Riccardo Calvani, Cristina Pais, Eleonora Meloni, Domenico Fusco, Maria Rita Lo Monaco and Maria Camilla Cipriani
Fondazione Policlinico Universitario "Agostino Gemelli" IRCCS, 00168 Rome, Italy

Daniela Ronconi and Hélio J. Coelho-Junior
Università Cattolica del Sacro Cuore, 00168 Rome, Italy

Federico Marini
Department of Chemistry, Sapienza Università di Roma, 00185 Rome, Italy

Alessandra Biancolillo
Department of Physical and Chemical Sciences, Università degli Studi dell'Aquila, 67100 L'Aquila, Italy

Jacopo Gervasoni, Aniello Primiano, Roberto Bernabei, Emanuele Marzetti and Rosa Liperoti
Fondazione Policlinico Universitario "Agostino Gemelli" IRCCS, 00168 Rome, Italy
Università Cattolica del Sacro Cuore, 00168 Rome, Italy

Md Shahjalal Hossain Khan and Vijay Hegde
Obesity and Metabolic Health Laboratory, Department of Nutritional Sciences, Texas Tech University, Lubbock, TX 79409, USA

Yu-Chia Kao
Institute of Clinical Medicine, College of Medicine, National Cheng Kung University, Tainan 704, Taiwan
Department of Pediatrics, E-Da Hospital, Kaohsiung 824, Taiwan

I-Fang Wang
Institute of Clinical Medicine, College of Medicine, National Cheng Kung University, Tainan 704, Taiwan
Institute of Molecular Biology, Academia Sinica, Taipei 115, Taiwan

Kuen-Jer Tsai
Institute of Clinical Medicine, College of Medicine, National Cheng Kung University, Tainan 704, Taiwan
Research Center of Clinical Medicine, National Cheng Kung University Hospital, College of Medicine, National Cheng Kung University, Tainan 704, Taiwan

Valeria Guglielmi and Davide Quaranta
Neurology Unit, Fondazione Policlinico Agostino Gemelli-IRCCS, 00168 Rome, Italy

Ilaria Mega, Emanuele Maria Costantini, Claudia Carrarini and Alice Innocenti
Department of Neuroscience, Catholic University of Sacred Heart, 00168 Rome, Italy

Camillo Marra
Department of Neuroscience, Catholic University of Sacred Heart, 00168 Rome, Italy
Memory Clinic, Fondazione Policlinico Universitario Agostino Gemelli-IRCCS, 00168 Rome, Italy

Yen Nhi Luu and Ian Macreadie
School of Science, RMIT University, Bundoora, VIC 3083, Australia

Efthalia Angelopoulou and Christina Piperi
Department of Biological Chemistry, Medical School, National and Kapodistrian University of Athens, Greece

Yam Nath Paudel and Mohd. Farooq Shaikh
Neuropharmacology Research Strength, Jeffrey Cheah School of Medicine and Health Sciences, Monash University Malaysia, Bandar Sunway 47500, Selangor, Malaysia

Cristina d'Abramo
The Litwin-Zucker Center for Alzheimer's Disease & Memory Disorders, Institute of Molecular Medicine, Feinstein Institutes for Medical Research, Northwell Health System, Manhasset, NY 11030, USA

Luciano D'Adamio
Rutgers Alzheimer's Disease & Dementia Research Center (RUADRC), Rutgers Brain Health Institute, Rutgers University, Piscataway, NJ 08854, USA

Luca Giliberto
The Litwin-Zucker Center for Alzheimer's Disease & Memory Disorders, Institute of Molecular Medicine, Feinstein Institutes for Medical Research, Northwell Health System, Manhasset, NY 11030, USA
Northwell Health Neuroscience Institute, Northwell Health System, Manhasset, NY 11030, USA
Donald and Barbara Zucker School of Medicine, Hofstra University, Hempstead, NY 11549, USA

Veronika Prikhodko
Laboratory of Molecular Neurodegeneration, Peter the Great St. Petersburg Polytechnic University, 195251 St. Petersburg, Russia
Department of Pharmacology and Clinical Pharmacology, Saint Petersburg State Chemical Pharmaceutical University, 197022 St. Petersburg, Russia
N.P. Bechtereva Institute of the Human Brain of the Russian Academy of Sciences, 197376 St. Petersburg, Russia

Daria Chernyuk, Nikita Zernov and Elena Popugaeva
Laboratory of Molecular Neurodegeneration, Peter the Great St. Petersburg Polytechnic University, 195251 St. Petersburg, Russia

Yurii Sysoev
Laboratory of Molecular Neurodegeneration, Peter the Great St. Petersburg Polytechnic University, 195251 St. Petersburg, Russia
Department of Pharmacology and Clinical Pharmacology, Saint Petersburg State Chemical Pharmaceutical University, 197022 St. Petersburg, Russia
N.P. Bechtereva Institute of the Human Brain of the Russian Academy of Sciences, 197376 St. Petersburg, Russia
Institute of Translational Biomedicine, Saint Petersburg State University, 199034 St. Petersburg, Russia

Sergey Okovityi
Department of Pharmacology and Clinical Pharmacology, Saint Petersburg State Chemical Pharmaceutical University, 197022 St. Petersburg, Russia
N.P. Bechtereva Institute of the Human Brain of the Russian Academy of Sciences, 197376 St. Petersburg, Russia

Eiko N. Minakawa and Keiji Wada
Department of Degenerative Neurological Diseases, National Institute of Neuroscience, National Center of Neurology and Psychiatry, Kodaira 187-8502, Japan

Yoshitaka Nagai
Department of Degenerative Neurological Diseases, National Institute of Neuroscience, National Center of Neurology and Psychiatry, Kodaira 187-8502, Japan
Department of Neurotherapeutics, Osaka University Graduate School of Medicine, Osaka 565-0871, Japan

John McDaid and Sarah Mustaly-Kalimi
Center for Neurodegenerative Disease and Therapeutics, Rosalind Franklin University of Medicine and Science, 3333 Green Bay Rd., North Chicago, IL 60064, USA
School of Graduate and Postdoctoral Studies, Rosalind Franklin University of Medicine and Science, 3333 Green Bay Rd., North Chicago, IL 60064, USA

Grace E. Stutzmann
Center for Neurodegenerative Disease and Therapeutics, Rosalind Franklin University of Medicine and Science, 3333 Green Bay Rd., North Chicago, IL 60064, USA
School of Graduate and Postdoctoral Studies, Rosalind Franklin University of Medicine and Science, 3333 Green Bay Rd., North Chicago, IL 60064, USA
Chicago Medical School, Rosalind Franklin University of Medicine and Science, 3333 Green Bay Rd., North Chicago, IL 60064, USA

Index

www.ingramcontent.com/pod-product-compliance
Lightning Source LLC
LaVergne TN
LVHW060547210926
848485LV00005B/1271

* 9 7 8 1 6 3 9 2 7 6 5 8 5 *